# Restoring Order in Health and Chinese Medicine

## STUDIES OF THE DEVELOPMENT AND USE OF QI AND THE CHANNELS

**Stephen Birch**
**Miguel Angel Cabrer Mir**
**Manuel Rodriguez Cuadras**

Foreword by Elisabeth Rochat de la Vallee

sayoshi BOOKS

**Restoring Order in Health and Chinese Medicine:**
**Studies of the Development and Use of Qi and the Channels**
**Second Edition**



Second edition published by Sayoshi Books

ISBN (Second Edition): 978-1-0683814-0-9

First edition published in May 2014 by La Liebre de Marzo, S.L.



Original cover design by Barbara Pardo
Revised cover design Formatted Books

Dear Reader,

Thank you for purchasing

**RESTORING ORDER IN HEALTH AND CHINESE MEDICINE**
(SECOND EDITION)

As a special thank-you gift, please download this extra free article by Stephen Birch and Miguel Cabrer Mir:

**Bringing Qi into Our Actions – Your Exclusive Free Download**

**How do we bring qi into everything we do?**

This short, insightful piece distils key lessons from our study and research, offering a practical take-home message on integrating qi into daily practice.

- ✓ **Understand how qi influences action and intent.**
- ✓ **Apply these insights to enhance your clinical skills.**
- ✓ **Explore a real-world example of qi in needling.**

**Get Your Free Resource Here!**

Scan the barcode with your mobile camera to access your free resource.
If you are unable to scan, simply visit the URL below.

**www.sayoshibooks.orankivity.com/restore**

# CONTENTS

# FOREWORD

Elisabeth Rochat de la Vallée

We wish there were more books like this. A book that goes deeply into the very substance of Chinese medicine, remaining not only readable but enjoyable. A book that assumes that the reader is capable of a real understanding and wants to go further than the surface in the comprehension of Chinese medicine.

A main feature is that it is not the work of one person or even of a group of people belonging to the same school. That fits well with a certain idea of what is a tradition and its transmission. It is always diversity that gives a dynamic richer that any specific teaching. In this diversity there is finally a kind of organic convergence, which is not made artificially, but appears as intrinsic. This does not prevent the book from offering a lot of comprehensive and detailed information and to provide materials and documents on many topics.

The beginners will not be lost and the seasoned practitioners will be surprised with all they learn and also how they deepen what they already know and practice. Indeed, this book can look like an amalgam. A constellation of seven people, coming from at least three different countries, sharing its authorship. In fact, it is necessary to see beyond appearances.

The chapters discuss different topics of which some are easily related to the usual study of Chinese medicine, and some others give the impression of treating topics not directly related to this medicine. In the ten chapters composing the book, we find studies on Qi and a choice of great concepts from Chinese medicine, consideration on the arrival of Qi during the treatment, study on meridians and points, techniques of puncture (including some Japanese ones), their history and their tools (the needles), herbs and herbal medicine. We find a reflection of Taijiquan, Qigong, Yiquan and Aikido, mainly focusing on their importance for those who wish to practice acupuncture and to cultivate their ability as well as their inner self. There is also a reflection on what it takes to be a true physician, and on research methods, and even an enlightening explanation of the first chapter of the Lingshu, etc.

Even in the chapters that seem devoted to a specific topic, like the meridians or the acupuncture techniques, several approaches are discussed, not in order to show erudition, but in order to guide on the way of a deeper understanding and a more efficient practice.

This book attends to history and transmission, to the various aspects of the practice of acupuncture and also to its language and the deep meaning of the concepts essential to the understanding of Chinese medicine, since this medicine was elaborated in China and in Chinese. It speaks of the inner state of the practitioner, the quality of his or her mind, and what makes it clear and profound, able to perceive the smallest sign and to penetrate its significance.

It also is concerned with relationship and interaction. It shows how body and mind are inseparable and how life is always the result of interaction within a person, between several persons, as between the authors of the book or as between patient and practitioner or any other human relationship. The interactions that exist between a human being and their surroundings, the social, familial, cultural context as well as the atmospheric conditions and the correlation with the whole cosmos.

Is this book simply several texts by different authors published together? Absolutely not. Only four chapters are signed by a single name, and even in these cases the others often gave their comments. The other chapters are signed by 2 or 3 authors. Still the book is a book, with its backbone, its purpose. The consistency and cohesion come from inside and the book is not disparate.

All the chapters answer one to the other and weave something between them. Exactly like in the Chinese model where all that exists is built through the continuous intertwining of the yin and yang qi. Reality is more likely to be approached by a movement of weaving and interaction than by the analysis, even a sharp one, of a single mind. Exchanges, in which each maintains one's own identity, with respect for the others and reference to common roots, lead to a composition naturally balanced.

The result is not a cacophony, but a song with several voices. There is a similarity between a canon, as musical canon or song and a canon as a classic book. Several different lines are possible; as long as they do not create a discordant mixture of sounds, unpleasant to the ear, they play together and it is their togetherness which gives the full score. Impossible to say that this line is better than this other, or that this one is good and the other wrong. Each of them has to take its place, its moment, its intensity. The result is a beautiful and meaningful symphony.

This way of thinking is well developed in the East, and the Chinese did not assume that if an approach were right, the other had to be wrong. As the authors point out, it is quite different from the emphasis put in the West on a kind of "objective truth" which is more often a delusion.

As they say:

> "Modern Western and scientific thinking has assumed that there is an objective truth out there that exists independently of any observers... Once this truth is established it will replace all other theories. Thinking in ancient China... was not concerned with trying to establish an objective truth. It has tended to see the individual always as part of a larger whole which is irreducible, the apparent parts of which are all interconnected and thus cannot be viewed independently... A natural consequence of these differences can be seen in how mind and body were seen."

There is no attempt to create an artificial unity, either in the chapters of the book or in the corpus of Chinese medicine. There is a constant attention to search for the meaning, a sense which is always both contextual and universal since every specific situation answers to the cosmic order.

To be able to seek out the significance of any situation implies an inner training, a self-cultivation, essential for anyone pretending to be a practitioner. Meaning, comprehension depends always on a given context. The plasticity of the notions is not because they are vague and imprecise, but because no English word (or word of any Western language) can have the same meaning and the same background as a Chinese character. The Chinese were able to focus and be specific when it was needed; but also to use general, non-specific words, or what appear for us to be like that, when they wanted to allude to a reality which is present, analogously, for instance in a human body, in the cosmos, in the society...

True knowledge is the art of life. To know is to know how to live, following and internalising the great rules of conduct, transmitted by the tradition, which are great and efficient because rooted in the cosmic order of life. So, any movement, action, behaviour becomes meaningful. To have a medical knowledge is to know how to act efficiently, to apply methods and techniques transmitted by lineages and masters and to find the deep meaning in following and internalising a theory which is a reflection of the cosmic order.

The authors do not try to simplify to the point to distort and disfigure the reality of Chinese medicine. Neither they do not make it more complicated; but they respect the intrinsic intricacy of life which transpires in the complexity of the texts and notions. Doing this, they make clear the differences between the Eastern and Western approaches.

There is a fundamental vision that is found in the great classical texts of China and for any great notion there is a bundle of meanings linked together and making sense. None is univocal, but a clear meaning emerges from their cultural background, from the context and from the association with other notions.

Likewise, the various possible ways in the theory as well as in the practice have a clear meaning and efficient use. Meanwhile, one has to pay attention not to mingle them without caution and the appropriate knowledge.

The basis of Chinese medicine is found in the medical classics as the Huangdi Neijing (Suwen and Lingshu), the Nanjing, the Jiayijing, texts specially investigated by the authors. But the roots are found in the classical texts written mainly before the end of the Han dynasty (circa 220 AD). Their knowledge is required to understand the great notions which are the pillars of the elaboration of the medical theory. These texts present a vision of the universe and the cosmic order, of the meaning of life and more especially of human life, the human mind and its awareness ; they belong to various streams in Chinese thought, different but not excluding others. Again, the bundle of the approaches built the understanding. It is like all the approaches forming a bundle were pointing at a center; this central place must remain empty to welcome the understanding of every one.

The texts of the book are acting the same way. They direct toward an empty place where the reader can put his or her own understanding, an understanding always evolving and changing, page after page, year after year, since it is a book which may be read several times and bring something new or deeper each time.

It is demanding. But without a sincere effort and a serious work, one cannot pretend to be an authentic practitioner of Chinese medicine. It takes time, a personal involvement, a bite of humility, a constant self-cultivation. But it is worth any hour spent to do it.

Finally, a last but not least quality of this book is to uphold that Chinese medicine is a true medicine, wholly able to rely on its own resources and without the need of a Western medicine either to evaluate its capacity or to give it help for diagnosis.

It is one of the targets of the authors :

> "to lay a foundation for establishing valid research approaches to acupuncture that attempt to investigate acupuncture more on the basis of the early descriptions of it and their modern practical applications."

A set of therapeutic techniques can be called a medicine only if it relies on its own corpus of knowledge and theory, has its own means of diagnosis and treatments, and is able to continue to evolve with its own researches.

Chinese medicine is grounded on a corpus of texts and on a variety of techniques and practice, with a transmission and a memory. It has to continue to progress, for example, through the constant and fruitful face to face (encounter) between its own theories and its own practices. The dialogue between both can be one of the foundations of a true research in Chinese medicine, allowing to enlarge its capacity and eventually to integrate some concepts of Western medicine. A medicine unable to evolve is a dead medicine. A medicine depending on something else than its own resources is not a medicine. Now we proclaim high and loud that the classical Chinese medicine that we practice is a wholly authentic medicine.

A dialogue between this classical Chinese medicine and the Western medicine can help to build the medicine for the future. This book is one of the foundations of such an appealing and needed project.

Elisabeth Rochat de la Vallée
Paris, March 2014

# PREFACE

Stephen Birch, Miguel Angel Cabrer Mir, Manuel Rodríguez Cuadras

In the field of traditional medicine from East Asia, qi [氣] and their channels in the body, the jingmai [經脈], have played important and unique roles in various health promotion and healing practices. An important use of these concepts can be seen in how they refer to or imply the natural order of things and how they can be used to restore a patient back into this state of natural order.

This edited book will explore how this came about by examining the development of the concepts of qi and jingmai (chapters one and two), the cultivated or "superior" practitioner (chapter three), how the concepts of qi and jingmai have been exploited in various health systems such as acupuncture (chapters four and five), herbal medicine (chapter six) and self- development methods like taijiquan, qigong and aikido (chapter seven). The concepts "qi" and "jingmai" are practical concepts and not just theoretical ideas. Thus in order to do justice to these ideas, we have added a practical section with a number of exercises that can be performed that help develop both an increased sensitivity to qi and an increased ability to use qi and the jingmai (chapter ten). The practical chapter is accompanied by an introduction (chapter nine) to help bridge between the theoretical parts of the book (chapters one to seven) and the practical chapter (ten). Further, since we are writing in the modern period where science has become the important language and method for establishment and acceptance of ideas, we also explore issues involved in valid scientific investigations of concepts like qi and the jingmai (chapter eight).

Fundamentally, like most ideas in classical China, the concepts of qi and jingmai are practical concepts (explored in chapters one and eight). Thus, like concepts used by artisans and practitioners of different arts and disciplines, these cannot only be understood intellectually, there is necessarily a different understanding that comes through experience. We often find people referring to ancient Chinese and traditional East Asian medical (TEAM) concepts like qi as being "philosophical", as though they refer to nothing but mere ideas and are not grounded in practical or real-world things. We can also find some referring to TEAM concepts like qi as though they had the same kind of status like the "cell", or "atom" or "liver" things that can be imaged or accessed with our senses and about which there is considerable consensus as to their existence (ontological status). Many people talk about things like "qi" with the same casualness as they might when they talk about electricity, rain or the metro. The status of the TEAM concept "qi" is neither a philosophical system or referential way of thinking, nor does it refer to things whose existence can be simply taken for granted. More care needs to be taken when we discuss such things since their nature is not captured well by casual ways of thinking such as these. Since these are fundamentally (but as we will see not exclusively) practical concepts grounded in experience and practical actions, it is there that we must look for a better understanding.

When the master pianist explains in words a difficult musical phrase and the methods of its expression to someone untrained in music, it may make no sense at all. To the beginning student his words may also have almost no meaning since their skills are not yet developed enough to grasp the meaning of the explanation. It is only to the more advanced and experienced musician that the language and concepts of the teacher make sense. This understanding is a hard-won thing that comes through years of repetitive practice and study, and even then may not be practically achievable without further practice. This is not only something related to the high arts of the master musician, it is involved in many if not most daily activities. Take for example the work of the carpenter or wood-worker. The fine details of wood working that a master carpenter or furniture-maker explains may not be understood by the beginner, but they make sense to the experienced apprentice or colleague, whether involved in creating things of beauty or function. While these words and explanations can serve as a backdrop for on-going education and practice to guide the developing experience of the beginner apprentice, as concepts they are not reproducible yet in their hands. It is only after more years of study and practice that the same apprentice starts being able to enact such words and explanations.

Thus in order to do justice to difficult and important concepts such as qi and the jingmai, it is not enough to simply read books, these ideas need practical expression and understanding which comes through the minds, hands and hearts of experienced practitioners. To be able to capture the range of meanings and understandings attached to words like 氣 [qi], we should look to the literature and interpret what we find not only on the basis of that and accompanying literature, but through the range of experiences that have come through years of working with qi. There is a well-established tradition in Asia of scholar-practitioners in the field of medicine, that is, practitioners who also spent considerable time reading, researching, interpreting and trying to explain the literature and concepts of their medicine. Over the centuries we find such scholar-practitioners mostly through their published works. Practitioners such as Sun Simiao, Hua Shuo, Li Shizhen, Yang Jizhou, Xu Dachun each spent years in their studies, investigations and writings. The works of these literate practitioners are not always easy to understand, but they help form the backbone of later practice systems of these medicines.

The authors of the chapters in this book are all practitioners who have turned their hands to scholarly investigations of the literature and practice methods. All of the authors have around 30 or more years of practical experience. Their interests in the literatures of their arts combined with their decades of experience using them have helped cultivate broader understandings of concepts like qi and jingmai.

The East Asian medical and health promoting disciplines of acupuncture, herbal medicine, Taiji quan, qigong, aikido are relatively new in the West. It is really only since the early 1970s that they have been developing in any substantial way. In Asia these disciplines have roots that go back for centuries, and it is here that we find the works of "scholar-practitioners". In the West, these different East Asian origin fields and disciplines have started maturing to a stage where it is now possible for scholar-practitioners to have developed and find their voices. Thus we wish to start exposing this scholar-practitioner tradition in the West as well. This book represents the first time that experienced scholar-practitioners have attempted such a book together so that these eminently practical ideas can be interpreted through the eyes and hands of practitioners who have cultivated a deep practical understanding of them.

The fields of investigation are huge, possibly more than anyone can handle. Fortunately though, in recent years, a large body of new scholarship has emerged of the period before and during the developments of medical thinking in Han dynasty China. This scholarship is largely unknown within the TEAM practitioner communities. The authors in this book have drawn from this literature to write these chapters. The authors help bring alive this scholarship for these practitioner communities with practical interpretations and applications. Included is also a chapter exploring for the first time how these practical concepts will need to be investigated in scientific studies. Thus the chapters in this book are mostly written following a broad reading of available scholarship, translations and at times interpretations of original texts. This is done to help reveal more of how the original authors of the time may have thought so that we can better contextualise how those and later authors thought about what they said.

In its scope we believe that this is a far ranging book covering ways of thinking before the medical traditions began to emerge in the Han dynasty, ways of thinking in the early medical and self-development literatures, how these ideas were applied in later medical and self-development practices, simple practical exercises that employ the earliest principles and finally how to grapple with these histories and methods in the modern scientific context.

STEPHEN BIRCH, Amsterdam,
MIGUEL ANGEL CABRER MIR, Barcelona
MANUEL RODRÍGUEZ CUADRAS, Barcelona
February 2014

# ACKNOWLEDGEMENTS

The writing of this book has taken over six years, during which time we have had the support of many different people. We are very grateful to Dianne Sommers, Chip Chace, Dan Bensky and Mark Bovey for their written contributions to this book and also to Steve Clavey for permission to reproduce the paper by Chace and Bensky from the journal he edits, "The Lantern". Chip, Dianne and Mark also gave much advice and support through many thought provoking conversations. We also would like to thank our families for their support and understanding while we worked on this book. A number of others have offered help and support as well in the actual preparation of the book, with talks, comments, feedback, editing. Thank you to Viv Manning, Damon Dunn, Ricard Fané and Rayén Antón. We would also like to thank our students who have seen us through some of the developments and breakthroughs that we have made

# CONTRIBUTORS

**Stephen Birch** has an early background in science and philosophy. He graduated the New England School of Acupuncture in Boston, Massachusetts in 1982. His early teachers included Tin Yau So, Ted Kaptchuk and Kiiko Matsumoto. Having developed an interest in Japanese acupuncture and the historical texts and traditions, he co-wrote "Five Elements and Ten Stems", "Extraordinary Vessels" and "Hara Diagnosis" with Ms. Matsumoto. In 1985 he met Dr Yoshio Manaka with whom he studied (1985-1989) and helped author the book "Chasing the Dragon's Tail". Dr Manaka inspired him to pursue scientific studies on acupuncture as well, leading to PhD work at Exeter University in the UK (1991-1997). Starting in 1988 he also studied with many other senior Japanese traditional acupuncture practitioners (more than a dozen with 45 or more years of experience each in the Toyohari Association –Kodo Fukushima, Toshio Yanagishita, Akihiro Takai, and so on). In 1998 he published the book "Japanese Acupuncture" with Junko Ida and in 1999 "Understanding Acupuncture" with Bob Felt. The most recent book "Shonishin" was authored by Dr Birch and released in 2011. He began teaching at the New England School in 1985 and since the late 1980s has taught many workshops on acupuncture in many countries, especially in Europe. He conducted his PhD research at a Harvard teaching hospital and also worked at Yale Medical School on research for 2 years (1995-7) and has collaborated on a number of other international research studies. He has published many papers on the history, nature and practice of acupuncture. He has also published many more scientific papers on acupuncture. He was founding co-president of the Society for Acupuncture Research in the US and has organized and been part of a number of research workshops on acupuncture, and co-founder of the International Committee or the Study of Traditional East Asian Medicine (ICS-TEAM). At present he is Associate Professor at the University College of Health Sciences –Campus Kristiania, Oslo, Norway and together with Dr Terje Alraek is collaborating with the Korean Institute of Oriental Medicine, Daejeon, Korea. Throughout this time, with the exception of holidays and study periods, he has maintained a practice in Japanese acupuncture (1982-present), currently in Amsterdam, the Netherlands.

**Miguel Angel Cabrer Mir** has studied and practiced Taiji quan for around thirty years, Yi quan around ten years and has been teaching Taiji quan twenty five years. He has studied with advanced practitioners in China and Canada (Sam Tam). He completed his studies in acupuncture thirteen years ago and has practiced in Barcelona and surrounds since then. He has been a student and practitioner of Japanese acupuncture methods, including Toyohari for over ten years, has been teaching Japanese acupuncture for several years and is starting to teach Toyohari. He has completed advanced trainings in Chinese medicine (2006) and Toyohari (2009). He has taught workshops in Spain, Holland and Germany on the art of sensitivity, training the body to increase sensitivity through touch. He has contributed several articles to journals since 2008.

**Manuel Rodríguez Cuadras** born in 1947, studied and practised Chemical Engineering, Management and Graphic Design. He also studied and practised several martial arts, especially Judo (15 years), Qigong (20 years), Aikido (30 years), and Iaido (15 years), and taught some of these, especially Aikido, for a number of years. More than 20 years ago he started studying Chinese medicine, both in Spain and in Beijing (living there for about 3 years), then teaching TCM in Spain for more than 10 years. After meeting S. Birch, he became adept at a different interpretation of this discipline, and consequently graduated in Shonishin, Manaka, Meridian Therapy and Toyohari systems. He published two books on Oriental style Paediatrics (2008), followed by another book on TCM theory (2010) and the terminology database for translating Chinese medicine into Spanish (2011). Currently a member of the ICS-TEAM and of the editorial board of the Journal of TCM (Spanish edition), he practices and teaches both in Barcelona and Madrid (Spain) and in Santiago (Chile).

**Dianne Sommers** studied philosophy (M.A. University of Amsterdam) and classical Chinese (Sinology department, University of Leiden). Her research interest focuses on the development of early Chinese Medicine. In 2007 she has published a translation and philosophical interpretation of the Neiye, an early Chinese text. She studied acupuncture, manual therapies and physiotherapy in the Netherlands, China and Japan and practices since 1983, currently in Amsterdam. She is also a member of the ICSTEAM.

**Mark Bovey** gained a MSc in animal breeding and worked as a geneticist for an international agri-business company. In 1983 he received his Licentiate from the College of Traditional Acupuncture in the UK, and has been in private practice in Oxford, where he lives since then. He divides his working week between practice and research: he is research manager for the British Acupuncture Council and has been the coordinator of the Acupuncture Research Resource Centre since 1998. He is the author of a number of acupuncture research articles and has been a co-investigator on studies of acupuncture use for fertility, acupuncture's effectiveness for Parkinson's Disease and the effects of cupping on inflammatory markers. He also teaches at the College of Integrated Chinese Medicine, Reading, where he helped to develop the research module. He is also a member of the ICSTEAM.

**Charles Chace** graduated from the New England School of Acupuncture in 1984 where he also began his study of Chinese Language. He has maintained a longstanding interest in the medical literature of China and is the translator of a wide variety of books and articles on pre-modern approaches to acupuncture and Chinese medicine including a translation of the first textbook of acupuncture from 100 C.E., The Yellow Emperor's Systematic Classic of Acupuncture and Moxibustion (Huang Di Zhen Jiu Jia Yi Jing), and Li Shizhen's Qi Jing Ba Mai Kao, the seminal text on the extraordinary vessels. He is also long time student of a broad range of palpation-based forms of practice in both the acupuncture and osteopathic traditions. Chip has practiced Chinese medicine for over twenty-five years and is on the faculty of the Seattle Institute of Oriental Medicine where he teaches palpatory approaches to acupuncture. He maintains a clinical practice in Boulder, Colorado.

**Dan Bensky** is a graduate of the Macau Institute of Chinese Medicine (Oriental Medicine Diploma, 1975), University of Michigan (B.A. in Chinese Language and Literature, 1978), Michigan State University College of Osteopathic Medicine (Doctor of Osteopathy, 1982), University of Washington (M.A. in Classical Chinese, 1996), and Chinese Academy of Traditional Chinese Medical Sciences (Ph.D. in Discussion of Cold Damage, 2006). He contributed to the translation and editing of "Acupuncture: A Comprehensive Text", "Chinese Herbal Medicine: Materia Medica", and "Chinese Herbal Medicine: Formulas & Strategies" and has also contributed to articles published in the Far Eastern Economic Review, European Journal of Oriental Medicine, Asian Medicine, and the Lantern, among others. Dr. Bensky helped found the Seattle Institute of Oriental Medicine in 1994 and has taught in North America, Europe, Australia, Japan, and China. In 2008, he was awarded the Wang Dingyi Cup International Prize for contributions to Chinese Medicine. He has lived and practiced in Seattle, Washington since 1985.

CHAPTER ONE

# QI, MIND AND BODY

## Explorations of the links between qi, the mind, mental and emotional states and the body[i]

**Stephen Birch, Miguel Angel Cabrer Mir, Manuel Rodríguez Cuadras**

"I have often heard the name of the Way, but have yet to hear its actuality.
May I ask to what this thing the Way refers?"
Master Jia replied: "This thing the Way, is what you follow
when you associate with the world of things. Its beginning
is called the undifferentiated, its endings are called techniques.
The undifferentiated refers to its essential subtlety;
it is plain and ordinary but one cannot act upon it.
Techniques refer to that by which one regulates the world of things;
the processes of movement and stillness. Both of these are the Way."

From the "Xinshu Jiaozhu", (second century BCE) [19:227]

若志，無聽之以耳而聽之以心，無聽之以心而聽之以氣。聽止於耳，
心止於符。氣也者，虛而待物者也。唯道集虛。虛者，心齋也
Make your will one! Don't listen with your ears, listen with your mind (心).
No, don't listen with your mind, but listen with your vital energy (氣).
Listening stops with the ears, the mind stops with recognition,
but vital energy is empty and waits on all things.
The Dao gathers in emptiness alone. Emptiness is the fasting of the mind.

From Zhuangzi (fourth century BCE) [136:93]

Thus by 350 (BCE), when philosophy began to be systematic, qi meant air, breath, vapor, and other pneumatic stuff. It might be congealed or compacted in liquid and solids. Qi also referred to the *balanced and ordered* vitalities or energies, partly derived from the air we breathe, that cause physical change and maintain life. [111:47]

气 気

i. We would like to thank Dianne Sommers, Mark Bovey for helpful feedback and comments on the chapter.

## Introduction

In order to understand the concept of "qi" [氣] particularly in traditional East Asian medicine (TEAM) it is necessary to look at premedical uses of the concept and trace how these uses gave rise to the formalized models of qi in the medical literature. The period from the late Spring and Autumn, through the Warring States to the early Han dynasty approximately 500-100 BCE was an important formative time when the foundations were laid for the medical literature. There has been a considerable increase in scholarship of this time which allows us to comment on the probable influences and relationships of concepts from this period into the medical literature. During this time concepts of the body, mind and qi were being developed and explored [1, 19, 62, 94, 98, 113, 128]. At this time, and generally since then, the mind and body were not generally thought of as being separate in Chinese thinking [1, 2, 18, 46, 47, 94, 98, 100]. The separateness of mind and body first arose in early Greek thinking and has dominated Western thinking especially since Rene Descartes famous "cogito ergo sum" –"I think therefore I am" [25]. There were also close links suggested between the mind (xin [心]) and qi as well that have been and remain influential, which have prompted modern scholars to suggest that it seems necessary to discuss qi when discussing the mind and vice versa [19:151].

The influence of the mind, emotions and different mental states on the qi were seen as key in the premedical and early medical literatures. Early physiological discussions intimated a clear link between the physical organs, their functions, specific mental states, specific emotions and qi [47, 78, 98, 128]. These were not only relevant for understanding etiology and treatment in the medical context, but these links are rooted in and provide an essential basis for understanding the meditative and movement cultivation traditions, yang sheng [養生] (nourishing life) practices, rulership, virtue and sagacity in both Confucian and Daoist traditions [1, 19, 62, 68, 94, 100]. These pre-medical discussions clearly influenced the early medical literature, and thus have exerted influence on the development of TEAM in formative and later stages. In recent years scholars have concluded that distinctions between the so-called "Confucian" and "Daoist" "schools" are increasingly inaccurate and not useful [19:10, 36:151-155, 44:3-11, 94:25, 115:3]. For example, while earlier scholars associated the concept of "wuwei" [無為] with the "Daoist" school [86], recent scholarship has shown its prevalence and importance across many of the so-called "schools" [115]. Even the classification of a "Daoist" "tradition" or "school" is questioned since there are competing threads of Daoist like thinking with different influences [94:25, 96, 100:5-9, 110]. Thus we mostly abandon this earlier attempt at classification by these "schools". We present ideas related to qi, mind and body mostly by textual tradition partly in chronological order and partly by association. The early medical literature drew from a wide variety of sources and shows influences from what have been known as "Confucian" [124] and "Daoist" thinking [38, 96], what we attempt to do is expose some of the variety of ideas that existed before the medical literature started appearing.

We will thus examine concepts of the mind and body and trace relationships between these and of both with the concept of qi through texts that discuss them. We will also argue that one of the important ways that the models of qi developed was out of experience –the mind experiences the world through sensory and non-sensory[1] input, the point of interaction of the mind with the world, where experience arises, is a place where we talk of qi. The mind experiences the world as an observer, and is also a participant in the world through that observation –the mind thus influences the world; the concept of qi captures that interaction and mutual influence.

## Qi –an overview

We start with a brief overview of the concept of qi. How is the term understood? How is it used? How has it developed? There have been not a few attempts to describe this term in different books dedicated to explaining it [53, 89, 98, 139]. It is clear that many different ideas have developed over time and that the "qi" has taken on many different meanings and is understood in many, often vastly different ways.[2]

The term "qi" has been through significant changes of meaning over time, bringing forward with it these various meanings [67]. Earlier forms are [气], [气] or [气]. Early references during the Shang period (1600-1046 BCE) give qi the meaning of "beseech", "end", "food donation" [38:77], but it is difficult to see how these relate to later meanings. By the mid-Warring states period (475-221 BCE) the term came to be associated with atmospheric and environmental conditions such as "vapours", "clouds", "mists" [67]. The Shuowen Jiezi [說文解字] (90 CE), the first etymological Chinese dictionary defines qi as "cloud vapour" [雲气] [1:88, 38:77].[3] By the fourth century BCE it became associated with "the fundamental stuff in nature which both promotes and indicates vitality in the phenomenal world" [67] and by the late Warring states period it had come to be associated with feelings and emotions, something inside the body, which gave the person attempting to control it, a new measure of control over their own bodies and health, exemplified by descriptions found in the important Neiye [內業] chapter of the Guanzi [管子] [67, 94]. The form established by the Han dynasty (206 BCE-220 CE) and in common use from that time was [氣]. Here the radical mi [米], "grain" was inserted into the character, thus giving the term qi [氣] the commonly associated meaning of the "vapors or steam rising from cooking rice" [98:10]. However, by the time of the earliest medical literatures (third to second centuries BCE) while it began to carry this meaning it also brought with it the older meanings, so that term had already become very complex. An old form of the character appears to have Daoist origins [炁] or [炁] [139], a modified form of which is used in the Guodian version of the Daodejing chapter fifty five [41:74 –see also 35]. Another modified form of the qi character is found on the "xingqi" [行氣], "moving qi" jade stone inscription which uses the fire [火] radical instead of the grain radical [米], see figure 1 [1:88]. The modern form of the "qi" character in China today is simplified to the earlier simple form [气], while in Japan the character was simplified by reducing the grain radical to an x [気], ki.

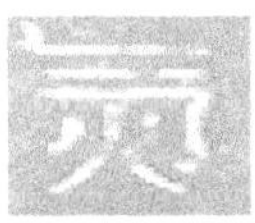

Figure 1

Today we find that the term "qi" [氣] has been rendered into various English words. English terms commonly found include "vapour", "energy", "breath", "vital" "force" or "energy", even "stuff". Box 1 gives many examples of how different translators and authors have approached the term. Perhaps the easiest approach we can take is to follow many other authors who have simply left the term "qi" untranslated as "qi".

It is easy for people to impose their own world views or culturally imbued perspectives on how they understand a concept like "qi". In the modern period "qi" (in Japanese "ki") has been used in China and Japan as a term to translate modern concepts, including and especially those that originated in the West, often in compound forms.[4] The term qi is widely used in daily life, we find many Chinese and Japanese uses.[5] For example in Japanese electricity is "denki"

[電気], weather is "tenki" [天気], energy is "kiryoku" [気力], health is "genki" [元気], anger is "doki" [怒気] and feeling/sensation is "kimochi" [気持], while in Chinese meteorology is "qì xiàng"'[气象], weather is "tianqi" [天气], electricity is "dianqi" [電气], complexion is "qì sè" [气色], breath is "qì xī" [气息], to vaporise is "qì huà" [气化], to hate is "qì hèn" [气恨] and strength, energy is "qì lì" [气力]. It is therefore not surprising that many people in China and Japan for example might tend to impose the implied meanings in these modern uses onto their understanding of the term "qi", uncritically overlaying that understanding onto older uses of the term. Similarly in the West, there has been a tendency to turn to the wisdom of ancient China for solutions to the perceived deficits of modern society and modern scientific thinking [12, 126, 127]. Qi has often been seen in "spiritual" and "energetic" terms as the individual searches for meaning in the ancient Chinese discourses. Indeed we see the qi character associated with the term "energy" in both China (qì lì) and Japan (kiryoku) as part of the modern translation of the Western concept of "energy". This suggests that there could have been a mutual influence (like Pickering's "mangle of practice" –see next section) from the West on Asia as to how "energy" should be understood and from Asia on the West in terms of how "energetic" medicine was sought. This tendency has often resulted in an uncritical imposition of modern thought processes onto an understanding of the idea of "qi", see examples in chapter eight, which explores qi, jingmai and their scientific investigation. We need to be careful to step aside from these thorny issues when we explore the meaning of the term "qi".

Sivin proposed that the term "qi" was used in three main streams of thinking in the period before the medical literatures started appearing in the early Han dynasty. One stream of meaning sees qi in relation to steam, vapor, clouds, breath and thus the vitality in us, the second as intangible but perceptible things like aromas, vapors, smoke, and the third rooted in cosmological thinking introducing the cycles and influences of yin-yang, the procession of the seasons, and through correlative thinking, the flavors of food, colours, musical modes [111:46], "qi had become the basic stuff of the cosmos, and the vitality that maintained processes and made change happen" [114:49]. Tang mentions a somewhat different threefold understanding of how the term qi can be interpreted, as "(a) material existence; (b) vitality and consciousness, as for instance in Mencius' and energetic and dynamic qi... or the Guanzi's essential qi; or (c) the ultimate, as for instance in the one evolved into three'... theme in Daoist thought" [122:38]. Examining other implications in the use of the term "qi", Daly draws out the analogized understanding of "qi" in hydrological, fluid metaphors, where "qi" was seen as a unidirectionally flowing thing like water [21]. Allan has also drawn attention to this [1].

**BOX 1 –qi in translation**

Early European encounters with the concept rendered qi into terms then familiar such as **“spirits”** (after Galen’s “animal spirits”) and “a circulation of the blood and humours” also akin to Galenic notions of the day [4:87]. Today, many terms can be found when searching through the literature, the following is a selection. We find for example: **“finest matter influences”** or **“influences”** [124:72], **“vapor”** [1, 38], **“hylozoistic vapors”** [2:62], **“breath”** [55:223,138:57], **“breaths”** [55:220], **“vital breath”** [55:266], **“breath/energy’** [62:61], **“pneuma’** [19, 40, 73:14-16], **“fluid’** [21:1], **“vitalizing fluids’** [31:260], **“the activating fluids in the atmosphere and the body”** [31:477], **“flow-event”** [Pfister in 61:103], **“subtle matter”** [86:228], **“spirit”** [55:174], **“energy”** [3, 42:77, 84, 135], **“matter-energy”** [59:14], **“energy flows”** [42:77, 132], **“internal energy”** [19], **“impulsions”** [46], **“psychophysical stuff”** [2:62], **“vital psychophysiological stuff”** [4:4], **“vital energy”** [1, 34:468, 62, 100, 121:88, 136:93, 138:57], **“vital force”** [96], **“vital forces”** [17:12], **“life force”** [121:57], the **“activity of life”** [65:9], **“vital energizing field”** [2:62]. Harper has a much more down to earth rendering of “qi” as “stuff” or “basic stuff” –“qi already referred to the ‘basic stuff’ of the phenomenal world” [38:77.][6] This seems to follow Sivin who discusses how qi can be thought of depending on context as **“what makes things happen in stuff”**, the **“stuff that makes things happen”** and the **“stuff in which things happen”** [111:47]. He goes on to discuss various terms people have used to render qi into English and his reasons for not using any of them [111: 47]. Ames and Hall have a similar usage with **“psychophysical stuff”** [2:62]. The analysis of Ames and Hall is similar to that of Sivin “Qi has to be distinguished from either ‘animating vapors’ or ‘basic matter’ because it cannot be resolved into any kind of spiritual-material dichotomy. **Qi is both the animating energy and that which is animated. There are no ‘things’ to be animated; there is only the vital energizing field and its focal manifestations”** [2:63]. Lo comments “early Chinese literature often invokes qi to explain the vitality and intensity of things” [67], and refers to it as “the fundamental stuff of life” [71:393] . Moeller discusses qi as follows: “Qi is a ‘something’ that streams through and blows through the whole world. Everything is made alive by Qi –not only humans, animals and plants, but also such things as paintings and stones. It is believed to be the kind of ‘vital force’ that is ‘breathing’ in everything that exists” [82:74], this is similar to the interpretation of qi as “stuff”–see below. Schwartz explains “Qi comes to embrace properties which we would call psychic, emotional, spiritual, numinous, and even ‘mystic.’ It is precisely at this point that Western definitions of ‘matter’ and the physical which systematically exclude these properties from their definitions do not at all correspond to qi… To the extent that the word ‘energy’ is used in the West to apply exclusively to a force that relates only entities described in terms of physical mass, it is as misleading as ‘matter’, I think, as an over-all name for qi” [Schwartz in 61:103].

These various streams of meaning and use are found in early and later medical literatures and can thus be seen to have been quite influential. In this chapter we will focus especially on exploring how the models of the mind, emotions and body developed around qi. We will also touch on the cosmological uses of the term qi. A number of generally accepted perspectives on how qi was used and understood have been proposed. It is thought to be associated with describing change "we can already see that ch'i (qi) provides a language for thinking about the stuff involved in change, as well as the energies that make change possible" [111:53], and some invisible, insubstantial or formless thing ("influences", "subtle matter", "psychophysical stuff") that is involved in those changes or which gives rise (for example by condensation) to the material forms of things and the actions of those things.

## Philosophical Perspectives

Before discussing the thematic concepts of this chapter, qi, mind and body, we feel it important to briefly mention underlying philosophical differences so as to help the reader put aside natural preconceptions and assumptions that can lead to misunderstanding the discussion of these themes.

Many people have written about the philosophical differences between Western and scientifically influenced world views and their assumptions and more traditional East Asian world views and assumptions [e.g. 36, 55, 94]. Paul Unschuld has nicely captured some of these issues especially as they pertain to understanding the medical literatures [124, 126, 127], Birch has recapitulated some of them [5, 6, 12, 13]. While there is a tendency to try to argue on the basis of "paradigmatic" differences between East and West [e.g. 5] following the arguments of Kuhn [54], there are counter arguments about the inadequacy of that approach [52, 102, 125]. Unschuld argues that "Thomas Kuhn's notions of 'scientific revolution' and 'periods of normal science' are hardly applicable to Chinese history of science" [125:6-7]. Scheid and others argue further that Pickering's "mangle of practice" model [92] is more suitable to understand how East and West differences can be examined [52, 69:63, 102]. We will thus not engage in arguments or discussions further about paradigmatic differences, instead focusing here on three major philosophical differences.

There has been a strong trend in Western and scientific thinking to try to establish an "objective" description of the world, one where the person observing and describing the world is able to separate himself from it and describe it independent of himself as observer [25]. This approach is based on the assumptions that the person observing does not influence what is observed and that they are able to separate themselves from their observations. The objective world is described once individual experiences of the world are superceded. This trend did not happen in East Asia [2:15, 66:192-193] until the adoption of Western ways of thinking in recent centuries [12, 13]. Instead, the observer was always placed at the center of observations and there was not a tendency to try to describe things objectively. The individual was conceived as part of a larger whole and thus individual experiences of the world could not be separated from the world that is experienced.[7] Kuriyama illustrates this well in his comparison of Greek pulse and Chinese "mo"[8] (pulse) diagnosis approaches [55]. The Greek model presages later Western approaches: "Greek pulse theory... sought strictly to segregate what a pulse is from how it feels, fact from perception" [55:95]. While in the Chinese model "the question of the identity of a mo blends indistinguishably into the issues of haptic technique... Each mo responds differently to the inquiring hand, and it is by their differing responses that one tells them apart" [55:96]. Kuriyama summarises this succinctly as "Asking 'what' was inseparable from asking 'how'?" [55:96]. We will see below that this characteristic of Chinese thinking has important implications.

A further important trend in Western and scientific thinking, which complements the first is that in order to describe a thing we can describe its parts and from the parts we can construct the larger picture of the whole thing, a process called "reductionism" [25]. The reductionist approach is based on the assumptions that any whole system properties of a thing are nothing more than the simple sum of the parts of that thing and that the reduction of the thing to its component parts does not diminish the thing or our understanding of the thing itself. The opposite tendency has dominated in East Asian thinking due largely to the tendency to think more "holistically", to see things as part of an inseparable whole [86].[9] While this model of holism has not been universal in pre-medical and medical traditions in East Asia [126, 127] it has certainly played very significant roles in how the mind and body were viewed and how they are seen in relation to the world and others.[10] Ames and Hall in a discussion of the "most crucial contribution of Chinese culture broadly" cite Tang Junyi saying it is "...the spirit of the symbiosis and mutuality between particular and totality. In terms of our understanding this means an unwillingness to isolate the particular from the totality, and in terms of feeling, it means the commitment of the particular to do its best to realize the totality" [2:11]. Reductionism is rather an antithesis to this basic approach. However to call the approach "holistic" can lead to much confusion and thus we avoid further use of this term.

The third important feature of Western-scientific thinking is the "either-or" logical assumptive approach. In the either-or assumptive model, one cannot accept the validity of competing ideas; if one idea is considered right a contradictory one must be wrong. The scientific method for establishing "truth" is a clear example of the either-or approach. Scientific truth is developed using methods that assume this to be axiomatic. While it has dominated modern Western scientific thinking, its virtual absence in ancient Asian philosophies is often overlooked. Evidence from the medical field clearly demonstrates a corpus of traditional literature that is full of contradictory ideas, even within the same texts, the absence of "either-or" thinking is normal [111:81].[11] TEAM was fundamentally syncretistic, it has always employed a strategy of merging disparate ways of thinking and acting. This was not a problem for early authors since they did not assume that if one approach was right the other had to be wrong. Rather ideas and assumptions of all kinds co-exist at many different "levels" of interpretation with no attempt or indeed any reason to derive an absolute truth [124, 126, 127].[12] This is reflected in acupuncture for example being more than a single uniform therapy, it is, and always has been, defined by diversity of ideas and methods [6, 12, 102, 103, 106]. The fact that these many different styles of acupuncture each has different theories also implies that the theories themselves are not simply descriptions of the processes thought to be occurring –a feature of objective descriptions of the world.[14] Theory in TEAM and traditional Asian thinking is about addressing the issues of how to solve problems or perform certain acts. Despite the beliefs of individuals using those theories, the theories cannot be thought of as describing the world in the same way that a scientist attempts to objectively describe the world. Scheid and Bensky state this quite clearly in a discussion of the dialectic between signification and method:[15] "In contradistinction to western positivist or realist accounts, this difference does not, however, derive from the difference between true and false knowledge but always remains grounded in the practice of signification. **Debates in Chinese medicine therefore are not concerned with the truth of a method but with its efficacy**" (emphasis added) [105:37].

If we are not aware of these differences we might assume when we read ancient Chinese texts or the literatures of TEAM that we are reading something familiar, when it is not at all so. Without realizing it we might superimpose our culturally imbued thinking patterns onto what we read and start interpreting it relative to those assumptions.[16] For example, one of the consequences of these differences lies in how we understand the models that are described in what we read. The Western tradition seeks to construct explanatory models, based on the idea of objectively describing the world; the observer separates himself from the observations [13, 25, 126, 127] then the descriptions if properly arrived at constitute "explanatory models", models of the world and body that exist independently of the individual describing them. The "explanatory model" describes cause-and-effect relationships or processes between phenomena or processes. We might read a description in a textbook of TEAM and unwittingly attribute the same cause-and-effect explanatory values to what we read. The idea that a patient has a problem of "stagnation of liver qi" also known as "binding depression of liver qi" might lead us to think that this is a causal description of the patient's condition. But since the Asian tradition is virtually devoid of attempts to reach objective descriptions, it did not construct models where the observer is separated from the observations. Instead what appear to be "explanatory models" are not "explanatory models" in the Western sense, they are rather practical descriptive models, placing the individual observer in a context where he acts on and is acted on by the world [13]. Some in the medical field aware of these differences make statements such as "diagnosis is treatment" [12, 85, 88]. The diagnostic labels refer to treatment selection, the theories behind them are related to problem solving or acting on the world, they do not objectively describe it, do not describe cause-and-effect relationships [12, 13] The diagnosis of "stagnant liver qi" or "binding depression of liver qi" means needle acupoints such as LV-2, LV-3, LV-8, LV-13, GB-40, GB-34 or take a certain herbal formula such as [柴胡疏肝丸] 'chai-hu shu gan tang' (bupleurum liver-coursing decoction) [133]. This is a clear example of how the "asking 'what' was inseparable from asking 'how'?" [55:96]. Even "why" type questions are answered by "how'" type answers.[17] A parallel to this can be seen in the Guodian texts (circa 300 BCE) which describe "Sages know the way of heaven. Knowing something and putting it into practice is righteousness. Practicing something with the appropriate timing is virtue (de [德])" [44:59]. Knowledge and practice are inextricably linked, knowledge is not seen here as of things themselves, but proper actions in relation to those things. Chunyu Yi of the mid second century BCE, a medical practitioner from before the Neijing corpus said of qi: "As for the so-called qi, one ought to harmonise drink and food, and choose clear days for coach rides and walks to broaden the mind in order to adjust the tendons, bones, flesh, blood and essel-pulses for bringing qi into flow" [45:76]. The "what" of qi is the "how" of its development and protection. We feel that it is thus necessary to suspend our usual Western or "scientific" ways of thinking about models when considering Asian premedical and medical models.

In summary, modern Western and scientific thinking has assumed that there is an objective truth out there that exists independently of any observers, we can break down the world into smaller and smaller parts in order to establish that truth as a reconstruction of the identified parts. Once this truth is established it will replace all other theories. Thinking in ancient China and thus through TEAM traditions before the modern period *and including mo-*

*dern TEAM texts and systems* was not concerned with trying to establish an objective truth. It has tended to see the individual always as part of a larger whole which is irreducible, the apparent parts of which are all interconnected and thus cannot be viewed independently. Logical cause-and-effect models were not proposed instead multi-faceted causality models were prevalent [86].[18] A natural consequence of these differences can be seen in how mind and body were seen.

## A contrast of mind-body perspectives

In 1644 the philosopher-mathematician Rene Descartes proposed that it is possible to view the mind and body separately with his famous "cogito ergo sum", "I think therefore I am", initiating the movement known as Descartian dualism [25]. This dualism did not start with Descartes, it had its origins with the ancient Greeks, further ramified by Christian theologians to become "one of the most influential problematics of modern philosophy" [36:29] following Descartes. This has been very influential in Western thinking since he first proposed it with a strong trend in the Western view and in science to see the mind and body as separate, creating a kind of dualism. This has become an embedded part of the Western world view that is difficult to dislodge despite growing evidence in science that it is invalid [25].

In contrast to this, the ancient Chinese and TEAM perspective tends to see the mind and body as being inseparable "the Chinese in contrast, accepted that the mind was part of the body, more refined and essentialized but of the same substance" [62:20]. While there have been occasional references that discussed mind and body as separate in the pre-medical [19:152] and early TEAM literature [18:165] and other discussions that seem to imply a similarity to the duality found in the West [55:180], the bulk of the pre-medical and medical literature discusses them as inseparable [1, 2, 19, 46, 47, 62, 94, 128]. We can thus reasonably take the continuity or inseparability of mind and body as typically but not exclusively representative of the early Chinese and TEAM traditions. Both are seen as different manifestations of qi. The character "xin"[心] that refers to mind itself is the same character for the heart so that it is often translated as the "heart/mind" [36:29] or "mind/heart" [1]. This is a clear example of how the mind and body were not separated. Hall and Ames state is thus "The most important inference about the meanings of xin is that none of them, even after the Buddhist incursion, suggests a basic mind-body dualism" [36:29]. Allan describes how qi as breath "is that which gives us our vitality. And as the vital energy of the mind/heart, it is that which controls our thoughts and emotions, the sources of our moral sensibilities" [1:92], while the "mind/heart is both a physical organ that circulates blood and the organ with which one thinks and feels" [1:89]. But the wealth of historical uses and descriptions that can be found in ancient Chinese writings make it difficult to make absolute statements on this issue of mind-body distinctions, Roth has summarised this problem very well: "Without engaging these problems in detail, suffice it to say that, in the early Chinese world view reflected in these early Taoist writings, such distinctions were not made with the same degree of concreteness and inflexibility that we are accustomed to" [100:41]. We will return to the details of this in the sections below.

There is thus a need to suspend our normal (cultural) Western assumptions about the nature of the mind and body [138:54-55]. Not only in the context of our discussions here, but also because there is a growing philosophical argument that the mind-body model of Descartian dualism is wrong [22, 25], a growing body of evidence from scientific studies of consciousness that reveal it to be wrong [48, 49, 95] and also strong evidence in modern physics that this is incorrect [9, 25, 30, 81].

In chapter eight we will return to a number of the issues raised here as they are important for an understanding of how one might try to use science to investigate qi and the jingmai.

## Emerging Asian models of the mind, body and qi

Bearing in mind the preceding discussions we now turn to an examination of how the mind, body and qi were discussed and used in important premedical and early medical literatures. Here we will discuss ideas that developed out of a number of influential texts and streams of thought: the "Confucian" texts (the Analects, Great Learning); the Wuxing texts; the Mencius (Mengzi); the Xunzi; the Chunqiu texts; the Neiye (a chapter of the Guanzi); the Daodejing; the Zhuangzi; the Huainanzi; the "yangsheng" nourishing life health extension traditions and the early medical literatures of the Mawangdui; finally the Neijing, reputedly the first main medical classic in China. Ordered and ordering models of the body and mind emerged out of the chaos of the Warring States period of Chinese history (475-221 BC), that influenced and were influenced by emerging models of the state, cosmos, morality, responsibility, self-development, health and disease [1, 19, 38, 47, 62, 94, 113, 124, 127]. A number of mutually interacting influences helped mould the various models of the mind and body that emerged out of this period. The theme of self-cultivation is found running through many of these textual traditions and practices, qi and its higher or more refined forms (jing [精] and shen [神]) play important roles in these various texts and traditions. If the individual can create sufficient order in himself to become someone connected with the virtue of heaven, can order himself so as to align himself with the ordering qualities of heaven, or import the higher qualities of heaven into himself, he can maintain himself in a higher ordered state, export that order to those around him, export it to the world around him or even (in some traditions) help order heaven.[19]

There is a significant body of scholarship of this period available today. As might be expected, the different scholars have focused on different aspects or particular perspectives in the thinking of the pre-Han and early Han Chinese, so that there are slightly variant interpretations or emphases in the reading and understanding of ideas and texts from that time. We hope that by compiling from these different approaches, emphases and perspectives the reader can gain a broader picture of how mind, body and qi were thought about as the medical literatures of the Han, the Huangdi Neijing corpus start to appear. But, as we find in much of the literature of the period, and even within the same text, apparent contradictions abound. Using fixed definitions and understandings of the concepts we discuss, especially from the modern TEAM literature will only serve to confuse the reader. Michael Puett demonstrates admirably that the term "shen" or "spirit" has multiple meanings depending on the precise tradition in which it was used [94, see also discussions in 11 and 43]. This kind of openness of meaning is common and must be grasped if we are to start to understand the concept of qi and its relation with the body, mind and emotions. We discuss the range of understandings and meanings of a number of important concepts in the next section "a further analysis of terms and concepts". Here we outline a number of traditional perspectives.

## *The works of Confucius* [孔夫子]

In general in the Confucian textual tradition, it was seen as vital that the individual strive to better himself so that all can benefit from that. The cultivation of virtue or "de" [德], variously translated as "virtue" [1, 19, 115], "inner power" [1], "this focus", "insistent particularity" [2:13-19], "potency" [1, 33],[20] was seen as very important, both in "Confucian" and "Daoist" texts. Through the proper cultivation of one's "de" one can positively affect others. The various methods and processes that describe how one cultivates one's virtue have been covered at great length by various authors [see 1, 19, 115], so we will not dwell on that here. Instead we will briefly examine how the works of Confucius relate the mind, emotions and qi.

The Great Learning, Daxue [大學] (circa 500 BCE) describes how if one is to be a proper ruler: "wishing to cultivate their persons, they first rectified their minds. Wishing to rectify their minds, they first sought absolute sincerity in their thoughts. Wishing for absolute sincerity in their thoughts, they first extended their knowledge..." [28:362]. Naturally as part of this process one must learn to control one's emotions. The passage continues "Only after things have been arrived at is knowledge perfect, and only then is there integrity of intention, and only then are heart correct, and only then are hearts cultivated, and only then are families regulated, and only then are states in order, and only then is the Empire at peace" [31:132-133].

In the Analects, Lunyu [論語] (circa 500 BCE) we find a discussion of different stages of life development where "qi is the source of emotional behaviour such as lust, aggressiveness and greed" [1:89]: "The person of superior cultivation guards against three things, the Master cautions: When he is young and the blood and qi are not yet settled, he guards against lust. When he matures, and the blood and qi are in full vigor, he guards against combativeness. When he is old, and the blood and qi have declined, he guards against covetousness" [55:103; see also 1:89]. This may be the first clear link between emotions and qi setting the stage for later discussions. Kuriyama notes that the Analects describe how qi and blood are associated with the "core aspects of a person's being" [55:103].

## *The Wuxing* [五行]

The Wuxing {five processes or five kinds of action} is a previously lost text dating from at least the early third and probably late fourth century BCE that was recently recovered in the Mawangdui archaelogical findings (1973) with an older version recovered even more recently in the Guodian tomb (1993) [19]. It appears to have been written around the same time or slightly before the Mencius and Mozi. Like both, it is a text about the cultivation of "de", virtue focusing especially on moral psychological considerations. It addresses how the cultivated virtue relates to bodily humors and describes the virtues in relation to qi. It thus seems to lay the foundations for some of the later medical ideas that emerged in the early Han dynasty with the Huangdi Neijing corpus.

The Wuxing has many discussions of the relationships between the mind, virtues and qi. For example the Mawangdui [馬王堆] Wuxing states:

> To see [the Gentleman's Way] and know it is wisdom... Wisdom is knowing what you have not seen from what you have seen. "To know it and bring settlement is

benevolence." What knows the Way laid out by the gentleman and warmly finds security in it is the benevolent qi. "To settle and enact it is righteousness." What, having settled it, applies it in a… manner is the righteousness qi. "To enact and show respect is ritual propriety." What having applied it is reverent in a "flapping manner" is the ritual propriety qi. What is settled, what is applied, and what is reverent, are all the human way [19:212].

Here we see the virtues related to forms or expressions of qi. In another chapter of the Wuxing sagely virtue is said to be "tian qi" heavenly qi [19:212] which we see again below in Dong Zhongshu's Chunqiu Fanlu discussions. The "de", virtue was seen as a property that comes from "tian" heaven, and by appropriate actions is cultivated in the individual. Yet another chapter of the Mawangdui Wuxing makes more explicit reference to the relationships between the state of mind of the person, the virtues they attain and their qi [19:330-331] concluding "It is this way on account of the body's qi".

The Guodian [郭店] Wuxing text also relates the emotions to the qi: "The qi of happiness, anger, sorrow, and grief is human nature" These "different kinds of affective qi" need to be balanced lest they disturb the qi and appear to be related to the "harm to the balance of qi that excess or depleted qi in the inner organs can cause" [19:210]. Since they are part of human nature they exist on the inside already so that "when it comes to their being manifested on the outside" (ie expressed) "it is because things have called them forth" [44:16].

The Wuxing helps understand and further explain other important texts like the Mencius and lays out the rudiments of a way of thinking about the emotions, the virtues and qi. It can also be seen as having been influential in the writing of the earliest medical texts in the Huangdi Neijing corpus [19].

## *The Chunqiu Zuozhuan* [春秋左傳]

The "Zuozhuan" probably of the early fourth century BCE is an important early historical record of the Warring States period and is thought to have introduced ideas that influenced the later medical traditions. It discusses the actions and rituals of the sage in relation to his body and their effects on his qi: "The sage respects the four moments of time. In the morning he holds an audience. During the day he collects information. In the evening he writes down the orders. During the night he rests. Doing that he is able to regulate the diffusion of his qi. Acting in such a way that the qi will not block or stagnate" [98:18-20] . Here we can see that qi was seen in relation to the actions of the sage as he considered tasks put before him to find solutions for them.

## *The Lushi Chunqiu* [呂氏春秋]

The Lushi Chunqiu circa 239 BCE has an important passage about the nature of health and pathology that may well have been influential in how the early medical literature approached the same theme. This passage discusses the role of qi:

> One wants the skin to be tight, the blood vessels to allow unimpeded motion, the sinews to be firm and the bones hard, the heart, mind and will to be concordant, the vital energies to flow. When this is happening, agents of disorder (bing) have nowhere to abide, and pathology has nowhere to be produced. The abiding of agents of disorder is the origin of pathology, blocking the flow of vital energies" [111:48].

Here Sivin translates "jing qi" [精氣] as "vital energies".[22]

A second passage cited by Sivin continues "Self-cultivation must begin with 'using the fresh and casting out the old, so there is a free flow within the interstices of the flesh (couli [腠理]). The vitalities (jingqi) are renewed daily, heteropathic qi (xieqi) [邪氣] is completely expelled, and a full span of life is attained'" [111:49]. This passage is important as it outlines the fundamental goal not only of health maintenance practices such as "yangshen'" [養生], but also the treatment systems that would soon develop in the Neijing [內經] tradition: If treatment can restore a free flow of the qi ("jingqi" in the Lushi Chunqiu), this helps the body expel influences that cause disease (xieqi). It is quite likely that such ideas helped lay the foundations for the Neijing's methods and theories and the model of founding health and disease in the concept of qi. We will come back to this idea below.

## *The Chunqiu Fanlu* [春秋繁露]

Dong Zhongshu's Chunqiu Fanlu of the early to mid Han dynasty extends the discussion of emotions and qi with reference to "tian qi" or "heaven qi" and the effects of the four seasons: "Human beings have contentment, anger, sadness, and happiness in the same way that tian has spring, summer, autumn, and winter. When contentment, anger sadness, and happiness arrive at the proper time and want to be expressed, it is like when spring, summer, autumn, and winter arrive at the proper time and want to be emitted-these are both the way they are because of tian's qi" [19:145]. Csikszentmihalyi goes on to explain how one can observe seasonal phenomena as a result of the qi of each season just as "the arousal of qi in one's nature by external things causes one to react in a way that expresses emotion" and that both are an expression of tianqi, the qi of heaven [19:145].[23] The Chunqiu Fanlu also describes the mutual influences of the qi of heaven, earth and man implying a fundamental interconnectedness "Heaven has yin and yang; humans also have yin and yang. When the yin qi of Heaven and Earth rise, the yin qi of humans responds to it and rises.[24] When the yin qi of humans rise, the yin qi of Heaven and Earth also properly responds to it and rises. Their way is one" [94:290-291]. Csikszentmihalyi discusses the opposite opinions of the later Han thinker Wang Chong who counter argued Dong Zhongshu's idea that through the principle of "tianren ganying" [天人感應] "heaven and human beings mutually respond to each other" human behaviour influences "tian" heaven and its effects on humanity (see below for further discussion of "resonance"). Wang Chong argued that "tian", heaven does not care about the actions of people, promoting a different understanding of the role and mechanisms by which qi acted [19:204-205].

## *The Mencius* [孟子]

The Mencius [Mengzi] of the late fourth-early third century BCE described the relation between the mind and qi in yet more detail. With the emphasis on self-cultivation that is found throughout the Mencius, it has been suggested that the author was influenced by other traditions such as we find in the Neiye, [19, 62, 94:134], a chapter from the Guanzi focusing on meditation and self-cultivation techniques and thought to be one of, if not the earliest Daoist texts [94, 96, 100]. We discuss the Neiye below and it is discussed further in other chapters. For the Mencius the "zhi" [志] or will governs and moves the qi: "the will (zhi) is the governor of the qi. Qi is what fills the limbs. Wherein the will arrives is wherein the qi lodges. Thus it is said, 'hold fast to your will and do not violate your qi'" [1:91, see also 62:26]. As clarification of the last sentence the Mencius comments "When the will is stopped up, then it makes qi move, when qi is blocked up, it makes the will move." [1:91].[26] The Mencius's use of the term "zhi" seems to imply a broader meaning of zhi beyond "will"; we discuss the meanings and translations of terms briefly in the next section. One of the main themes of the Mencius was the development of virtue. He saw a clear relationship between qi and the virtue of the sage "This is a qi which is extremely vast and unyielding. Nourished with integrity and unhindered it fills the spaces between Heaven and earth. Qi unites yi (morality) and dao (Ways)" [37:175].[27] According to Mencius it is by the importation of tianqi [天氣] heaven's qi into the body that sets the stage for the person to become virtuous [19:156]. In his comments on the Mencius, Csikszentmihalyi describes how the "Mencius introduces qi... into the process of cultivating the virtues" and that self cultivation results in physical changes in the body [19:102]. This links developing conceptions of the body with qi and with the development of virtue. Lewis states it thus: the Mencius "insists that qi, as something controlled by the mind, can only flourish when fed on the moral virtues" [62:26] and goes on: "Identifying the vital energies (qi) that form the body with moral virtues" the Mencius argues "that the virtues are consequently part of the body" [62:27].[28] The Mencius also outlines ways of observing the inner state of the body through visual inspection of its surface, including both emotional and the state of one's qi and thus physiological condition [19:135-6]. In what is probably a forerunner of later medical descriptions, the Mencius discusses how we can observe the "se" [色] or facial colouration of a person through visual inspection to assess both the state of moral development and state of health [19:138-9]. Interestingly the first etymological dictionary, the Shuowen jiezi (circa 90 CE) defines "se" (facial coloration) as "the qi of the forehead" [19:135]. The Mencius also discusses the effects of self-cultivation on one's appearance essentially explaining that one can see the resultant "healthy jing 'essence' and qi" in the person's face, especially in the eyes [19:127].

Csikszentmihalyi also argues that the Mencius "believes qi cannot flourish without mind" and since "qi is what 'the body is full of', it would not make sense to talk about it independently of the mind" [19:151], thus in Mencius's perspective one cannot really talk about qi without talking about the mind and vice versa. Quoting Chinese scholar, Yang Zebo, Csikszentmihalyi says "From Mengzi's point of view, the mind is the foundation of the qi. Without it, the qi will have no foundation, and so will have no source" [19:151]. While not all scholars would agree with such a perspective, it seems to fit with a wide range of textual sources about the mind, perception, cognition and qi (see below).

## *The Xunzi* [荀子]

The Xunzi of the mid-third century BCE describes the relationships between the mind, emotions and desires [28:289-291]. It is natural for people to have emotions and desires, but they must learn to restrain them so as not to produce undesirable consequences. The Xunzi also saw a clear relationship between qi, the mind and different living creatures "Water and fire possess qi, but they do not have life. Plants and trees possess life but do not possess awareness. Birds and beasts possess awareness but do not possess the sense of duty [ie a sense of what is right and appropriate]. Human beings possess qi, life and awareness, and add to them a sense of duty" [98:46] and again "Among all the living beings between heaven and earth, those having blood and qi possess awareness" [98:47]. Using language and descriptions similar to that found in the Daodejing and the Neiye the Xunzi describes how one must use emptiness and stillness for the mind to function well [28:290], also stating "the art of controlling the qi and nurturing the heart/mind: if the blood and qi are firm and strong, then soften them with balance and harmony" [1:89-90]. Here the Xunzi parallels the Daodejing with reference to the "soft" [1:90]. The Xunzi advocates the use of ritual to guide the individual, and although the Xunzi was clearly influenced by and used concepts from Daoist sources [115], it changes them to suit its arguments [28]. The Xunzi describes methods intended to change the very physiological basis of the individual so that they will naturally accord with proper behaviour without the need to be forced into that behaviour [115:247].[29]

## *The Neiye* [內業]

The late fourth century BCE text the Neiye, "Inward training", a chapter found in the Guanzi [管子], is thought by some to be older than and the precursor of the Daodejing and the Zhuangzi [100]. Dianne Sommers recently published an annotated and commented Dutch translation of the Neiye [116] and discusses the influences of the text in chapter three [117], so we will not discuss it much here. The treatise of the Neiye is one of several treatises in the Guanzi on the art of the mind (the "Xinshu" [心術]), similar and parallel discussions being found in those chapters. Additional later texts such as the "Shiwen" [十問] offer similar parallel discussions [94:208]. The Neiye is seen as influential for later conceptions of the body [62:24]. It is further seen as being influential on the development of the medical literature and systems as it articulates a model of qi-jing-shen and the body that is a precursor of the medical literature, [38, 96]. Rickett argues that the stream of Daoist thinking exemplified in the Neiye was likely to be the stream that most influenced the Huangdi Neijing corpus [96:31]. Chace has shown that passages about needling in the Huangdi Neijing Lingshu [黃帝內經靈樞] are likely based on ideas and practices found in the Neiye [15, 16]. The Neiye is thus a pivotal text in our understanding of how the mind, body and qi were conceived in the early TEAM literature. We mention some of the implications of this below.

The Neiye articulates a system of inner training or self-cultivation. Self cultivation had become an important feature in Chinese thinking by the Warring States period, with the impetus to develop the individual by bringing shen (the most refined form of qi) into the body and thus cultivate the person [94]. Puett suggests this was done in order to help relocate power away from a not well functioning centralized political power [94]. Self cultivation methods were also developing in order to help instill virtue and proper moral conduct in more people –an important concept with the chaos and lack of morality exemplified during the Warring States period. The Neiye is a pivotal text marking the transition out of the chaotic Warring states period of the Zhou dynasty followed by the more orderly Han dynasty [94].

In the Neiye qi is linked with jing and shen in a mutual relationship. Jing [精] (essence) is a more concentrated and refined form of qi, and shen [神] (spirit) is a higher, purer and more concentrated form of both. The three exist in a continuum, Puett describes this continuum thus: "Qi, which I leave here untranslated, is the energy and substance of all things. In its most refined form, qi becomes essence: 'essence is the essence of qi'. Spirit is then defined as refined qi as well... it becomes another name for essential qi" [94:109].[30]

Basically the Neiye describes a model of how consciousness or the mind is influenced by internal and external events, describing the importance of calming/controlling the emotions, quietness, stillness, proper alignment of the body in self-cultivation and how this affects the person practising. In these descriptions we can see that the mind is seen as integral to how the qi, jing and shen are to be grasped and developed. The following quotes exemplify this relationship. Roth translates jing as vital essence and qi as vital energy:

> All the forms of the mind are naturally infused and filled with it (the vital essence), are naturally generated and developed (because of) it. It is lost inevitably because of sorrow, happiness, joy, anger, desire and profit seeking. If you are able to cast off sorrow, happiness, joy, anger, desire and profit-seeking your mind will revert to equanimity. The true condition of the mind is that it finds calmness beneficial and, by it, attains repose. Do not disturb it, do not disrupt it and harmony will naturally develop [100:50].

And:

> If you can be aligned and be tranquil only then can you be stable. With a stable mind at your core, with the eyes and ears acute and clear, and with the four limbs firm and fixed, you can thereby make a lodging place for the vital essence (jing qi). The vital essence: it is the essence of the vital energy (qi). When the vital energy is guided, it (the vital essence) is generated. But when it is generated, there is thought, when there is thought there is knowledge, but when there is knowledge, then you must stop. Whenever the forms of the mind have excessive knowledge, you lose your vitality" [100:60].

The accumulation and development of qi, jing and shen is also described as having beneficial effects on the health of the body and the clarity of the mind, presaging medical discussions of these concepts in relation to health and disease: "If people can be aligned and tranquil, their skin will be ample and smooth, their ears and eyes will be acute and clear, their muscles will be supple and their bones will be strong...They will mirror things with great purity and will perceive things with great clarity" [100:76]. It also allows the individual to develop certain powers and abilities: if the adept can align themselves correctly ("align your body, assist the inner power" [100:66]) and calm their emotions completely ("if you are able to cast off sorrow, happiness, joy, anger, desire, and profit-seeking" [100:50]) using proper breathing and other techniques then they can activate "the mind within the mind" which is "an awareness that precedes words" [100:72]. With this they "can be aligned and tranquil" allowing them to "perceive things with great clarity" [100:76]. In that state "the myriad things will be seen in their proper perspective" [100:70], they will be grasped "to the last one" [100:48], "harmony will naturally develop" [100:50], "even the far-off will seem close at hand" [100:82] and "Once this flow of vital energy is achieved, All under the heavens will submit" [100:80]. The relationships between qi, the body, the mind, health, disease, self cultivation and virtue becomes clear with the Neiye. The consolidation of qi-jing-shen in the body through these practices helps develop the mind bringing knowledge, wisdom, inner power and even what we might call "paranormal" abilities.

One final but very important passage guides our understanding of how one "welcomes" the qi: "Therefore this vital energy cannot be halted by force, yet can be secured by inner power, cannot be summoned by speech, yet can be welcomed by awareness"[31] [100:48]. The important sentence for us here is "yet can be welcomed by awareness." The term awareness is the Chinese term "yi" [意]. Only when the mind manifests itself in the proper state "yi" (brought about through calming the mind, aligning the body, etc), can the qi be "welcomed" –brought into the body or into action. Qi is moved and affected positively by certain mental states, here awareness, "yi", and in the Mencius will, "zhi", while the emotions disturb the qi. We will come back to this below.

## *The Daodejing* [道德經]

The Daodejing has little direct discussion of qi or qi and the mind. The term "qi" only occurs three times throughout the Daodejing text, which is perhaps a little surprising. The text covers a broad range of important issues of rulership and philosophy. There are a number of themes that run throughout, a Daoist vision of cosmology; how the soft and weak can wear down the hard and strong; how non-action, the quiet and passive can be powerful tools for creating change. On cosmological thinking chapter forty two discusses the fundamental place of qi: "The Way gives birth to the one, the one gives birth to the two. The two give birth to the three, the three give birth to the myriad things. The myriad things carry the yin and embrace the yang, and blend vapors (qi) so as to become harmonized" [94:165].[32]

Following the focus on not striving, not forcing, not acting, chapter fifty five has an important discussion in relation to the mind and qi. While it is translated differently by different Western translators, the basic idea is the same: "The heart puts qi into action as envoy" which Rochat de la Vallee describes as "the heart is making the qi too active and the result is violence" [98:21]. Ames and Hall render this passage thus: "While allowing the heart-mind to use up the qi one has, is to overdo things" [2:163]. Moeller renders it thus: "If the heart directs the Qi, this is called: forcing" [83:38]. In the Daodejing the caution appears to be to not try to move the qi or force the qi with the xin, heart/mind. This appears to parallel the Neiye's emphasis on how a quiet reflective aware state "yi" can "welcome" the qi. We will return to this again below.

Chapter ten of the Daodejing has further discussion of how the mind influences the qi. This is the third occurrence of the term qi in the Daodejing. The text specifically discusses qi zhi [氣至], translated by many as "concentrating your qi" [1, 2:90, 115:93]) in other contexts translated as the "arrival of qi" or simply "qi arrival". Qi zhi occurs as a result of the internal state of the individual, presumably triggered by quiet meditation [2:90]. Certainly the passage mirrors passages found in the Neiye, the Zhuangzi and elsewhere, using similar metaphors associated with meditation "In carrying about your more spiritual and more physical aspects and embracing their oneness, are you able to keep them from separating? In concentrating your qi (qi zhi) and making it pliant, are you able to become the newborn babe? In scrubbing and cleansing your profound mirror[33], are you able to rid it of imperfections?" [2:90]. Here we see a clear association of the action of the mind on the qi which recurs importantly in the early acupuncture literature. In the Huangdi Neijing Lingshu chapter one, "qi zhi" is a prerequisite for effective needling. More recent analyses support an interpretation of this that strongly parallels this usage in the Daodejing [8, 15, 16]. We will return to this several times below and in other chapters.

## *The Zhuangzi* [莊子]

In the Zhuangzi qi is clearly seen in relation to the mind, for it is through cultivating the mind that the qi is cultivated and effective in its influence on others. What is needed is to achieve the right state of mind "Let your mind/heart roam in the flavorless, blend your breath (qi) with the featureless and accord with the manner in which living things are so of themselves, not leaving room for self interest, and all under heaven will be in order" [1:116]. Zhuangzi's approach was to avoid the highly structured and heavily ruled approaches of the Confucian traditions. He describes the application of the principle of "wuwei" [無為]: "if they rest, then they become empty; if they become empty then they are filled and that which fills them becomes ordered. If they are empty then they are still; if they are still then they move; if they move then they succeed. If they are still then they do nothing (wuwei)" [1:84].[34] Zhuangzi was clearly interested in how one can help create a more ordered state within the body:

> Don't look and don't listen; embrace the spirit by means of stillness and the physical form will correct itself. You must be still and pure; do not belabor your physical form and do not agitate your quintessential. Only then can you live a long life. When the eye does not see, the ear does not hear, and the heart/mind does not know, then your spirit will protect the body, and the body will enjoy long life [115:201].

Here we see ideas that presage the medical literature,[35] engaging in this action of calming the mind and reducing sensory stimulation,[36] helps keep the body in a more ordered state "the physical form will correct itself" which allows a cultivation of the spirit which protects the body.[37] These practices allow more contact to the spirit which naturally brings a state of higher order.

In a famous passage about the "fasting of the mind", Zhuangzi makes the following distinctions in a hypothetical discussion between Yanhui and Confucius "Make your will one! Don't listen with your ears, listen with your mind (xin). No, don't listen with your mind, but listen with your vital energy (qi). Listening stops with the ears, the mind stops with recognition, but vital energy is empty and waits on all things. The Dao gathers in emptiness alone. Emptiness is the fasting of the mind" [136:93]. Yang analyses this passage to help us understand Zhuangzi's "three-stage doctrine of listening with the ears, the mind and the vital energy". According to Yang, Zhuangzi is describing the various stages of how a person embodies the dao to achieve knowledge. With each stage different methods of perceiving and knowing are involved: the first employing the sense organs, which produce a limited grasp of things, conditioned by the limitations of how they work and the physical body through which they act; the second coming through a deeper more unitary form of perception, the "common sense", which arises directly through the heart-mind, where different sensory organ perceptions are indistinguishable and a more immediate perception of a thing may be possible;[39] the third is a direct perception through one's qi, which opens one to a much broader perceptive depth and perceptive field, since the qi is everything and everywhere, thus allowing a form of perception and knowledge to the heart of the thing [136]. Yang sees the two transitions between the three steps in the following terms:

> 1. The body merges with the mind: that is, the body loses its independent, perceptual significance and is completely transformed by the mind.
> 2. The mind merges with the vital energy: the mind loses its function as lord of the body; it is no longer the "heavenly ruler", but rather melds into the midst of the body's vital energy so that the entire mind becomes vital energy [136:103].

We will see below and in later chapters how the description of Zhuangzi's three stages and different forms of perception and knowledge give us important ways of understanding the nature of qi in relation to mind and specific types of actions and processes to aid in further developing and investigating qi.

Zhuangzi like many other authors was concerned with the development of "de" [德], virtue, without which self cultivation cannot really proceed:

> Our body can be produced only by the dao, and our life can shine only through virtue (de). One who conserves life and reaches the fullness of his days is one who –upon the foundation of virtue– has caused the way (dao) to gleam. Isn't that the royal virtue? Majestically one emerges from the indistinct; he advances full of power, and the ten thousand beings follow in his wake [98:21].

Zhuangzi also gives us a clear understanding of the relationship between qi and life: "Life is the follower of death and death is the predecessor of life, but who knows their cycles? Man's life is due to the conglomeration of the qi, and when they are dispersed, death occurs" [86:76]. This last sentence is rendered as: "Qi gathered together is life; qi dispersed is death" by Kuriyama [55:223]. The intimate relationship between qi and life was expressed by Zhuangzi in the famous story of his wife's death:

> She began and yet at the source she had no life. Not only did she have no life, but at the source she had no form. Not only did she have no form, at the source she had no vitality. When mingled in the amorphous, something changed and there was vital energy (qi). The vital energy changed and there was form. The form changed and there was life. Now once again, it has changed and there is death [1:145].

In one passage the Zhuangzi describes how the optimal state of a person is to lack feelings since the emotions can cause injury[40]

> "Hui Shi said to Zhuangzi 'Can someone be a person without feelings?' 'Not a problem' replied Zhuangzi. 'But how can someone be called a person' asked Hui Shi 'if they don't have feelings?' Zhuangzi said 'Their context provides them with the appearance and shape of a person why wouldn't we call them such?' 'Since we are calling them persons' asked Hui Shi 'how could it be that they are lacking feelings?' 'This is not what I meant by feelings' replied Zhuangzi 'what I meant when I say that they are 'wuqing' (literally 'without feelings') is that they do not injure their own persons with likes and dislikes and are always responsive to what is natural without trying to increase life" [2:47].

This parallels ideas found in the medical literature about how the emotions can cause injury.

## *The Huainanzi* [淮南子]

The Huainanzi is an important early text from around 122 BCE with clear Daoist influences, clearly elaborating older and current ideas of the time. It describes a number of important ideas that set the stage for understanding how qi, the mind and body were conceived by the early Han dynasty. In one passage there is an unequivocal statement about the relationship of the "xin" or heart/mind to the qi, "the heart/mind is the master of the five depots. It is the means of commanding the four limbs, and of causing the blood and energy (qi) to flow" [62:324-325]. Similar passages can be found establishing the heart/mind at the center of the body and how it expresses itself in the world:

> Heaven has the four seasons, the five phases, the nine sections, and 366 days. People also have the four limbs, five depots, nine openings, and 366 bodily segments. Heaven has wind, rain, cold, and heat. People also have taking, giving, happiness and anger. Therefore the stomach is the clouds, the lungs are the breath/energy (qi), the liver is the wind, the kidneys are the rain, and the spleen is the thunder. In this way the body can be a third with Heaven and Earth, and the heart/mind is its master [62:324].

The Huainanzi discusses qi in relation to how humans are formed and in part in distinction to how animals are formed: "coarse qi forms animals, refined qi forms humans" [119:74]. Sterckz goes on to describe how in the Huainanzi the juxtaposition of coarse and refined qi "indicates that the physiological basis of animals and humans was perceived to be made up from the same basic stuff, while physical and behavioural differences were thought to originate primarily from the way in which the creature's qi is structured" [119:74].[41] Like the Mencius, the Huainanzi saw the "possession of tian's qi by human being as a prerequisite for attaining the status of a spirit" [19:158], by importing tianqi [天氣] heaven's qi into the body one attains a more refined form or status. Also in the cosmology of the Huainanzi, humans by their nature possess the more refined qi and arc thus naturally aligned with heaven "This is the reason that the essence and spirit are possessions of Heaven, whereas bones and limbs are the possessions of earth" [94:271]. Thus "the sage models himself on heaven and follows his disposition" [94:271]. By becoming more refined the sage aligns himself with the original spirits that ordered the cosmos and thus enables the same ordering qualities of those spirits.

The Huainanzi has discussions of how the body can be maintained in a healthier more pure state such that xieqi [邪氣], "perverse" or "depraved" qi cannot affect it adversely, this parallels the ideas we saw above in the Lushi Chunqiu. These descriptions probably helped lay the foundation for the medical descriptions of the role of qi in health and the focus on the xieqi in disease and as a target of treatment. "For [one with] the dao stores his essence within, perches his spirit in his mind, is quiet, tranquil and placid, and pleased and harmonious within his breast. Depraved energy (xieqi) has nowhere to stick, and in the four limbs and many joints, sweats out through the pores and discharges within" [136:100].

The qi was also seen in relation to one's self cultivation, to become like shen (spirit). The Jingshen chapter of the Huainanzi describes this process in the following terms:

> Blood and qi are the flowering of humanity, and the five repositories are the essence of humanity. Now, when the blood and qi are concentrated by the five repositories and do not fall away in excess, then the chest and stomach will be full, and lust and desires will be reduced. If the chest and stomach are full and lust and desires are reduced, then the ears and eyes will be clear, and one's hearing and seeing will connect with their objects. When the ears and eyes are clear, and ones' hearing and seeing connect with their objects, we call this clarity. If the five repositories can be gathered by the mind, and there is no deviation, then distracted attention will be overcome and the movements will not be corrupt. When distracted attention is overcome and

> the movements not corrupt, then the essence and the spirit will flourish and the qi will not dissipate. When the essence and spirit flourish and the qi is not dissipating, then one will be patterned. When one is patterned, one will be balanced. When one is balanced, one will penetrate. When one penetrates, one will be a spirit (shen). When one is a spirit, one will thereby see without anything not being seen, one will thereby hear without anything not being heard, and one will thereby act without anything not being completed [94:275].

The Huainanzi also describes a cosmological model with qi at the center. We find a description that parallels Daodejing forty two: "The way, that is to say, the law, begins with one. One [alone] does not give life. Hence it parted and became yin and yang. Through the union of yin and yang, the myriad beings came to life. Hence it is said 'one generates two, two generates three, three generates the myriad things'" [128:34]. In this cosmology qi lies at the core since "everything is made of qi." "Qi is both process and substance, and comes into being as the concrete manifestation of spacetime; differentiating into the light and clear, the heavy and turbid, qi (now describable in terms of yin and yang) becomes the basic stuff of the visible universe" [75:27]:

> When Heaven and Earth were not yet formed, all was ascending and flying, diving and delving. Thus it was called the Great Inception. The Dao began in the Nebulous void. The Nebulous void produced spacetime[42]; spacetime produced the primordial qi (yuan qi). A shoreline (divided) the primordial qi, that which was pure and bright spread out to form Heaven. The heavy and turbid congealed to form Earth [75:62].

Le Blanc summarises one of the core messages of the Huainanzi as follows: "As far as the Huainanzi is concerned, the teachings of the schools of yin-yang and five elements may be reduced to four basic ideas: –the idea of qi (matter-energy); –the idea of resonance (ganying –see below) between different formations, configurations and categories of qi; –the idea of an alternating principle of change, yin and yang, and; –a sequence of phases relating the foregoing 'principle' to concrete things and making it possible to classify the latter into systems of correspondence" [59:197]. The cosmological influences in the understanding and modeling of qi that are found in the early medical Neijing corpus are likely to have been influenced by the stream of thinking we find in the Huainanzi.

There were many expressions of this cosmological view of the role of qi. For example the "zhengqi song" of the Wentian Xiang (before 200 BCE). "Heaven and Earth have correct qi; its form is flexible and fluid. In the lower parts it is in the rivers and mountains on earth; in the upper parts it is in the sun and the stars in the sky; the human being is overwhelmingly and universally soaked in it" [76:5].

## *Yangsheng* [養生] *and other early physiological discussions*

The term yangsheng refers to a number of different practices used to systematically help cultivate the body, promote health and thus the ability for more efficacious action. We have seen numerous references to the idea of using techniques for the cultivation of virtue, cultivation of qi, etc. The yangsheng is a further development of these self cultivation practices, of which by the the time of the late Warring states, early Han, there were many.[43] A number of tombs have been unearthed in recent decades exposing a wealth of new texts describing self-cultivation practices such that it has been necessary to update opinions of received traditions [34:460]. Among these tomb findings the manuscripts from the Mawangdui [馬王堆] and Zhangjiashan [張家山] tombs give some of the first clear discussions of qi in reference to the physiology of the body. According to Harper the first reference to qi as flowing in the vessels (mai) [脈]can be found in the Guanzi from before the third century BCE, "water is the blood and vapor (qi) of the earth –like what flows through the muscles and vessels" [38:77]. The Mawangdui texts (circa 168 BCE) the "Yinyang Shiyimai Jiujing" [陰陽十一脈灸經] and the "Zubi Shiyimai Jiujing" [足臂十一脈灸經], the "Maifa" [脈法] and the "Yinyang mai sihou" [陰陽脈死候] and the Zhangjiashan text, the 'Maishu' [脈書] (circa mid second century BCE) elaborate on this in what maybe the earliest physiological models of the body in China [38, 46]. The early Han physician Chunyu Yi [淳于意] whose case histories from around 154 BCE are recorded in the "Shiji" [史記] of circa 90 BCE also discusses the vessels and their associations with qi [38, 46][44] see also the next and later chapters in this volume. The Shiwen [十問] from the Mawangdui tomb offers a description of how qi is brought into the body, preserved and refined to become jing [精] and ultimately shen [神] that is similar to that of the Neiye, but with some interesting differences [94:208-214].[45]

The physiological details of these texts are nowhere near as precise as the later Huangdi Neijing corpus and subsequent texts, and the qi in the vessels is not seen to circulate as we find starting in the Neijing [21, 38, 125, 128].[46] The inseparability of qi and mind starts to become central in these early discussions of health and physiology and qi starts to become more discussed in terms of flow. Although we have seen Zhuangzi already stating that emotional expression can cause injury, discussions of how the qi in the vessels becomes disturbed are not yet generally found, instead ailments ("bing") associated with each vessel and how to treat them are given [46]. Most of the symptomatology of the vessels described in the Mawangdui and Zhangjiashan texts relate to physical problems [38:73], such as "neck pain; throat numbness; shoulder pain; pain in the outer part of the elbow... deafness with blurring; swelling in the throat" [38:207]. However there are a few references to more psychological or emotional symptoms such as "when hearing the sound of wood, panicked alarm... the desire to close doors and windows and dwell in isolation... the desire to mount high and sing, and to cast off clothing and run" [38:206], "a tendency to become angry; panicky heart with the fear that one is about to be seized by someone" [38:210]. Chunyu Yi mentioned grief and anger in relation to the heart and liver organs as an outgrowth of vessel theory [46]. These occasional references to what we might consider as mental and emotional "ailments" provides further evidence of the link between qi, the correct movements of qi and the mind and emotions. However, these links, like the texts themselves, provide only tentative insights into how the more developed Huangdi Neijing traditions began. Hsu demonstrates that these texts do not show signs of the later models of the "five natural inclinations" or the seven emotions that are characteristic of the Neijing [46]. But they do imply a possible reason for the developing link between the jingmai and the zang organs [46]: the zang organs were seen as the seat of the emotions; emotions cause disturbances of the qi; qi was seen to be contained in the mai (and the later "jingmai"); one palpated the mai (and jingmai) in order to understand the state of the qi and emotional effects on the organs. Hence one can suggest a linking of these ideas in the development of "vessel theory" and the interlinking of qi, emotions, mai/jingmai and the zang, as increasing emphasis was placed on the emotions in disease in the Neijing, following statements about the emotions we have seen in for example the Analects, Neiye, Guodian Wuxing and the Chunqiu Fanlu.

There is an interesting passage in the Heyinyang [和陰陽], "Harmonising yin-yang" sexual cultivation text from the Mawangdui about what happens when the "qi arrives": "The qi arrives, blood and qi flow freely, the ears and eyes are keen and bright, the skin gleams, the voice is clear, and the back, thighs and buttocks are sturdy, so that one 'attains divine illumination' (tong shenming [通神明])" [72:381].[47] The "arrival of qi" is an important concept in the literature describing therapeutic needling.[48] We have here a precedent for understanding what is the importance of needling to gain the arrival of qi: the blood and qi flow freely, perceptions become clearer, the skin more lustrous and the body stronger. This is an important concept for understanding potential therapeutic effects of needling. The passage also ends with the statement to "attain divine illumination", which is a reference to a heightened spiritual state, an important goal in the cultivation literatures.

The Tianxia zhidao tan [天下室道談] "discussion of the culminant way in under heaven" from the Mawangdui texts, describes further sexual cultivation techniques.[49] It describes seven "detriments" [七損] or ways of diminishing qi and eight "benefits" [八益] or ways ways of increasing qi [38:429-432, 61:152-153]. Avoiding the seven detriments and implementing the eight benefits are done for the purposes of improving longevity. The specific details intended to improve one's qi condition involve a series of simple actions. The first of the eight "benefits" is described: "To rise at dawn, sit upright, straighten the spne, open the buttocks, suck in the anus, and press it down is 'cultivating vapor'" [38:430]. The text describes similar actions both during and outside of sexual intercourse.

## *The Huangdi Neijing* [黃帝內經]

The Neijing texts as we know them today have been compiled over several centuries. The earliest portions probably date from the second century BCE. The received Neijing introduces more formal descriptions of the body in health and disease, how to identify the nature of the problems that cause the disease or result in symptoms and methods for addressing those problems with appropriate treatments. In the stages of development of the Neijing corpus [51] qi becomes very important. There are thought to be approximately 50,000 characters that make up the text the Huangdi Neijing Suwen [黃帝內經素問], over 1,100 of which (more than 1/50) is the term "qi" [76:5].[50] More than fifty kinds of qi in the body and in nature are mentioned in the Huangdi Neijing Suwen [61:105], Porkert lists thirty-two types of qi [93:167-173]. Obviously with such common usage, the concept "qi" had become very important.

Evidence suggests that initial attempts at describing physiology and treatment tended to focus more on older blood circulation based models and that later, qi based descriptions develop to become dominant [24, 128]. As the medical authors began describing health, disease, diagnosis and treatment within the framework of this qi-based model, it naturally became necessary to differentiate qi (which was largely undifferentiated by that point) into discrete subdivisions thus allowing authors to classify functions and systems in ways that relate to diagnosis and treatment strategies [18, 58:42, 98:58-59, 111:51].[51] We find very general discussions involving qi and very specific references and discussions involving qi. For example in Lingshu chapter eight we find that life results from the descent of "de", virtue from heaven and the streaming up of "qi" from earth: "Heaven within me is virtue (de). Earth within me is the breaths (qi). Virtue flows down, the breaths expand, and there is life." [56:16]. We found numerous discussions in the pre-medical literatures about the development of "de", virtue in humans and how this comes from "tian" or heaven. In this passage we see a clear expression of this idea. While in many other passages and references we find more focused discussions resulting in the introduction of multiple forms of qi [93, 133, 134] each labeled according to where it is and/or what it is doing (such as "spleen qi", "source qi", "defensive qi", "yin qi", etc).

Qi was seen as that which kept you healthy and able to resist disease. Lingshu sixty-six states this principle quite clearly in a quite novel way: "If wind, rain, cold or heat don't encounter a depletion [of bodily vitality (qi)], their xieqi alone can't harm people... Only when a depleting wind encounters a depletion within the body can [the wind] possess the body" [55:222, see also 63:1120 and 111:100]. Disease results from the disturbance of the body triggered by the xieqi, pathological qi. If the body's qi is intact and shows no sign of weakness, even with exposure to circumstances that can make one sick, sickness does not occur.

Qi started to be seen in relation to all the anatomical structures and their functions, both as material substrate of those structures and as functional expressions associated with them. It was described as residing within certain trajectories or pathways (such as the "jingmai" and "luomai") and then to be circulating within them in a continuous circuit –the circulation of qi through the twelve jingmai said to occur fifty times per day [Lingshu fifteen, Nanjing one –see 78:77, 125:65-66]. It was described in relation to the blood, such that somehow the jingmai circulates both qi and blood. We saw above the association of qi and blood in the compound term "xueqi", blood and qi. This is not only a physiological or physical reference, it also implies an association with mental functions such as "the heart-mind and spiritual awareness" and a possible association to the emotions [119:75] –see discussions below. Qi became the basis for describing how treatment with a needle was to be conducted –one should focus on the qi and attempt to get "qi zhi" [氣至], the "qi arrival". Acupuncture focused on influencing this circulating qi in the "jingmai" or channels by targeting the "xue" [穴] or acupoints that lie along the trajectories of these channels. The Neijing represents the culmination of development of many streams of thinking (some of which we have seen above) in order to allow its readers to apply theory, diagnosis and treatment for the help of people with different health problems.

The Neijing marks a clear beginning of explicit discussions of how qi is related to the emotions and how emotions relate to the internal organs (zang) and internal physiological states.[52] When a specific organ has a dysfunction it can result in the expression of a specific emotion, so that we see how problems of the liver can result in the expression of anger, problems of the lung in the expression of grief. The organs produce through transformation the qi that manifests as the five emotions, Suwen five tells us "Man has five (zang) and through transformation, five qi to produce elation, anger, sadness, oppression and fear" [57:27-8, 128:228]. There are commonly associated correspondences between emotions and organs, for example in Suwen chapter five we find reference to how the emotions can injure specific organs, such as "anger injures the liver", "sorrow injures the lung," "fear injures the kidney" [57, 78:43]. While there are commonly accepted associations, different descriptions can be found in the medical literature that are contradictory. For example in Lingshu chapter two we find discussion of how sorrow affects the liver: "As for the liver system, if sorrow disturbs a person's interior, then this injures the hun. If the hun is injured, then (the person becomes) (wild), forgetful and unable to concentrate." [18:46]. Suwen twenty-one implies that fear is associated with the lung and liver (the usual association of fear is to the kidney) "when something makes one stumble [causing] fear [that one may fall] the [resulting] panting originates from the liver... when something makes on feel frightened [causing] fear, the [resulting] panting originates from the lung" [128:234]. Lingshu chapter four describes how "worry and fear result in damage to the heart" [63:1119]. While there is not complete consistency in these descriptions,[53] we find a relatively clear model of relationships between various organ functions, emotions and the mind.

These can be seen further in relation to qi: in Suwen thirty-nine, Huangdi describes how each emotion affects qi in the body "when one is angry, then the qi rises. When one is happy then the qi relaxes. When one is sad, then the qi dissipates. When one is in fear, then the qi moves down... When one is frightened, then the qi is in disorder." [128:161-162]. He then asks Qibo what diseases generate these states, in answer to which Qibo describes specific mechanisms associated with each emotion, for example: "when one is in fear, then the essence withdraws. When it withdraws, then the upper burner becomes closed. When it is closed, then the qi turns around. When it turns around, then the lower burner becomes distended. Hence, the qi does not move" [128:162]. These descriptions clearly link emotions to qi and its movements and to specific organs. Each emotion is capable of injuring an organ, each emotion is characterized as a specific disturbance in movement of qi. But, as is typical in ancient Chinese and TEAM thinking, these are not simple cause-effect relationships, they are mutually causal, influencing both ways. One is to understand that if a specific organ has a problem it can result in the expression of an emotion, that emotion is simultaneously a specific set of disturbances of qi movements triggering other problems and can re-injure the specific organ it is associated with. Further, if the qi moves in a particular disordered way it can manifest as or trigger the specific associated emotional expression, which itself can then injure the associated organ. Conversely, if (following the ideals of both Confucian and Daoist thinking) one is able to control or regulate one's emotions, one necessarily regulates one's qi and thus physiology.

The Neijing literature brought together a range of ideas around the theme of health, disease and treatment. There were various discussions about how lifestyle habits, not taking proper care of oneself and or not regulating one's emotions can cause internal injury or vacuity [虛]. As mentioned already, in Lingshu sixty-six we find the revolutionary idea about how the external factors from the environment can only cause disease if there is first an internal weakness. Another important idea was the role of "wuxing" [五行] or five-phase or five processes theory in medical discourse [21]. Also here there is a linking of the "wuxing' with qi. The Baihutong [白虎通] of 80 CE stated: "when we say hsing (xing) the meaning we wish to express is that it is the activity of ch'i (qi) [as maintained] by the natural order" and the Shiming [釋名] of 100 CE "asserts that hsing (xing) is what ch'i (qi) does "wu hsing (xing) means what is carried out by the five ch'i (qi), each in its own domain" [111:74-45]. By the second half of the Han dynasty qi had become ubiquitous and its divisions-classifications in terms of yin-yang and the five phases likewise very common. It is possible to say many more things here about qi and how these ideas are brought into the Neijing and subsequent medical treatises (some aspects are covered in later chapters in this volume), such as an elaboration of the relationship to the functional systems, the organs, the zangfu [臟腑],[54] the nature and influences of the perverse qi, xieqi [邪氣] climatic influences, seasonal cycles and the role and implications of cosmological thinking[55] and contradictory statements that we find there and in later texts, But we finish discussions of the development of qi concepts in relation to mind and body here.[56]

### *Summary of historical survey*

In the discussions above we can see that qi has been used by different authors in many different ways. Often the authors cite or implicitly include earlier meanings and uses (even though some may appear contradictory) and then add their own modifications, extensions, new meanings.[57] Regardless of this variety, there do seem to be certain common features that emerge and which can be found manifesting by the time of the medical tradition of the Huangdi

Neijing of the second century BCE. Qi appears to have become central to an understanding of the body and the mind. Mark Lewis argues that the relations between the mind and body established around the time of the Neiye were fundamental for understanding how both were conceived: "the Chinese in contrast, accepted that the mind was part of the body, more refined and essentialized but of the same substance" [62:20]. Further "Crucial to this new explanation of cosmic patterns was the vision of the mind and body as composites of the same energies that formed Heaven, Earth and everything within them. Through the new version of qi and the integrated cosmos articulated in the "Neiye", the Mencius and the Zuozhuan, the human body came to occupy the center of the Warring States visions of ordered space" [62:36].

In the above historical overview we see that as the concept and role of qi developed in different traditions it has been related closely with the emotions, the mind and body. This can be found manifest in many different ways both in the emergent medical literature and later texts. Models of the body, mind and qi as a continuum of similar influences can be found in numerous places. For example the Huainanzi of 122 BCE tells us: "the form is the dwelling of life, qi is the filling of life, and spirit (shen) is the regulator of life"[58] [94:265]. In the later Han dynasty, the Lunheng [論衡] (circa 90 CE) describes a kind of continuum of qi in more dense forms to more rarified forms: "qi creates the person, water makes ice; water becomes solid making ice, qi becomes solid making the person [body]" [78:114]. We also see a maturation of how emotions and the mind are related to qi from the early Confucian writings through to the early medical writings. Suwen five tells us: "man has the five depots (zang organs) they transform the five qi, thereby generating joy, anger, sadness, anxiety and fear" [128:228].

We would like to finish this brief historical survey of what different traditions have said about qi and turn now to looking at the implications of this. In the final sections of this chapter we will briefly examine the following three areas: i) further elaboration of the relations of the mind and emotions to qi and especially how certain states of the mind are involved in influencing, regulating or welcoming the qi; ii) mechanisms that were proposed of how to access qi and of how qi might act in the world and finally iii) implications of these in how qi (especially the qi of the individual as mind-body) is an active agent that acts upon the world. The early models of qi-mind-body have certain common themes that we will see emerging in later chapters of this book and which have important implications for our understanding and investigations of, for example, acupuncture, taijiquan, qigong and herbal medicine.

## A further analysis of terms and concepts, xin, yi, zhi 心意志

Although all mental and emotional states are related to "xin" [心], "heart", "mind" or "heart-and-mind", it is useful to draw the distinction between emotions, affects and different mental, cognitive states or functions since they have different kinds of effects on the qi.[59]

Emotions are all intimately related to the xin, heart-and-mind [2, 91, 138:40]. Modern scholars have described or characterized this in different ways. Sarah Allan has expressed the intimate relationship between the xin, emotions and qi very clearly: "The primary image for the xin is that of a pool of water which is clear and reflective when still. When sympathetic emotion is stirred, the heart has a responding resonance. Violent emotion is the stirring up of the xin –the calm pool– thus causing one's perceptions of reality –the reflection– to be blurred whereas the still, undisturbed mind, contemplates with clarity. This disturbance is described in terms of qi 'vapor' or 'vital energy'" [1:86]. Slingerland states that the xin has "in the Chinese view both cognitive and affective capacities and tendencies, and in addition serves as a 'container' for settled dispositions to act in a certain way, thereby including what we might refer to as the 'will'" [115:139]. Ames and Hall discuss this: "It is significant that xin –a stylized drawing of the aorta–[60] precludes the assumption of distinctions between thinking and feeling, or idea and affect. Xin is frequently translated as 'heart', but since it is the seat of thinking and judgement, the notion of mind must be included in its characterization if the term is to be properly understood. Indeed, the functional equivalent of what we often think of as 'purpose' or 'intention' is also implicit in the notion of xin" [2:100]. Roth states the nature of xin thus: xin is "for the early Chinese, the locus of the entire range of conscious experience, including perception, thought, emotion, desire and intuition" [100:42]. The xin has both affective and cognitive aspects. Based on all the above considerations we can say that the affective, emotional related aspects of the xin are by nature disturbing to the proper or higher functioning of the xin, heart-and-mind. While the cognitive and dispositional aspects of the xin heart-and-mind, especially the higher mental/consciousness functions (yi, zhi, hun, po, shen), often have more of a regulating influence than a disturbing influence.

Several passages in the pre-medical literature make clear statements about the importance of the heart in our life and growth. The Xunzi tells us:

> How can a person know the dao? By the heart. How can the heart know? By emptiness, the pure attention that unifies being and quietude. The heart is never without treasure yet it is called empty. The heart is never not completely filled, yet it is called

unified. The heart is never without movement, yet it is called quiet. Man lives and possesses knowledge: he knows and through knowledge possesses will. [56:48].

Similarly the Liji [禮記] says of the heart: "By nature man possesses blood and breaths (qi), and a heart that allows knowledge. Grief as well as joy and elation as well as anger do not exist permanently in him; they are reactions to the incitement of objects. It is then that the Art of the Heart intervenes." And:

> From the first moment of his existence, a man's heart is in a place of absolute calm (it is free of all desire); Heaven creates it in this state. Soon external objects act on it and produce diverse movements; these are desires that add themselves to its nature (to its original state). In the presence of external objects, man has the faculty (or desire) to know them; when he knows them, he experiences feelings of attraction for some and feelings of revulsion for others. If he does not master these feelings, he lets himself be drawn towards external things and becomes incapable of returning within himself (and regulating the movements within his heart); he loses the good tendencies he has received from heaven [56:47].

These and other passages such as "The qi of happiness, anger, sorrow, and grief is human nature" from the Guodian Wuxing text [19:210] make it clear that the emotions were intimately linked to qi [1, 19, 56, 57, 78, 128]. We saw how the Analects cautioned to guard against the emotions that arise during different stages of one's life (development of qi and blood) and how the Chunqiu Fanlu describes how the proper expression of the emotions is related to tian qi like the arrival of each of the seasons at their proper time. The Xunzi expressed the need to regulate one's emotions in order to be able to assist in one's self cultivation and development of proper virtue. The Neiye *explicitly* discusses how emotions are disruptive to the functioning of the mind and how the mind is cultivated through proper practices, including the regulation of one's emotions. The cultivated mind, through its accumulation of ever more refined qi and thus shen or spirit then holds influence or control over less highly developed forms [34, 94, 100]. The Daodejing and Zhuangzi both echo these sentiments with various discussions of how one must regulate or control one's emotions. Ames and Hall in their commentary on the Daodejing state it thus: "The optimum posture of the heart-and-mind (xin) is to achieve and sustain an emptiness and equilibrium that will enable it to take in the world as it is without imposing its own suppositions upon it, and without allowing the world to cause it agitation" [2:100].[61] Kuriyama states this principle simply: "somatic integrity and emotional self-mastery coalesced in health" [55:223].

In the premedical contexts, the expression of emotions was seen as being disruptive to the process of self cultivation and development of virtue, sometimes with explicit mention of how the qi is disturbed in relation to this. It is thus natural that the medical literature should clearly describe how emotions disturb the qi in the body and how they can injure particular systems [56, 78, 128, 133].[62] Emotions were seen as disturbances to one's self-cultivation practices, they negatively impacted on one's ability to regulate the qi of one's body. Thus it is natural as the medical corpus takes form, with physiological and pathophysiological descriptions starting to be elaborated, emotions would follow this trend. They both result from internal disturbances and result in those internal disturbances. The medium through which they were described as manifesting and acting was primarily the qi: organ functional disturbances result in emotional manifestations; emotional manifestations result in distur-bances of qi movements and organ functioning; disturbances of qi movements result in emotional manifestations. These are not so much causal relations as forms of synchronistic manifestations. We thus take as a core understanding of the emotions that: "the arousal of qi in one's nature by external things causes one to react in a way that expresses emotion" [19:145] and that "emotions are disturbances of one's qi" [1:90], that emotions result in "a distortion in the good circulation of qi" [57:62].[63]

The non-affective mental states to do with perception, cognition, thinking, planning, acting are represented by a number of different terms in the premedical and TEAM literatures. While not consistently used among different texts, they have, for the most part not been seen as triggering or resulting from disturbances of one's qi. Instead, they have mostly been seen in a more positive light in their effect on the qi [56, 78].[64] They are sometimes described as having more of a regulatory effect rather than simply being a manifestation of the qi systems or causing automatic disturbance in those systems. We saw above passages from the Huainanzi such as "the heart/mind is the master of the five depots. It is the means of commanding the four limbs, and of causing the blood and energy to flow" [62:324-5] that establish the heart/mind has having rulership over the body. We find similar passages in pre-medical texts such as the Liji [禮記]: "The heart/mind in the body has the position as ruler" [62:37] and the Xinshu shang [心術上] chapter of the Guanzi "The heart/mind in the body has the position of the ruler" [62:37]. The early medical literature has parallel statements. Lingshu [靈樞] chapter eight describes how the "xin" or heart-mind "is the controller of the body" [78:37] while Suwen chapter eight describes "the heart/mind has the office of the ruler" [62:38] while Suwen chapter nine says "The heart is the rooting of life, the place where changes are made by the spirits."[56:32]. The xin, heart/mind was seen as lying at the center of how one regulates oneself and how the body regulates itself. The centrality of the xin or heart/mind is clearly stated in Suwen thirty-four: "when a person's body and mind have no mutual [relationship], this is to say death" [128:228].

Lingshu chapter forty-seven describes the role of "zhi" or "will" and "yi" or "intention", "attention", "awareness" in overall regulation: "If the intent and ideas (yi and zhi) are harmonized, then the essential spirit energies will be concentrated and straight, the hunpo will not scatter, resentment and anger will not arise, and the five depots will receive no pernicious energies" [62:331, see also 78:37].[66] This is an important passage as it brings together themes we found in Mencius regarding the relation of zhi [志] to the qi, the Neiye of yi [意] to the qi. This is elaborated below and reemerges in various chapters in this book.

The Chinese character or term for "heart" is "xin" [心], the same term that is used in Chinese to refer to the "mind" [2, 18, 78]. In fact, in the historical Chinese literature, it is often difficult to separate "mind" and "heart" when the "xin" is discussed leading some to suggest a compound translation of "xin" as the "heart/mind" or "mind/heart" [1, 2, 36, 138]. There is an interesting story in the Liezi [列子], circa 300 CE about how two people have their hearts exchanged and each returns to the home of the person from whom the received heart came. Each person now believed that they were the other person [32:106-107]. This allegorical tale informs us about a profound linking between what we call "heart" and "mind" and shows a clear understanding of the two as one. Virtually all emotional, feeling and cognitive states described in the historical Chinese literature employ characters that include "xin" or "heart" as a radical in the character [2, 91, 138]. The "xin""heart-mind was also described in relation to a "somato-psychic-social process" [138:41] in Lingshu eight:

> What responds to environment is called xin [心] (heart-mind). What xin brings out is called yi [意] (imagery). What yi stores is called zhi [志] (memory, memorization). Because of zhi, knowledge is reorganized. This is called si [思] (thinking, reflection). Because of si, one thinks for the future. This is called lu [慮] (strategy, plan). Because of lu, one makes decisions and takes actions. This is called zhi [知] (wise, wisdom). [138:41].[67]

Early literature and scholarship of this literature clearly support the interpretation of what is called separately the "heart" and "mind" as a compound interactive unit. This matches ideas in other cultures including our own that places the emotions (mind) as seated in the heart [2]; in classical Greek thought (around 400-200 BCE) feelings were located in the heart [55]. It is also interesting to note further correlations. The "xin" or "heart/mind" is involved in producing what Hall and Ames have characterized as "focal awareness" and "field awareness" [2]. "Focal awareness" is the action of the "xin" or "heart/mind" while focusing on something. "Field awareness" is the action of the "xin" or "heart/mind" while taking in something in the context of the total field of experience or background against which all focal events occur. Ideally one maintains field awareness while focusing on something. We will return to the implications and applications of this in the next section.

The Guanzi contains not only the "Neiye" which discusses xin but three additional chapters specifically about the "art of the heart-mind" the "Xinshu shang" [心術上], "Xinshu xia" [心術下] and the "Baixin" [白心] [see 96]. We cited briefly from the Xinshu shang above, but here include a more extensive quote to illustrate further how the xin or heart-mind was conceived.

> In the body, the heart holds the position of the ruler. The functions of the nine apertures correspond to the separate responsibilities of officials. The eyes and ears are the organs for seeing and hearing. If the heart does not interfere with the activities of seeing and hearing, the organs will be able to maintain their separate functions. Now if the heart is full of desires, the eyes will not see when things pass by nor will the ears hear when there are sounds. Therefore it is said: "if the person on high departs from the way (dao), those below will be lax in their work." Therefore it is said: "The art of the heart lies in controlling the apertures by non-action" [82:74, see also 96:71].

Clearly xin was seen to be responsible for the correct functioning of the parts of the body, optimally achieved through "non-action". The stillness of "xin" is essential for this.

We find important discussions about the nature of the heart/mind in other historical sources which extend the idea of the stillness of the xin and are helpful to a broader grasp of the concept of the xin and its relation to qi. Allan demonstrates that it is common in ancient texts to use analogies to the nature and properties of water to understand important concepts such as the "dao" (way), "de" (virtue) "qi", "xin" heart-and-mind [1]. Other authors have picked up on this as well [e.g. 115]. One of the properties of water is that if you let it sit still for a while, it settles and clears [1:49-53], the Xunzi describes this property thus: "the human heart/mind is like a bowl of water. If it is placed on a level surface and not moved, the impurities will settle to the bottom and the surface will be so clear and bright" [115:228]; the Zhuangzi thus:

> When water is still, it reflects one's beard and moustache clearly. Its levelness corresponds to the carpenter's level and the great craftsman takes his standard from it. If water when still is so clear, then how much more the quintessential spirit (jings-

hen). The mind/heart (xin) of the sage is clear! It is the jian-mirror of heaven and earth and the jian-mirror of the myriad living things [1:53].

These discussions illustrate an important property of the heart/mind: in stillness comes clarity. The achieving of stillness comes through calming the emotions and aligning the body –a model explicitly articulated in the Neiye [94, 96, 100]. The Zhuangzi also warns us of what happens when water stagnates: "the nature of water is to become clear when it is not disturbed, to become level when nothing moves it. But when it is blocked up and cannot flow, it also cannot become clear" [1:51].[68] Ishida captures this analogy between water and the mind very well when in a discussion of Asian conceptions of the mind, he talks of "the flowing mind" [47]. Just as water flows and needs to flow, so too does the mind. But we can suggest taking this analogy a little further, water is analogised also with qi. The medical literature has many discussions of the consequences of what happens when qi does not flow properly [134]. The close relationship between the heart/mind and qi can also, we suggest, be understood in the similarities of analogy. The Zhuangzi tells us: "Make your will one! Don't listen with your ears, listen with your mind (xin). No, don't listen with your mind, but listen with your vital energy (qi). Listening stops with the ears, the mind stops with recognition, **but vital energy is empty and waits on all things. The Dao gathers in emptiness alone. Emptiness is the fasting of the mind** (emphasis added)" [136:93]. By the time of the Neiye, qi "is thus the very substance of our physical and mental functioning" [34:472].

Traditionally there are a number of concepts that refer to non-affective mental functions such as the five "shen" the "shen", "hun", "po", "yi" and "zhi" each of which has over time accumulated various related meanings.

"Shen" [神] is more commonly translated as "spirit" [38, 62, 94, 96, 100, 123, 128, 134], sometimes as "spirits" [28, 56], "numen" [62:22], "god, divinity or divine" [75:18], "daemon, daemonic" [33], "vitality" [138:37][69] and often seen in relation to the mind itself. It is also sometimes translated as "knack" [16, 26].[70] In some descriptions it is that which animates the body during life. We find in the Huainanzi (circa 122 BCE) a description of how shen acts to transform formlessness to create the form of the animated tree, and that at the death of the tree the shen departs and ceases its transformations [78:91]. While this is not by any means an exclusive meaning and usage for the term "shen" [94] it does highlight an important way that the term has been used and understood in medical contexts. For example in the Huangdi Neijing Lingshu we find "the one who loses his shen dies; the one who obtains his shen lives" [62:54]. Clearly "shen", "spirit" is associated with being alive.

In the Neiye tradition, the "shen" is seen as one of three basic entities; qi, jing [精] (essence) and shen, which are of the same nature only jing is more concentrated and pure than qi and shen is more concentrated and pure than jing [62, 94, 96, 100].[72] The purpose of the practices described in the Neiye was to invite shen to take residence in the body so as to gradually accumulate shen in the body. As Puett states it: "Thus since all things consist of qi, that which possesses the most refined qi (as do the spirits) possesses both knowledge about and power over that which possesses less refined qi. By accumulating essence within himself, man becomes like a spirit; able to understand the changes of forms, avoid being harmed by them, and even gain control over them" [94:115]. This idea implies an ability to influence one's physiology by one's actions and even to influence whether and how outside influences might affect one so that one is not harmed by them. From this we can expect that this idea was carried forward into the yangsheng tradition and from there into the early medical literature.

The early medical literature seems to have also understood shen as an entity that slowly accumulates in the body and that can travel within, in and out of the body [69].[73] Ishida talks of the "flowing mind", the idea that the mind is not fixed but can flow within the body [47], we find passages in the Neijing that describe a free flowing of shen as well; Lingshu chapter one, in a brief discussion of the nature of acupoints describes them as "places 'where the jie (joints) intersect, where the qi of the shen (or alternatively qi and shen) travels in and out'" [69:88].[74] Slingerland in a discussion of the passage from Zhuangzi discussing cook Ding, suggests a link between qi and shen thus: "it might be appropriate to view spirit as the dynamic aspect of qi –as the tenuous qi in motion within a human being and issuing forth to interact with things" [115:201].

"Hun" [魂] and "po" [魄] are variously translated as "hun-soul", "po-soul" [123], "ethereal-spirit" and "earthly-spirit" [38:122] or "ethereal and corporeal souls" [15]. While there have been tendencies to try and see these in relation to Greek or Judeo-Christian ideas of the "soul" when we find for example ideas in the Liji of how they leave the body at death to return the heaven and earth [62:333, 78:20] or in the Hou Hanshu [後 漢 書] of how the hun leaves at death and disperses [62:54, 78:84], however, this can be misleading. Recent scholarship has characterized them as "refined bodily substances associated with mental faculties" [62:55, 69].[75] We must be careful not to project our own ideas onto these two concepts, because they could be seen in relation to similar sounding Judeo-Christian concepts, with which they have no relationship.

We need to explore the terms "yi" and "zhi" further since, as we have seen, they have been described explicitly in relation to how we influence qi. These descriptions are important for a deeper understanding of the early acupuncture

**BOX 2 –yi [意] in translation**

"Yi" [意] is translated as **"thought"** [111:287, 115:123, 123], **"idea"** [31, 36:38,62:331, 82:57], **"imagery"** [138:41], **"intellect"** [74:63], **"purpose"** [57:42], **"sentiment"** [125:361], **"meaning"** [36:38, 56:176, 82:56, 123, 138:59], **"attention"** [16, 96:51, 102:176], **"judgment"**[77] [29:143-144, 104:44], **"intelligence"** [105:35], **"significance"** [56:176], **"signification"** [105:35] and more commonly as **"intention"** [31, 47, 56:176, 69:83, 123, 128], **"desire"** [59:171, 82:56], **"wish"** [82:56]. It is also translated as **"awareness"** [62:23, 96, 100] or **"power of awareness"**, a **"basic mental capacity that precedes thought"** [96:31], **"the unexpressed thoughts of the mind"** [78:37], **"an understanding that can be unfolded in practice but is not limited to representational knowledge"** [102:177], **"the image rather than the concept of a thing, and the movement to action with which one responds to it"** [31:501]. Lingshu chapter eight talks of yi: Larre and Rochat de la Vallee render this as: "when the heart applies itself, we speak of intent (yi)" [56:51].[78] Scheid and Bensky have a nuanced variation: "That which takes responsibility for things is called the heart. The heart has a place to focus its attention, which is called intention," [105:35]. We feel Rickett's characterization as "basic mental capacity that precedes thought" [96:31] and Scheid's "an understanding that can be unfolded in practice but is not limited to representational knowledge" [102:177] are insightful. As we have seen in the Neiye, the "yi" manifesting in a very quiet passive properly aligned state "welcomes" the qi [96:39-40, 100:48].[79] The Huangdi Neijing Lingshu text also discusses how the interaction with qi is brought about via one's yi "attention": "Whether meeting it or following it, by means of one's attention, one harmonizes it" [16]. This usage seems to be a direct parallel of the Neiye's discussion of how one "welcomes" the qi through one's "yi", a quiescent attention or awareness.[80]

**BOX 3 –zhi [志] in translation**

"Zhi" [志] is most commonly translated as **"will"** [1:90-1, 19, 68, 98:34, 123] or **"willpower"** [74:67]. It is sometimes translated as **"intention"** [1:86, 62:26, 98:34, 111:287, 115:123 & 154-5], **"intent"** [31], **"ambition"** [69:83], **"mind"** [1:87, 123, 134:395], **"aims"** [123], **"aspirations"** [2:81-82], **"memory"** [28:291, 138:41], **"attention"** [31], and **"emotion"** [113]. Hall and Ames describe how zhi is a combination of "heart-and-mind" with "to go to" or "to abide in", giving it the meaning of "**to have in mind**", or **"to set one's heart on"** [36:38]. The use of "zhi" to refer to emotion is interesting since we find the "five zhi" as a general label to refer to five emotions in for example the Suwen and Taisu (of circa 610 CE) [18:120-1]. Rochat de la Vallee characterizes "zhi" as the will or intent "the inner orientation of the mind" [98:34], the "will, or intent guides the qi through the inner orientation coming from the heart" [98:35]. Graham describes "zhi" as "sustained attention to something and the orientation of action towards it" [31:478]. In Lingshu chapter eight we find "when intent (yi) becomes permanent, we speak of will (zhi)" [56:53].[81] As we have seen in the Mencius, the "zhi" governs and moves the qi [1:91, 62:26].[82]

literature, cultivation and martial arts literatures. The terms "yi" and "zhi" have been translated variously by different authors, sometimes using a translation that is common for one term (i.e. "yi" as "intention") as the translation for the other term (i.e. "zhi" as "intention"). Perhaps this confusion is natural given what the Shuowen Jiezi (circa 90 CE) says of "yi" and "zhi" that they are the same [2:38, 78:37].[76] Thus as we have seen above, we find the terms "yi" and "zhi" sometimes used interchangeably and both sometimes to refer to the more general concept for which the term "xin" is more commonly used. We find a variety of ideas expressed in the historical literature that each gives us a flavor of how to understand these terms. However it is also useful to remember the point raised by Kuriyama, that in answer to a "what" question we usually find a "how" response [55:96]. The more useful understanding of these two terms lies in how we apply them. Box 2 and Box 3 give many examples of how the two terms have been translated into English by different authors.

There are some important distinctions between these two terms that can be highlighted in relation to how we use the heart/mind. Of the "zhi", Mencius said "The will is the governor of qi. Qi is what fills the limbs. Wherein the will arrives is where the qi lodges" [1:91]. The will (or mind) directs the qi in this model. The "zhi" moves the "xin" in a certain direction so as to create the focus necessary to achieve certain actions [1:86-87]. Of the "yi" the Neiye describes how the qi cannot be moved by force, yet it can be "welcomed by the awareness" (yi) [100:48], a quiet awareness when the emotions are calmed can welcome the qi. In this sense of the term, the "yi" as a quiescent manifestation of the mind influences or welcomes the qi. The role of this yi, as a quiescent focused awareness that "welcomes" the qi is hinted at in various places in the medical literature. Chapter sixty-two of the Huangdi Neijing Suwen talks about the importance of the yi in relation to correct needling [128:281]. This soft focus approach to influencing the qi is also echoed in the Daodejing which states: "If the heart directs the Qi, this is called: forcing" [83:38]. The effect of the heart/mind on the qi is forced if the heart/mind tries deliberately to direct it, coercion is not used instead a quiet focus or awareness is used, labelled as "yi", awareness, in the Neiye [100:48].[83] The yi and zhi feature in an additional passage from Lingshu forty-seven which further extend how we can see the yi and zhi: "Intent (zhi) and ideas (yi) are the means of directing the essential spirit (jing-shen) and of concentrating the hunpo" [62:332]. The shen, spirit is directed by the yi and zhi, different aspects of how the mind manifests itself. While "yi" is important in how an acupuncturist can influence the qi of the patient following the ideas we have discussed here,[84] yi was also discussed much more widely in medicine.

In the medical traditions of China "yi" was seen as being essential to the practice of medicine. The Han dynasty physician Guoyu [郭玉] (circa 100 CE) is quoted in the Hou Hanshu, as saying: "Medicine is attention (yi). The regions of the skin are very finely divided. Following the flow of qi requires consummate skill. When inserting needles, an error of a hair's breadth will mean failure. A kind of spirit connects the physician's heart with his hand, and that is something I can know but not explain" [102:177].[85] Attention (yi) relates to how we perform our actions and is hard to capture in words. Expressing a similar understanding, other medical authors have discussed "yi" in a similar vein. Sun Simiao of 652 CE stated "medicine is yi", adding "'those who are proficient at using yi are good doctors' and 'those who match [the correct type of medicine with the appropriate condition]... can be considered superior craftsmen. So it is said 'Medicine is yi,'" [105:35]. The later physician Zhao Xuemin (1719-1805) said "Medicine is yi. It is not as good to use medicinals as it is to use yi. Whether or not a treatment works is based on yi. If yi can enter into the fundamental subtleties [of the illness] one can achieve a penetrating understanding," [105:35]. Yi as a state of mind not only was seen as being important for how one "welcomes" the qi and is thus essential in needling, it is also involved in how the practitioner achieves a penetrating understanding so that the correct diagnosis and treatment selection is made in herbal medicine.[86] In chapter six, the chapter discussing herbal medicine, qi and jingmai [99], we will see that this extension of how yi was understood and used in medicine provides a further link for the manifestation and use of yi and consequently qi in herbal medical practice.

We would like to extend the understanding of the term yi [意] through incorporation of the three stages of perceiving and knowing that are described in Zhuangzi.

> Make your will one! Don't listen with your ears, listen with your mind (心). No, don't listen with your mind, but listen with your vital energy (氣). Listening stops with the ears, the mind stops with recognition, but vital energy is empty and waits on all things. The Dao gathers in emptiness alone. Emptiness is the fasting of the mind. [136:93].

We mentioned above that Yang presented evidence for how this can be seen as a three stage process: perceiving/knowing through the sense organs; perceiving/knowing through the mind; perceiving/knowing through the qi. As further evidence for this three stage process Yang also cites the Wenzi [文子] (probably circa fourth century CE [100:7], but with older portions certainly predating 55 BCE [101:1041], possibly from the early Han [23]) "The highest learning listens with the spirit, the middle learning listens with the mind and the lowest learning listens with the ears"[136:95] and the Huainanzi:

> My body merges with my mind, my mind merges with my vital energy, my vital energy merges with my spirit and my spirit merges with nothingness. If the slightest something or the smallest sound comes to disturb me –whether it be as far outside the eight wilds or as close as between my eyebrows and lashes– I invariably perceive it. [136:96].

Slingerland discusses the same three stages in relation to a parallel passage in Mencius [115:183-184] and points out, following commentary by Pang Pu that Zhuangzi's cook Ding story gives a further parallel "What I care about is the way, which goes beyond mere technique. When I first began cutting up oxen, all I could see was the ox itself. After three years, I no longer saw the ox as a whole. And now –now I meet it with my spirit and don't look with my eyes. My sensory knowledge is restrained and my spiritual desires are allowed to move/act. I follow the heavenly pattern…" the three stages are "sensory perception (looking with the eye)", "use of knowledge (no longer seeing the ox as a whole)" and "guided by spirit (meeting it with the spirit)" [115:199-201]. There are several passages in the historical literatures that can be seen to propose three stages of perception as a kind of progressive development.

We think it possible to understand and interpret the concept "yi" in a similar three stage manner. At first "yi" is like "intention", as a beginner at something one can intend that thing to happen, one can direct one's physical actions to try to help it happen, but one can only involuntarily work with the qi to make it happen, or at least only sporadically do so. It does not yet come naturally, it takes work and concentration. Such actions are *not* without effort (not "wuwei" [無爲]).

With further experience and training the "yi" gradually develops so that it is less of an effort, one starts to work more quietly and easily with the qi. Here the mind rather than the physical body is involved and "yi" is more like "attention", a consciously held focus. But at this stage, there is a risk, described in the Daodejing as "forcing": "If the heart directs the Qi, this is called: forcing" [83:38]. One has to be careful to not force this attention, but so long as one does not try forcing the change, one can engage the qi more easily and consistently than in the first stage.

In the third stage, after a lot more experience and/or training, the yi acts naturally without conscious intervention, here it is like simply drawing "awareness" of the thing on which one wants to act or the act one wants to accomplish. The qi is not only involved, as the Neiye says, it is "welcomed by one's yi", it is automatically engaged and involved, as a matter of course, with minimal or no effort ("wuwei") and no longer any risk of "forcing". Of this the Zhuangzi comments: "when you have the method, will you find it easy to practise it? He who thinks it easy will be disapproved of by the bright Heaven," [60]. Sharf citing Le Blanc discusses how in the Huainanzi the concept of "wuwei" "is explained as the source of the creative and transformative power of the sage-king. Non-action is the means by which the sage-king attains perfect resonance between himself and the masses" [107:91]. We find a clear discussion about how the special abilities of the "sage-king" (or advanced practitioner), utilizes ganying (see the next section) in conjunction with wuwei to attain his effects. This third stage, "yi" as "awareness" also captures the use of the term "shen" as "knack" as used by Zhuangzi in his discussion of the skills of cook Ding [26:212, see also 16]. The third stage also naturally brings order. The cook Ding passage cited above ended with "I follow the heavenly pattern" [115:200]. The term "heavenly pattern' is [天理] which implies a kind of natural order.

In Taijiquan [太極拳], the first stage (yi as "intention") is like the novitiate learning and practicing the form, it is an effort, it is not yet natural or embodied and working with qi is more limited.

In the second stage (yi as "attention"), the experienced practitioner more naturally performs, but still needs to retain a focus of his actions in order to engage the qi. In this second stage the ability to call upon and utilise qi is greater than in the first stage.

In the third stage (yi as "awareness") the master simply acts and performs naturally, his actions are embodied through the qi, this is "effortless action" [無爲]. The ability to merge and flow with and thus call upon and utilise qi is much greater then in the two previous stages and requires considerable training and or experience to develop.

These stages of development are important for an understanding of not only taijiquan, which we will see in the chapters on taijiquan [14], acupuncture [8], research [10] and the practical sections of this book in the last chapter, this is an important and useful three-fold distinction to draw. Training, actions and effects are different according to what stages of development the person practicing is at. This affects how we can expect people to perform or practice according to where they are at in their stage of development. It also means we must pay more attention to these distinctions when we try to investigate for example qi and how people engage or influence qi in their practice.

Now that we have established an at least tripartite understanding of the term "yi", we can look at usages of the term that can be found in early Han cultivation literature. The Yinshu [引書] from the Zhangjiashan site has discussions of how the person should place their "yi" in certain parts of the body or an activity in order to achieve certain actions [71:406]. This gives us additional hints on how the "yi" might be acting and, we feel, further support for our notion of the "yi" in a several leveled understanding.

The "yi" can be distracted or agitated so that its proper actions do not occur, which is corrected by certain actions to recreate the "concentrating attention" [71:406]:

> Pulling incipient exhaustion illness. The intention (yi) is agitatedly set on pacing around, the body hurts more and more. At this moment you must treat it with the pull of the eight warps; quickly breathe out (dry breath) and quickly exhale (warm breath), pull yin. Soak the space between the eyebrows in cold water for the time it takes to eat bowl of rice...

Placing the intention (yi) at certain sites also helps treat problems [71:407]: "incipient illness in the bowel. Invariably there will be swelling at the front. When there is swelling, apply the intention (yi) to the lesser abdomen and concentrate on puffing out (moist breath). Stop after one hundred times." Lo goes on to describe how with such technique the sites "become the location for concentrated attention, presumably achieved with increased awareness of that area of the body; then with the measured manipulation of the breath function, perhaps even with the imagination of comfort through conscious projection of qi, after a prescribed time a sequence of therapeutic events unfolds of its own accord" [71:407]. One's yi [意] is moved around as a kind of attention or greater awareness to create changes in the qi, especially when additional actions are engaged in, such as breathing (as we find in the Yinshu and the Neiye) and later needling (as we find in the medical classics of the Huangdi Neijing). Lo describes this further in a kind of anthropological language, she refers to the "intentional body" which is linked with a multiplicity of bodies ("the manifestation of his sick body, its biology and its biological processes, the experience of the sick body and the imagination of a well ordered body, its idealized social identity, its social projection –the body that can be affected by breathing– a body infused with qi") [71:407]. Citing a passage on breath and sexual cultivation from the Mawangdui Hanmu boshu Lo describes how the "intention" (yi) activates potential influences in the body to create a change for the better:

> Be careful, do not drink wine and eat the five flavours; put the qi in order with intent and the eye will be bright and the ear keen, the skin will gleam, the one hundred mai will be full and the yin will rise again. From this you will be able to stand for a long time, go a long way, and live for (ever)" [71:408].

These examples, we feel, support our thesis for how the yi positively influences the qi in the body. The more adept one is at engaging such influences, the more change one can produce. This theme is discussed further in chapter four where the influence of the practitioner, especially through their mental state, their yi is examined in depth.

While the natures of the xin, shen, hun, po, yi and zhi are generally understood, and a deeper understanding of them continues to evolve, they, like the emotions, are intimately related to the qi: qi "is that which gives us our vitality. And as the vital energy of the mind/heart, it is that which controls our thoughts and emotions" [1:92]. For Mencius "the mind is the foundation of the qi. Without it, the qi will have no foundation, and so will have no source" [19:151]. In general these higher mental functions tend to have regulatory influences on the qi while the emotions have disruptive influences.

## Probing deeper –exploring mechanisms of qi action

### Qi as resonances, ying, ganying 應 感應

Interesting and important concepts for grasping something of the nature of qi are the concepts "ying" [應] –"respond" or "response" [59:87 + 253], "responding to" [31], "responding" [26:220, 115:248] and the equivalent term "ganying" [感應], "resonance" [18, 59, 75, 86:281], "sympathetic resonance" [107:78], "cosmic resonance" [40:20], "stimulus and response" [59, 107:78, 113], "encounter" [87:407].[87] The terms "ying" and "ganying" refer to the influence of things upon each other [40:22-28, 75:28], and, we feel provide further insights into the linking of qi with the mind and emotions. "Ying" seems more related to how one thing responds to another[88] while "ganying" seems more related to a kind of mutual influence of one thing upon another, like influences like. But the use of these two related terms ("ying" and "ganying") by different writers makes it difficult at times to draw this kind of distinction, often they are used in the same way. A less commonly used term is [相應], "xiangying", "complementary response" [107:84] or "mutual influence" which can be found in the Huainanzi [59:118 (see text on page 212)]. A later term that is used to describe "qi interactions" in the medical literature is "qijiao" [氣交] which Unschuld calls "qi interaction". This term is found in later chapters of the Suwen in Wang Bing's eight century edition in the context of "wuyun liuqi" [五 運六氣] discussions of "the sphere where the qi of heaven and of earth interact; it is the space where man resides" [128:484]. Suwen chapter sixty-eight states: "What is… 'qi interaction'?" Qibo responds 'Amidst the interaction of the qi of the positions of above and below, that is where man resides…' What is above the heavenly axis, the heavenly qi rules it. What is below the heavenly axis, the qi of earth rules it. The sphere of qi interaction, the human qi follows it, the myriad beings originate from it" [128:484]. Wang Bing expands "Hence all transformations and generations, as well as changes, take place in the [sphere of the] qi interaction" [128:484]. While a different kind of qi interaction than "ying", response, "ganying", resonance or "xiangying", mutual influence, the term "qijiao" attempts to capture something of how the human being is a product of his environment (qi of heaven and qi of earth) and the mutual interactions these have around and through him. Since the primary discussions of the influences of qi and how one interacts with it seem to utilize the terms "ying" and "ganying", we will focus on these terms here.

One would suppose that in the correlative cosmological thinking of wuxing, (five phase) and yinyang theories, that the term ganying might be used[89], but interestingly a different term is often used Henderson argues that "ganying" is not intrinsic to correlative thinking, but that it does play a role in some cosmological models, such as that of the Huainanzi: "the conception of gan-ying was important in the operation of two basic modes of correlative thought sketched above, man-cosmos and state-cosmos correspondence" [40:22].[90]

Various uses and passages clearly link ying/ganying with qi starting with the Zuoyan of the third century BCE [75:30]: "All things are the same as their qi; all things respond to their own class" [Huainanzi quoted in 75:28]. The Lushi Chunqiu (239 BCE) says "[Things of the same] category are certain to attract each other; when their qi is the same they are in harmony; when sounds are matched they resonate" [113]. The principle of ying or ganying is important in the establishment of correlative thinking or what has been called the theory of systematic correspondence that became dominant during the Han dynasty and forms the basis of medical models (yin-yang, five phases).[91] It also helps explain how the sage or leader can influence others [19:183-192], how nature (heaven and earth) can influence people [75:28-32] and how people can influence nature [113]. Recall the quote above from the Chunqiu Fanlu "Heaven has yin and yang; humans also have yin and yang. When the yin qi of Heaven and Earth rise, the yin qi of humans *responds* to it and rises. When the yin qi of humans rise, the yin qi of Heaven and Earth also properly *responds* to it and rises. Their way is one" [94:290-291]. Sivin summarises these influences thus: "The political and somatic microcosms resonate in harmony with the macrocosm because the ensemble of dynamic processes circulate qi... throughout all three. The influence runs not only downward but upward, and between state and body as well" [113]. At the end of the second century BCE there was a debate about how heaven and man influenced each other. Two distinctly different models of the resonance between heaven and man "tianren ganying" [天人 感應] can be found. Dong in his Chunqiu Fanlu "strongly opposes all interpretations of cosmos as a natural or physical order free from moral intention. From Zhou theology he revives the idea of Heaven as an anthropomorphic deity... Heaven manifests its will in omens, warning the ruler of the human world" [130:186] While the Huainanzi "replaces Dong's cosmology of the moral intention of heaven with a physical cosmology of resonance' –"resonance within the same category' or 'resonance with the same qi'" [130:186].[92] While there were different political models interpreting how ganying operates each saw ying or ganying in relation to qi.

Ying/ganying is a phenomenon that is observable in nature, for example when a bell is struck one can see a mutual resonance or vibration of the jade stone or other bells nearby [19:182-6]. The striking of a note on a stringed instrument is observed to cause resonant vibrations on strings of nearby instruments [86:281-282]. The terms ying or ganying are used to describe these invisible mutual influences. This mutual influence is given as an analogized explanation of the nature of qi [86]. As the model of qi was developing, "various groups used qi to explain 'invisible' concepts such as action at a distance or disease processes" [19:145]. Major explains it thus: "Resonance (ganying) between or among things within a class is conveyed through qi, conceived of as both the basic stuff of concrete phenomena and as an intangible vibrating medium pervading empty space" [75:28], qi is both the medium of these interactions and the constituent of the things in interaction [75:30].

It is therefore natural that the terms "ying" or "ganying" might also be used in reference to properties of the mind. In his exploration of Huainanzi chapter six, Le Blanc says and then quotes "The perfect ruler needs to be one with Tao in order to govern through mutual resonance 'It follows that he who relies on knowledge to rule will hardly be able to sustain the state. Only he who is merged with Great Harmony and holds fast to the **Responses of the Natural** has the capacity for such things'" (emphasis added) [59:136]. Zhuangzi used the term ying (to respond) as a property of the perfected person: "The Perfected Person in using his heart/mind is like a mirror: he does not lead, nor does he welcome; he responds (ying) but does not store. This is why he is able to win over things and not be harmed" [115:192].[93] Csikszentmihalyi demonstrates that the resonance of ganying was analogized from the influence of metal bells on the jade stone in Mencius to concepts of virtue and morals in the self cultivation literature: "virtue was thought to create a sympathetic moral influence likened to resonance" [19:183]. The Mozi [墨子] of the early third century BCE states: "The appearance of one's intention (zhi –志) and qi, causing others to be like one. It is as unavoidable as a metal bell sounding and a jade stone vibrating" [19:187]. Likewise the Wuxing of the late fourth early third century BCE similarly uses the analogy of the vibration of the jade stone with the sounding of the metal bell as how the virtue of the sage acts upon others "'A metal bell sounding and a jade stone causing it to vibrate,' is the presence of virtue'. 'A metal bell sounding,' is good. 'A jade stone causing it to vibrate' is sage. Good is the human Way, and virtue is tian's Way. Only once virtue is present can there be 'a metal bell sounding and a jade stone causing it to vibrate'" [19:178].[94] These references to the metal bell and the jade stone are references to the concept of response or resonance (ying –ganying). The Mozi passage also discusses the "ability to transform others through one's zhi and qi (intention and pneuma)" [19:188]. We saw above how concepts of qi, mind and body were influenced and partially developed out of the literature on virtue and moral development, several authors have described these connections [19, 113].

Le Blanc proposes a classification of "ganying" (and its associated term "ying"), resonance into two subtypes: "simple" or "relative resonance" and "total resonance" [59:139-142] Examples of "simple resonance" are the striking of one string and having the same string on other instruments vibrate or the response of the horses after mounting the chariot and grasping the reins to direct them [59:140]. Examples of "total resonance" are the striking of an untuned string on an instrument and having all strings vibrate and the response of the horses as a result of simply mounting the chariot without direction from the riders [59:140], "that which causes the twenty-five strings to resound is not a particular sound belonging to either the yang or to the yin category. It transcends all categories of sound" [59:141]. The example from Zhuangzi above of "The Perfected Person in using his heart/mind is like a mirror: he does not lead, nor does he welcome; he responds (ying) but does not store. This is why he is able to win over things and not be harmed" [115:192] is another example of "total resonance" as is the following from Zhuangzi: "Once the pivot is centered in its socket, it is able to respond (ying) inexhaustibly" [26:215].

This subclassification of types of "resonance" distinguishes between resonance or response that is more related to yin-yang, five phase type influences, on the one hand and a more complete "total resonance" that has a more Daoist influence. In the first we can say that the responses are due to more local interactions, that is, interactions directly between one thing and another. While in the second the responses are due to a broader interaction with environmental or contextual aspects. Practically, in terms of how an individual can utilize these two types of response, the first will require less development, skill or training, the second is something only the true expert or "sage" can accomplish.

This discussion of the concepts of ying and ganying is not to esoteric or strange ideas, these are ideas that can easily be seen to have arisen out of daily experience. We are all familiar with the emotional atmosphere or tension we can feel upon entering a room, or when we talk of feeling another's emotions or being sympathetic to another person's feelings. This kind of emotional sympathetic resonance is not something special it is a part of our daily lives. So it probably was in ancient China. The fact that this analogized understanding of the nature of qi as "ganying" a kind of mutual resonance or sympathy implies in the use of the term in relation to feelings, emotions and the mind that they can be seen in relation to qi. Perhaps, the act of observing something with a quiet mind, places the observer in a "ganying" with the observed thing. There is a mutual influence of observer and thing observed. We can suggest that this may be the principle at work when medical authors stated that "medicine is yi", where the ability to achieve a penetrating insight allows for the proper matching of the herb to the patient. Perhaps the principle is to match the functional aspects of the herb to the physiological state of the patient to create a resonance between the herb and patient? This is discussed further in chapter six.

Le Blanc, who has made a thorough analysis of "ganying" concluded ganying "may be defined, in the final analysis, as the power of things to affect and to be affected in such a way as **to bring about harmony** (emphasis added). This power is based on the persistent affinity and attraction of things that were originally one, but that became scattered when the world began" [59:209]. If we accept this conclusion, we can see that ganying is not only related to how "qi" functions or behaves, but also in the ability of someone to engage the qi using "ganying", they may bring about "harmony", an important concept in for example, the medical tradition. The more advanced the person, the greater their ability (relative resonance versus total resonance) to engage qi and the greater the harmonizing effects. This is an important notion that is discussed further in later chapters.

## Dynamic engagement of qi-ji 機

Another important concept that helps us deepen our understanding of qi and its relationships is the concept "ji" [機], translated variously as "mechanism" [19:215, 97], "subtle mechanism (of life)" [56:31], "activating force" [97], "dynamic" [16], "germ" [33, 78:85, 86:79], "turning point", "pivot", "first stirring" [36:231], "trigger" [2:58], "wellspring" [Mair in 16], "impulse" –"that from which movement starts" [31], "thing which makes it go" [33]. Robinet describes ji as "the spring of the world, its activating force... the extreme degree of quiescence and purity which is on the verge of changing into movement" [97]. It is an ancient term for the firing mechanism of a crossbow [97] and "by extension, it is the crux or hinge of a thing" [16]. Commonly "ji" is seen as the dynamic or mechanism by which things happen. It is said to be "the dynamic aspect of the Dao, the motive force of the world that never ceases to function and originates in the tension between the opposites –yin and yang... It is also the point of junction between them, the mechanism of transformation" [97]. This concept is discussed extensively by Chace and Bensky in this volume, so we will not discuss it here much. But as a pivotal concept for understanding the mechanism of qi's actions it is important we outline here some meanings and uses of this term in relation to qi.

It exerts its influence at the start of an action or event. It is used in various ways to describe this characteristic. There is "heavenly mechanism" (tianji) a kind of cosmic influence that is seen as a kind of trigger or cause of things happening.[95] A cognate of the term "ji" is "ji" [幾] variously translated as "first inklings or stirrings" [36:230-1], "incipience" [16], "inchoate" [2:58]. These two terms are often used synonymously or interchangeably. Ji –incipience/first inklings has very old uses and meanings that are influential. One finds it in the Yijing [易經] (earliest datings from ninth to seventh centuries BCE [50:342]) in a discussion of the importance of ji relative to the hua [化] or active transformations which lie at the heart of change. In the Xici [繫辭] commentary of the Yijing (probably late third century BCE) it says "the changes are the means by which the sages searched the profound and examined incipience. Only by the profound can one penetrate to the purpose under heaven; only by incipience can one perfect the tasks under heaven" [16]. The Yijing commentary continues "To understand the first inklings (ji) this is spiritual understanding (shen)... The first inklings are the suggestion of movement" [36:231].[96] This establishes the concept of ji - incipience as fundamental for understanding the way of heaven, and how changes, movements occur. It also links the concept with shen –spirit [36:31, 115:199]. This shows up in a number of different ways. Those involved in internal cultivation or alchemy practices aim at uniting their human ji with heavenly ji [97] so that they may have greater insight into the world around them. The Huainanzi tells us how "The realized man (the sage) is able to attach or connect to "tianji" [天機] [heaven's loom, heaven's germ (sic)] inside the body" [78:85]. These meanings and uses extend to the term ji –dynamic or mechanism. We find important uses of this concept in the early medical literature of the Huangdi Neijing relative to how to apply needling and influence the qi [16]. The superior physician is cautioned to "attend to the dynamic" and "those who understand the way of the dynamic, will not impede it and it thus manifests" [16]. This is part of a discussion of the essential subtleties of needling and how to needle so as to activate and work with the qi.

The Zhuangzi and then later the Liezi [列子] discuss how the "myriad things come out from the ji and re-enter at the ji" [78:85]. Needham uses the term "germ" to refer to this usage arguing that is it a precursor of germ theory [86:79], however this approach to understanding the term can be misleading. Mair renders the same passage as "The ten thousand things all come out from the wellsprings and all reenter the wellsprings" [16]. However one chooses to interpret this passage, it is clear the Zhuangzi is using the term to refer to the beginnings of things.

Other uses of the term ji (dynamic) imply it lies not just at the start of change/events but also at the center. Ji "is associated with the empty spaces or intervals between phases of activity" [16]. In Lingshu chapter one it states: "the movement of the dynamic is not separate from its empty spaces; the dynamic within this empty space is clear, still and subtle" [16]. Suwen chapter fifteen describes the ji in the following: "the way [道] is in the unity, and the spirits [神] imprint a rotating movement without ever bringing up the rear. If they were in the rear they would no longer guarantee the rotations; the subtle mechanism (of life) [機] would be lost" [56:31]. The ji is wholly involved in all movements and transformations in nature. Robinet describes it as "the wondrous movement that unites movement and quiescence, the true spring that moves spontaneously by itself (ziran [自然]) and without intention (wuxin [無心] –Robinet gives a different translation for "xin' than is usually encountered) and acts without action and interference (wuwei [無為])" [97]. We have seen extensive discussions above of how we cannot force the qi to react, it is by a quiet awareness (yi) that we can welcome the qi (Neiye); we cannot force the qi with our mind (Daodejing), it is through non-action (wuwei) and quiet focus that we try to grasp the subtle spaces through which change/action arises and through this influence that change/action. We try to change ourselves through various practices and disciplines (Neiye, Mozi) so that we can do this spontaneously (ziran) as a natural expression of ourselves. It is here that the term ji is important. Robinet also argues that the term ji –dynamic/mechanism is synonymous with the heart-mind (xin) and spirit (shen).[98] She states "physiologically, ji is located in the center of the body which in turn is related to yi intention and to the spleen, or it can be identified with the interval between breathing in and out, corresponding with the closing and opening of the world in the instant that preceded the movement of breath" [97].

Given these important early historical uses of the term ji –dynamic/mechanism and its early cognate ji –incipience and a clear articulation of how they are accessed via one's internal state of mind it is not surprising that we find a key passage from the Lingshu discussing the importance of ji for the proper application of needling to influence the qi and create maximal change. Chapter five by Chace and Bensky discusses this in greater detail with a full annotated and explanatory translation of the Lingshu passage. Together, these various uses help us expand further our understanding of the important and vital relationships between qi and the mind. It is only through a properly developed understanding developed via correct postures and mental practices that one can truly influence the qi to maximum effect. The term ji –dynamic/mechanism helps us understand further the process for doing this just as the terms ying and ganying help us understand further the possible mechanisms by which these things might occur.

## Speculations on the nature of qi in relation to consciousness

Qi is not just an abstract concept, it is fundamentally an everyday thing related to our experiences of the world. Nor is it a purely invisible or imperceptible thing. Qi is also directly perceptible, since it is a concept that arises out of our experiences and thus perceptions of the world and others. Kuriyama discusses how qi was perceptible stating: "At the same time, however –and this point merits emphasis– the experience of qi was never purely internal. Qi was subjectively felt, but it was also perceptible from without" [55:103-4] as in palpating the pulses or observing the facial complexion to observe the qi directly. Hsu also argues that the qi was palpable, something directly perceived by the hands [46]. In more broad discussions of Chinese thinking and especially so-called "Daoist cosmology", Ames and Hall explicitly acknowledge the centrality of "experience" to understanding Chinese thinking [2:15-18].[99]

On the basis of the above discussions we propose that one of the important ways that qi was discussed was in relation to experience of the world. The xin (heart/mind) interacts with the world through the senses (and non-sensory experiences). Since the world was not described independently of the experiences of it (the non-objectivity of traditional perspectives) the mind was seen as an active player within the world, interacting with it in many ways. In the ideal, the cultivated person has a quietly focused mind that (inter)acts on the world. At the interface of this interaction, we find qi (the Neiye is clear on this). However, experiences of the world trigger emotional reactions which disturb this interface,[100] hence since the development of virtue, "de" is related to one's qi [see 19:210-211], then in various traditions it is almost a moral imperative to regulate one's emotions. In the Neiye one must calm the emotions in order to expand the cultivation of qi (and thus jing-shen) and in the Neijing we see the clinical manifestations of not controlling one's emotions –various qi disturbances that cause physiological changes and thus bodily symptoms, disturbances of higher mental functions such as the yi or zhi.

As further examples of the links between qi and the mind we cite additional texts and draw together the argument that to talk of qi we must talk about the mind [19:151]. One of the important ways that qi was conceived was through the mind's experiences, including all sensory experiences of the world. In a very important way, qi is the mind and its sensory experiences of the world. The mind is a construct of qi, in higher forms. Material objects are constructs, condensations of qi. When the mind observes things, the experiences themselves are seen in terms of qi.

We have already discussed xin, heart/mind above but add here a short quote from Mencius: "The organs of the ears and eyes do not think (si [思]) and they are beguiled by [living] things. When living things have contact with one another, they simply attract each other. As for the organ of the mind/heart, it thinks" [1:85]. Here the xin, heart/mind is seen to be responsible for thinking, the sense organs (attached to the brain) and thus the brain were seen to be easily distracted. The Daodejing discusses the problem of being distracted by the outer world differently: "The five colors blind the eye. The hard riding of the hunt addles both heart and mind. Property hard to come by subverts proper conduct. The five flavors destroy the palate. And the five notes impair the ear" [2:92]. While the expression is different than that of the Mencius, the basic idea is similar, the mind, which has an intimate relationship with the qi is easily distracted or disturbed by its experiences of things, due to the effects on the qi.

In the modern period such passages as these from the Mencius and the Daodejing may seem mystical or quaint, but there is a wealth of related concepts and understandings that are part of an extended model. In the pre-medical corpus, one of the concerns of writers was of how virtue could be cultivated. This was a specific concern of Confucius, the Daodejing, Mencius and various other authors [1, 19, 115].

The Chunqiu Zuozhuan [春秋左傳] (of circa 200 BCE) states "Heaven has six qi which descending generate five tastes, issue as five colours, are evidenced by five sounds, and in excess they generate six diseases" [98:13], similarly "the six qi are generated using the five processes (wu xing). The qi become the five tastes, issue as the five colours, and are proclaimed as the five sounds" [98:24]. Here we see the idea that the various sensory experiences of the world (tastes, colours and sounds) are all qi based derived from the "six qi" of heaven. These six qi were further discussed in the Zuozhuan "In mankind the likes and dislikes, elation and anger, sorrow and joy are generated from the six qi. Therefore take care to model yourself on appropriate categories in order to control the six inclinations or wills (zhi)" [98:23]. Various other sources support this interpretation of qi as the mind and its experiences. The Guoyu [國語](possibly fifth century BCE) describes "the mouth draws in taste and the ear sounds. Sounds and taste generate qi. The qi in the mouth becomes speech and in the eyes becomes light" [98:26]. Nylan writing of the Huainanzi (circa 122 BCE) describes "qi in the Huainanzi functions as the subtle sensory medium permitting connections to be made between discrete things" [87:402].

The material world is seen through the eyes of qi. In a model of the body and mind where everything is qi, how would the world be experienced? When one perceives things, everything can be understood in terms of qi: Qi is the experience (sensations), the thing experienced and the person/mind doing the experiencing. We can see this very clearly in the historical literature from China. For example the qualities of food that are used to create and support the body are the five tastes. Food was not seen as being broken down into constituent parts or substances, but was seen in terms of the five tastes. [70].[101] Each of the five tastes was associated with particular properties and effects on the body and related to a specific organ. The flavour itself was seen as a form of "qi" [70]. The stomach was thought to mulch the food so that the nutrition, the qi associated with five tastes can be extracted by the spleen; quoting the Suwen, Wiseman et al. inform us "The spleen, stomach, small and large intestines... having the ability to transform the five sapors (tastes) entering, and the waste leaving the body" [133:74]. Suwen nineteen describes the source of man's nutrition from food via the five tastes "The herbs generate the five flavors; the delicacies of the five flavors exceed one's perception... Heaven feeds man with five qi, the earth feeds man with the five flavors" [128:111]. The material substance of the body is constructed (at least in part) from the combination of the five tastes [70]. This brought nutrition into the larger framework of the five phases "By attributing a quality of qi to every foodstuff, medical authors embraced nutrition within a larger framework of knowledge, thereby providing the rationale for what became an enormous and influential tradition of food combinations and prohibitions" [70].[102] We can see this for example in how foods were taken into the political arena. The Chunqiu Zuozhuan says "flavor serves to enhance the circulation of qi. Qi serves to give fullness to the mind, the mind is used to fix words and words are used to issue commands", here "political commands are induced by the intake of flavor through the medium of qi" [120:45]. The role of the flavours becomes encoded and even more important in the early herbal medial literature. As we will see in chapter six, the Bencao herbal tradition codified the properties of each herb not in terms of the substance itself rather in terms of the observed effects it had on the body and sometimes discussed in terms of qi. Here the five flavours became instrumental for understanding how to select and use the herbal substances in therapy. While the codification of qi-related herbal properties in terms of subjective sensory experiences represents a similar linking of mind and qi it possibly also made it difficult for the Bencao tradition to absorb the emerging systematic theories of medicine (the theory of "correspondences"). It was many centuries before the Bencao herbal tradition had developed or absorbed a systematic theory of practice, however, another use of the theory of correspondences is found in the Shanghanlun and traditions that follow it [see 99].

Similarly with vision we perceive the five colours. The term colour is "se" [色] explained in the Shuowen Jiezi to be the "qi of the forehead" [19:135, 55:174, 46].[103] The act of looking is not limited to looking at and seeing the physical body, one can observe the qi of the person examined. When we visually observe a person we observe the qi of the five colors. This qi was classified in the medical literature (Suwen chapters ten and seventeen) in terms of whether it was bright, lustrous or flat and lustreless [27] giving the ability to judge whether the person is healthy or very ill, will live or die [55:188]; color "is the flower (or flowering) of the spirit (qi)" [55:188].

Additionally minerals were seen to be formed from the "qi of the five colors" [75:27], the physical object, the mineral, is constructed from qi (of non-material experiences) associated with colours. The experience of an object (its colour) is a form of qi, the object is a construction from the different qi of those experiences. The relevant point here is not a philosophy of matter, but the fact that it is through the qi of sensory experiences (here colours, in the body, tastes) that the material object is constructed.

There are also extensive discussions of how sounds can transform the listener [19:178 & ff]. Here various different sounds (often classified in terms of the five phases) are used to trigger "resonant" (ying/ganying) reactions that can transform the listener [19:185]. Sounds, bells, chanting have a long history of use because of these transformative resonant properties in ancient China and were put to use to help create or spread virtue among people [19]. Xunzi commented on these properties with respect to the effects on the qi: "whenever depraved sounds arouse man discordant ch'i (qi) responds to it, and modeling itself disorder is generated; when correct sounds arouse man, accordant ch'i (qi) responds to it, and as it takes form, order is created" [31:260] and similarly "Hence with the performing of music intent clarifies, with training in ceremony, conduct matures. Ear and eye hear and see more clearly, the blood and ch'i (qi) are harmonious and calm," [31:261]. Xunzi also focused on how music affects the mind "The gentleman uses the bells and drums to guide intent (yi), the zithers to delight the heart (xin)" [31:260].[104]

In discussing the role of palpation and tactile experiences of the body, Hsu examines early medical discussions of pulse diagnosis in the case histories of Chunyu Yi found in the Shiji (circa 90 BCE) [46]. After discussing the relationships between the pulses and qi she concludes "In other words Chunyu Yi would touch the mai and feel qi. So qi was not an entity that could not be seen, but one that could be felt... Chunyu Yi could tactually perceive qi in the mai" [46:21-22]. Here the sensory experience of touch is described in terms of qi.

In the sexual cultivation literature of the yangsheng traditions, there are discussions of how qi is moved and of the "arrival of qi". Lo highlights a parallel usage of the term "qi zhi" [氣至] "arrival of qi" in the Mawangdui text, "Heyinyang" [和陰陽] and the later medical treatises of the Neijing [68]. She concludes "The common features of all these references to the "arrival" or "obtaining" of qi is certainly the climax of a change in inner body sensation" [68:44].[105] There are somatic sensations associated with qi in both the sexual and acupuncture literature. The somatic experiences are described in terms of qi. Lo also describes how the term qi came to be used with reference to sensation within the body "In literature of the late third and early second centuries BC, qi very often describes an intensification of sensation experienced within the body" [67].

In all these instances of using the sense organs the acts of observing are classified not into objective observations but subjective sensations that interact with the person thus making the observations and simultaneously triggering changes in the state of qi (and thus virtue, health, etc) of that person. In food it is not the physical constituents that nourish the body but the tastes and their proper balance. In looking, one experiences the five colors as expressions of states of the thing observed (in terms of five phase characteristics and overall qi quality); in models of how objects are formed, the colours can be sufficient to form physical objects such as minerals. In listening the qi of the five sound qualities can influence the person who listens. In palpating the pulses it is not so much the vibrations and movements of the arteries that are palpated as the qi that is perceived. In sex the feelings of orgasm herald the arrival of qi just as the needling of acupuncture can trigger sensations that are associated with the arrival of qi "like the wind blowing away the clouds to reveal the blue sky". In acupuncture, more recent descriptions of "deqi" [得氣], while different are still based in bodily sensations "soreness, heaviness, numbness, heaviness and distension around the point" [68:44]. In these examples we can see how qi is also tied to perceptual experience and the mind of the person having those experiences.

## Conclusion: Implications in the pre-medical and medical literatures

There are a number of important implications of this model of understanding the world, the body and the mind. All are seen as mutually interacting, in order to capture this one cannot describe observer and the thing observed as distinct separate things it is necessary to find a language for capturing that mutual influence. This is one of the ways that qi can be seen and understood: it is a concept that can capture the mutual interactions of observer and observed, the mind, the experiences of the things that the mind has and those things that are experienced. One of the important implications of this is that the individual person is seen as both influenced by the world and capable of influencing the world. In the traditions that emerged out of the fifth to first centuries BCE, self development and the development of virtue were strongly stressed. The individual that develops their "de" [德] is capable of ruling the people creating positive influences throughout the world. This thematic stream of the development of "de", virtue, runs through many of the traditions that we have examined, whether it be the various Confucian or Daoist models. Stepping aside from these socio-political understandings and influences, there is an important implication that can be drawn and that is especially relevant in the medical traditions. With the commonality of qi in how the mind expresses itself, experiences the world and constructs those objects that are observed, we see the idea that the mind can influence the world. This is explicit in certain contexts. We have seen above that there are various ideas expressing how the cultivated person can influence the world in the Neiye. It is especially in a quiet, focused emotionally regulated state of mind that the qi is most accessed (see the acupuncture chapter by Birch below). The Neiye tells us that it is the "yi" or awareness/attention/intention that is responsible for this. The Mencius tells us that qi is controlled and moved by the "zhi" or will. In the early medical literature of the Neijing, the act of needling involves the same quiet focus of the mind, and again it is the "yi" awareness/attention/intention of the practitioner that is involved in the correct influences of the needle upon the qi: Lingshu chapter one instructs us "Whether meeting it or following it, by means of one's attention (yi), one harmonizes it" [Chace, Bensky chapter five in the volume], see also chapter four below for further discussions of this.

In modern parlance, we call these "mind-matter" interactions [49, 95]. There is a wealth of highly significant research on how the mind can and does influence the material world. These ideas about qi and its relationship with the mind that we see in Chinese thinking from the late Warring states to early Han dynasty period appear to match the findings that have emerged through hundreds of studies on consciousness and its effects on the material world. In modern China we find a sudden interest in "qigong" [氣功] and demonstrating extraordinary qigong feats and effects. Among the publications since the early 1980s we find many examples of non-explainable phenomena (the "Extraordinary Powers") that were related to qi effects that would in Western terms be examples of paranormal effects [64, 90]. This focus is discussed in chapter seven where there is an examination of research on qigong. What is significant here is that these unusual events, including mind-matter interactions are treated as special qi-related phenomena. While research on mind-matter and other consciousness related phenomena in Western groups was focusing on convincing skeptics and demonstrating special properties of the mind, the same phenomena were being drawn into the public domain in China with claims about the extraordinary powers of qigong [90].

The models and methods of inquiry that have emerged in this work may be instructive when we try to come to grips with how to investigate qi and the jingmai scientifically (see chapter eight). But equally, we can now understand the kinds of emphases that we find emerging in studies of acupuncture and qi and the jingmai (see chapter four), the martial arts, qi and the jingmai (see chapter seven). In both, the early literature is quite clear about the importance of a kind of quiet, non-active or non-concentrated mental focus, paying attention or giving awareness to rather than actively focusing. This, probably more than any other characterises the early Chinese discussions of how the mind can influence the qi. We can also speculate that this kind of understanding about qi and how to influence it may be what tended to keep or contribute to the distancing of early herbal medical literature and theories from qi based models [see 99]. The herb was thought of as the vehicle for what was doing the healing so that the herbal medicine was seen as doing the work of healing, while in acupuncture and various internal cultivation traditions it is the practitioner that does the work through their own internal training and changes. Although, as Scheid has shown [102:176-177], later herbal medical authors have incorporated this idea of how the practitioner's inner state influences treatment and the patient, it appears not to have held such influence within the herbal traditions in earlier periods, rather it is related to the process of selecting the herbs.

Another important implication from what we have examined in this chapter is that we can see that qi is not a magical mystical thing it is related to our every day experiences of the world and our attempts to explain these experiences. There have been attempts on the part of many people to stress that qi is some special thing –most visible in the kind of fantasy martial arts movies with people flying through the air, performing super-human feats. We are not saying that qi is unimportant or not special, quite the contrary, that it is an essential part of our daily lives, but already as an everyday thing. When we choose to focus on doing something with it, as occurs for example with more traditional forms of acupuncture, the recognition of the role of the inner state of the practitioner in relation to the ability to influence the qi changes the way many have thought about acupuncture.

We have found a very good summary from Lloyd and Sivin which captures much that can be said about qi, we cite the passage here: "There we have it: the cosmos, heaven and humanity's surroundings on earth and its parts, the state, the emperor who personifies it, the body that physicians treated and in which philosophers found correspondences, each organism sharing the universal qi, all resonating with the others – these ideas took shape during the mighty efforts to end the chaos of the Warring States. They came together in complex synthetic visions as society reached stability in the Han, and they added to that stability" [66:226].

## Bibliography

1- Allan S. *The Way of Water and Sprouts of Virtue*. Albany, State University of New York, 1997.

2- Ames RT, Hall DL. *A Philosophical Translation: Dao De Jing –making this life significant*, New York, Ballantine Books, 2003.
3- Anon. *Energy Fields in Medicine*, Kalamazoo, Michigan, John E. Fetzer Foundation, 1989
4- Barnes LL. *Needles, Herbs, Gods and Ghosts*, Cambridge, Harvard University Press, 2005.
5- Birch S. Introduction. In Manaka Y, Itaya K, Birch S. *Chasing the Dragon's Tail*, Brookline, Paradigm Publications, 1995:ix-xxvii.
6- Birch S. Diversity and acupuncture: Acupuncture is not a coherent or historically stable tradition. in AJ. Vickers (ed.) *Examining Complementary Medicine: The Sceptical Holist*. Cheltenham: Stanley Thomas, 1998, pp. 45-63.
7- Birch S. Filling the whole in acupuncture. Part 1: What are we doing in the supplementation needle technique? *EJOM*, 2009:6(2):25-35 (part 1); 2009:6(3):18-27 (part 2).
8- Birch S. Chapter four: The Jingmai and qi –acupuncture perspectives. In this volume.
9- Birch S. (In preparation-a). Filling the whole in acupuncture. Part 2: The "treatment space"–modeling the treatment process in acupuncture.
10- Birch S, Bovey M. Chapter eight –Qi, Jingmai: Scientific investigation of concepts based in traditional East Asian medicine: challenges to cross-paradigm research. In this volume.
11- Birch S, Dhaenens C, et al. Questions of Shen. *Thieme Almanac 2008: Acupuncture and Chinese Medicine*. Stuttgart, George Thieme Verlag, 2008:267-289.
12- Birch S, Felt R. *Understanding Acupuncture*, Edinburgh, Churchill Livingstone, 1999.
13- Birch S, Lewith G. Acupuncture research, the story so far. In MacPherson H, Hammerschlag.R, Lewith G, Schnyer R (eds). *Acupuncture Research: Strategies for Building an Evidence Base*. London, Elsevier, 2007:15-35.
14- Cabrer Mir MA. Chapter seven: Qi and stillness –Taijiquan, qigong and acupuncture. In this volume.
15- Chace C. On greeting a friend, an approach to needle technique. *Lantern*. 2006:3(3):4-7.
16- Chace C, Bensky D. Chapter five: An axis of efficacy. The range of meaning in chapter one of the Lingshu. In this volume.
17- Cheng CY. On human consciousness in classical Chinese philosophy: developing onto-hermeneutics of the human person. In Lai KL (ed). New interdisciplinary perspectives in Chinese philosophy. *J Chinese Philosophy –Book Supplement*, 2007, pages 9-32.
18- Chiu ML. *Mind, body, and illness in a Chinese medical tradition*. Ph.D. thesis, Harvard University, 1986.

19- Csikszentmihalyi M. *Material Virtue: ethics and the body in early China*. Brill, Leiden, 2004.
20- Dalai Lama. *An Open Heart*, Sydney, Hodder, 2001.
21- Daly NP. *Hybridizing the human body: The hydrological development of acupuncture in early Imperial China*. Masters thesis, Department of East Asian Studies, McGill University, 1999.
22- Damasio A. *The Feeling of What Happens –body, emotion and the making of consciousness*. London, Vintage books, 2000.
23- van Els P. The Wenzi: creation and manipulation of a Chinese philosophical text, PhD thesis, Leiden University, 2006.
24- Epler DC. Bloodletting in early Chinese medicine and its relation to the origin of acupuncture. *Bull Hist Med*; 1980; 54:337-367.
25- Foss L, Rothenberg K. *The Second Medical Revolution*, Boston, Shambhala Publications, 1987.
26- Fox A. Reflex and reflectivity: Wuwei in the Zhuangzi. In Cook S (ed). *Hiding the World in the World*. Albany, State University of New York, 2003: 207-225.
27- Fukushima K. *Meridian Therapy*, Tokyo, Toyo Hari Medical Association, 1991.
28- Fung Yulan. *A History of Chinese Philosophy*, Princeton, Princeton University Press, 1952.
29- Furth C. Producing medical knowledge through cases: history, evidence and action. In Furth C, Zeitlin JT, Hsiung PC. (eds). *Thinking with Cases*, 2007, Honolulu, University of Hawai'i Press pages 125-151.
30- Goswami A. *The Self-Aware Universe*, New York, Jeremy P. Tarcher, 1993.
31- Graham AC. *Disputers of the Tao: Philosophical Argument in Ancient China*, Illinois, Open Court, 1989.
32- Graham AC. (Trans). *The Book of Lieh-tzu: a classic of tao*. New York, Columbia University Press, 1990.
33- Graham AC. *Chuang Tzu: the inner chapters*. Indianapolis, Hackett Publishing Company, 2001.
34- Graziani R. The subject and the soverign, exploring the self in early Chinese cultivation. In J. Lagerwey, M, Kalinowski (eds). *Early Chinese Religion*. Leiden, Brill 2009, pages 459-517,
35- *Guodian Daodejing* chapter fifty five. To see this text see the following link: http://daoisopen.com/A17toA18Chapters5544.html
36- Hall DL, Ames RT. *Thinking from the Han*, Albany, State University of New York Press, 1998.
37- Hanson C. *A Daoist Theory of Chinese Thought*, Oxford, Oxford University Press, 1992.
38- Harper D. *Early Chinese Medical Literature: the Mawangdui Medical Manuscripts*. London, Kegan Paul, 1998.

39- Helms JM. *Acupuncture Energetics*, Berkeley, Medical Acupuncture Publishers, 1995.
40- Henderson JB. *The Development and Decline of Chinese Cosmology*, New York, Columbia University Press, 1984.
41- Henricks RG. *Lao Tzu's Tao Te Ching*. New York, Columbia University Press, 2000.
42- Herfel W, Rodrigues D, Gao Y. Chinese medicine and the dynamic conceptions of health and disease. In Lai KL (ed). New interdisciplinary perspectives in Chinese philosophy. *J Chinese Philosophy –Book Supplement*, 2007, pages 57-79.
43- Hertzer D. *Das Leuchten der Geistes und die Erkenntnis der Seele –The shining of the spirit and the understanding of the soul.* Frankfurt, Verlag fur Akademische Schritten, 2006.
44- Holloway KW. *Guodian –the newly discovered seeds of Chinese religious and political philosophy*, Oxford, Oxford University Press 2009.
45- Hsu E. Pulse diagnostics in the Western Han: how mai and qi determine bing. In Hsu E, (ed). *Innovation in Chinese Medicine*, Cambridge, Cambridge University Press, 2001:51-91.
46- Hsu E. Tactility and the body in early Chinese medicine. *Science in Context*, 2005:18(1):7-34.
47- Ishida H. Body and mind: the Chinese perspective. In Kohn L (Ed). *Taoist Meditation and Longevity Techniques*, Ann Arbor, Center for Chinese studies, University of Michigan, 1989, pages 41-71.
48- Jahn R, Dunne B. *Margins of Reality: The Role of Consciousness in the Physical World*, Harcourt Brace Jovanovich, New York, 1987.
49- Jonas WB, Crawford CC (eds). *Healing, Intention and Energy Medicine*, Edinburgh, Churchill Livingstone, 2003.
50- Kalinowski M. Diviners and astrologers under the Eastern Zhou: transmitted texts and received archaeological findings. In J. Lagerwey, M, Kalinowski (eds). *Early Chinese Religion*. Leiden, Brill 2009, pages 341-396,
51- Keegan J. *The Huang-ti nei-ching: the Structure of the Compilation; the Significance of the Structure*, doctoral diss. Berkeley; University of California, 1988.
52- Kim JY. Beyond paradigm: Making transcultural connections in a scientific translation of acupuncture. *Soc Sci Med*. 2006:62(12):2960-72.
53- Kubny M. *Qi Lebenskraftkonzepte in China: Definition, Theorien und Grundlagen*. Heidelberg, K.F. Haug and Scheid, 1997.
54- Kuhn T. *The Structure of Scientific Revolution*, Chicago, University of Chicago Press, 1970.
55- Kuriyama S. *The Expressiveness of the Body and the Divergence of Greek and Chinese Medicine*, New York, Zone Books 1999.
56- Larre C, Rochat de la Vallee. *Rooted in Spirit*, New York, Station Hill Press, 1995.

57- Larre C, Rochat de la Vallee. *The Seven Emotions.* London, Monkey Press, 1996.
58- Larre C, Rochat de la Vallee E. *Essence, Spirit, Blood and Qi*, London, Monkey Press, 1999.
59- Le Blanc C. *Huai-Nan Tzu –Philosophical Synthesis in Early Han Thought.* Hong Kong, Hong Kong University Press 1985.
60- Legge J, "The Writings of Chuang Tzu", 1891, text found at: http://chinese.dsturgeon.net/text.pl?node=2712&if=en
61- Leo J. *Sex in the Yellow Emperor's Basic Questions*.Dunedin, Three Pines Press, 2011.
62- Lewis ME. *The Construction of Space in Early China.* Albany, SUNY Press, 2006.
63- Li Jianmin. They shall expel demons: etiology, the medical canon and the transformation of medical techniques before the Tang. In J Langerwey, M Kalinowski (eds). *Early Chinese Religion*, Leiden, Brill, 2009, pages 1103-1150.
64- Lin ZX, Yu L, Guo ZY, Shen ZY, Zhang HL, Zhang TL. *Qigong: Chinese Medicine or Pseudoscience?* New York, Prometheus Books, 2000.
65- Liu YC. *The Essential Book of Traditional Chinese Medicine*; volume one. New York Coumbia University Press, 1988.
66- Lloyd G, Sivin N. *The Way and the Word*, New Haven, Yale University Press, 2002.
67- Lo V. Tracking the Pain: Jue and the Formation of a Theory of Circulating Qi through the Channels. *Sudhoffs Archiv*, 1999, pages 191-211.
68- Lo V. The influence of nurturing life culture on the development of Western Han acumoxa therapy. In Hsu E, (ed). *Innovation in Chinese Medicine*, Cambridge, Cambridge University Press, 2001:19-50.
69- Lo V. Huangdi Hama jing 'The Yellow Emperor's Toad Manual' in a special edition of Asia Major, 2001;14(2):61-99, edited by Nathan Sivin: Essays Contributed in Honour of Michael Loewe [published in Spring, 2004]. See also http://www.ihp.sinica.edu.tw/~medicine/ashm/lectures/Lo.pdf.
70- Lo V. Reflex and reflectivity: Pleasure, prohibition and pain: food and medicine in traditional China. In Cook S (ed). *Hiding the World in the World.* Albany, State University of New York, 2005: 163-185.
71- Lo V. Imagining Practice: Sense and Sensuality in Early Chinese Medical Illustration. In: Bray F, Dorofeeva-Lichtmann V, Métailié G, (eds). *The Warp and the Weft: Graphics and Text in the Production of Technical Knowledge in China.* Leiden, Brill; 2007, pages 383–424.
72- Lo V, Li Jianmin. Manuscripts, received texts and the healing arts. In Nylan M, Loewe M (eds). *China's Early Empires –A Re-appraisal*, Cambridge, Cambridge University Press, 2010, pages 367-397.
73- Lu GD, Needham J. *Celestial Lancets*; Cambridge, Cambridge University Press, 1980.
74- Maciocia G. *The Psyche in Chinese Medicine*, Edinburgh, Churchill Livingstone, 2009.

75- Major JS. *Heaven and Easrth in Easrly Han Thought*. Albany, State University of New York Press, 1993.
76- Manaka Y, Itaya K, Birch S. *Chasing the Dragon's Tail*, Brookline, Paradigm Publications, 1995.
77- Matsumoto K, Birch S. *Five Elements and Ten Stems*, Brookline, Paradigm Publications, 1983.
78- Matsumoto K, Birch S. *Hara Diagnosis Reflections on the Sea*; Brookline, Paradigm Publications, 1988.
79- McCraty R, Atkinson M, Bradley RT. Electrophysiological evidence of intuition: Part I. The surprising role of the heart. *J Alt Complem Med*, 2004:10, 1:133-143.
80- McCraty R, Atkinson M, Bradley RT. Electrophysiological evidence of intuition: Part II. A system-wide process? *J Alt Complem Med*, 2004:10, 2:325-336.
81- McTaggart L. *The Field*, London, Element Publishers, 2001.
82- Moeller HG. *Daoism Explained*, Chicago, Open Court, 2004.
83- Moeller HG. *The Philosophy of the Daodejing*, New York, Columbia University Press, 2006.
84- Motoyama H. A biophysical elucidation of the meridian and ki energy. What is ki energy and how does it flow? *Research Relig. & Parapsych*. 1981:7:1.
85- Murakami M. Lecture given in Newton, Massachusetts, September 1998.
86- Needham J. *Science and Civilisation in China –Volume II*, Cambridge, Cambridge University Press, 1956.
87- Nylan M. Yin-yang, five phases and qi. In Nylan M, Loewe M (eds). *China's early empires –a re-appraisa*l. Cambridge, Cambridge university press, 2010, pages 398-414.
88- Ogawa T. Workshop given at the New England School of Acupuncture, Watertown, MA., April, 1996.
89- Onozawa K. *Ki no Shiso*, Tokyo, Tokyo University Publishing company 1980.
90- Palmer DA. *Qigong Fever –Body, Science and Utopia in China*. New York, Columbia University Press, 2007.
91- Pao B. *Mental health implications of the Chinese linguistic concept of "hsin" (heart)*. PhD thesis. Boston University, 1985.
92- Pickering A. T*he Mangle of Practice*, Chicago, University of Chicago Press, 1995.
93- Porkert M. *The Theoretical Foundations of Chinese Medicine*. Cambridge, MIT Press, 1974.
94- Puett MJ. *To Become a God: cosmology, sacrifice, and self-divination in early China*. Cambridge, Harvard University Asia Center, 2002.
95- Radin D. *Entangled Minds*, New York, Paraview Pocket Books, 2006.
96- Rickett A. Nei Ye. Inner workings and introduction to the four "xin shu" chapters. In *Guanzi, Volume Two*. Princeton, Pinceton University Press, 1998:15-55.
97- Robinet I. Ji. In Pregadio F (ed) *Encyclopedia of Taoism*, Oxford, Rutledge, 2008, pages 536-537.

98- Rochat de la Vallee E. *A Study of Qi in Classical Texts*, London, Monkey Press, 2006.
99- Rodriguez M. Chapter six: Qi, jingmai, yaoyi –a study of their relationships. In this volume.
100- Roth HD. *Original Tao –Inward Training* (Nei Yeh). New York, Columbia University Press, 1999.
101- Sakade Y. "Wenzi," in Fabrizio Pregadio (ed) *The Encyclopedia of Taoism*. Routledge, 2007, pages 1041-1042.
102- Scheid V. *Chinese Medicine in Contemporary China*, Durham, Duke University press, 2002.
103- Scheid V. Not very traditional, nor exactly Chinese, so what kind of medicine is it? TCM's discourse on menopause and its implications for practice, teaching and research. *J Chin Med.* 2006, 82:5-20.
104- Scheid V. *Currents of Tradition in Chinese Medicine 1626-2006*. Seattle, Eastland Press, 2007.
105- Scheid V, Bensky D. Medicine as signification. *European J Orien Med*, 1999:2, 6:32-40.
106- Schnyer R, Birch S, MacPherson H. Acupuncture practice as the foundation for clinical evaluation. In MacPherson H, Hammerschlag. R, Lewith G, Schnyer R (eds). *Acupuncture Research: Strategies for Building an Evidence Base*. London, Elsevier, 2007:153-179.
107- Sharf RH. *Coming to Terms with Chinese Buddhism*, Hawai, Kuroda Institute and University of Hawaii Press, 2002.
108- Sheldrake R. *The Sense of Being Stared At*, London, Arrow Books, 2003.
109- Shudo D. *Introduction to Meridian Therapy*, Seattle, Eastland Press, 1990.
110- Sivin N. 1978. On the Word "Taoism" as a Source of Perplexity: With Special Reference to the Relations of Science and Religion in Traditional China. *History of Religions* 1978;17:303-330.
111- Sivin N. *Traditional Medicine in Contemporary China*, Ann Arbor, Centre for Chinese Studies, University of Michigan, 1987.
112- Sivin N. "Huang di nei ching." In Loewe M. (Ed). *Early Chinese Texts: A Bibliographical Guide*. Early China Special Monograph Series number 2, Berkeley, Society for the study of early China and Institute of Asian studies, University of California, 1993:196-215.
113- Sivin N. State, cosmos and body in the last three centuries BC. *Harvard J. Asiatic* Studies. 1995:55(1):5-37.
114- Sivin N. Drawing insights from Chinese medicine. In Lai KL (ed). New interdisciplinary perspectives in Chinese philosophy. *J Chinese Philosophy –Book Supplement*, 2007, pages 43-55.

115- Slingerland E. *Effortless Action*, Oxford, Oxford University Press, 2003.
116- Sommers D. De *Chinese Fascinatie Voor de Geest (The Chinese fascination with the spirit)*, Amsterdam, Uitgeverij Libra & Libris, 2007.
117- Sommers S. Chapter three: How to become a shang yi or "superior physician," An exploration on the influence of the practitioner in early China. In this volume.
118- Stapp HP. *Mindful Universe: Quantum mechanics and the participating observer*, Berlin, Springer, 2007.
119 - Sterckx R. *The Animal and the Daemon in Early China*, Albany, State University of New York, 2002.
120- Sterckx R. Food and philosophy in Early China. In Sterckx R (ed) *Of Tripod and Palate*, New York, Palgrave, MacMillan, 2005, pages 34-61.
121- Stux G. Background and theory of traditional Chinese medicine. In Stux G, Berman B, Pomeranz B (eds). *Basics of Acupuncture*, Berlin, Springer Verlag, 2003, pages 87-122.
122- Tang YJ. Constructing "Chinese philosophy" in Sino-European cultural exchange. In Lai KL (ed). New interdisciplinary perspectives in Chinese philosophy. *J Chinese Philosophy –Book Supplement*, 2007, pages 33-42.
123- Tessenow H, Unschuld PU. *A Dictionary of the Huangdi Neijing Suwen*, Berkeley, University of California Press, 2008.
124- Unschuld PU. *Medicine in China: A History of Ideas*, Berkeley, University of California Press, 1985.
125- Unschuld PU. *Nan Ching: The Classic of Difficult Issues*, Berkeley, University of California Press, 1986.
126- Unschuld PU. Traditional Chinese medicine; some historical and epistemological reflections. *Soc Sci Med*; 1987:24, 12:1023-1029.
127- Unschuld PU. Epistemological issues and changing legitimation: Traditional Chinese medicine in the twentieth century. In Leslie C, Young A, (eds) *Paths to Asian Medical Knowledge*; Berkeley, University of California Press, 1992, pp. 44-61.
128- Unschuld PU. *Huang Di Nei Jing Su Wen –nature, knowledge, imagery in an ancient Chinese medical text.* Berkeley, University of California Press, 2003.
129- Unschuld PU, Tessenow H, Jinsheng Z. *Huang Di nei jing su wen: An annotated translation of Huang Di's Inner Classic –Basic Questions*; volume 1 and volume 2. Berkeley, University of California Press, 2011.
130- Wang AH. *Cosmology and Political Culture in Early Culture*, Cambridge, Cambridge University Press, 2000.
131- Wang JY. *Applied Channel Theory in Chinese Medicine.* Seattle, Eastland Press, 2008.
132- Wikipedia. Qi. http://en.wikipedia.org/wiki/Qi accessed 29 August, 2008.
133- Wiseman N, Ellis A. *Fundamentals of Chinese Medicine*; Brookline, Massachusetts, Paradigm Publications, 1985.

134- Wiseman N, Feng Y. *A Practical Dictionary of Chinese Medicine*, Brookline, Paradigm Publications, 1997.
135- Wolpe PR. The maintenance of professional authority: Acupuncture and the American physician. *Social Problems*; 1985:32(5):409-424.
136- Yang RB. From "merging the body with the mind" to "wandering in unitary qi": a discussion of Zhuangzi's realm of the true man and its corporeal basis. In Cook S (ed). *Hiding the World in the World.* Albany, State University of New York, 2003:88-127.
137- Yang ZY. On presence of mind and subtle sensations. *Lantern*, 2007; IV:2:28-30.
138- Zhang YH. *Transforming Emotions with Chinese Medicine.* Albany, State University of New York Press, 2007.
139- Zhang YH, Rose K. , Brookline, *A Brief History of Qi*, Paradigm Publications, 2001.

## Endnotes

1. By non-sensory we mean the making of observations that do not utilise the sensory organs but which might arise as for example "intuition", a felt sense of something. Non-sensory experiences and observations of the world have been extensively studied and documented in recent years [see e.g. 49, 79, 80, 95, 108].

2. We will not attempt to resolve differences or perform the needed scholarship [67], rather we will catalogue a large range of opinions from various scholars and sources to illustrate both the range of meanings and lay the groundwork for later chapters that explore how the term has been used in different traditions of practice. We will offer some syntheses to help understand some of what we document.

3. Zhang and Rose describe a somewhat different origin to the qi character [139:3-4]. Citing the Qing scholar Duan Yucai, they describe how before the Zhou dynasty (1066-770 BCE), the term was like the character for three, san [三], referring to the "shape of rising clouds". Then in the Zhou dynasty, probably to distinguish it from the character "san" a small hook was added to the top line, extending the meaning from "cloud qi" to include to "give", to "beg", to "take" or to "save", This was followed later by the extension of the bottom line to create [气], which among other things started attaching the meaning of "breathing in and out" [139:3-4]. This later modification is now the form to which the Shuowen Jiezi text refers. Allan expresses a similar idea with her pictograms of the "earliest forms" of the character [1:88]. Harper explains "It is not clear whether qi originated as a word for atmospheric vapors (clouds, steam, etc.) which was generalized to encompass the source of human vitality and everything else; or whether qi was a term for the life-sustaining stuff received from food, drink, and arir or breath, which was extended to the natural world" [38:77].

4. In Japanese there are over 11,000 known compound terms that use ki [http://www.answers.com/topic/qi-1].

5. Zhang and Rose have a good discussion of examples of the use of "qi" in daily life, [139:161-167.]

6. Although he chooses to use the term "vapor" [38:77-78], one has the feeling that he prefers the much less loaded term "stuff".

7. Ames and Hall state it thus "The field of experience is always construed from one perspective or another. There is no view from nowhere, no external perspective, no decontextualized vantage point" [2:18].

8. The term "mo" is an alternate pronunciation for the term "mai". The term mai/mo refers to the (blood) vessels, it also refers to the early stage formulation of the channel system as the "11 vessels" in the Mawangdui and Zhangjiashan texts to which treatment in the form of moxibustion and bleeding can be applied [38, 55]. In the first formalized medical literature, the Huangdi Neijing corpus, the term is used in several different ways. It is used to refer to the vessels, functional structures associated with blood and regulated by the heart; it is used to refer to the pulses, which are palpated in order to make diagnoses, these pulses are located in multiple locations on the body with several different systems of assessment described. The pulses for diagnosis were later systematized to the radial arteries at the "cunkou" in the Nanjing [55:37-40, 125]; The term "mai" is also used with the term "jing" as the jingmai", referring to the more developed model of the 12 channels of acupuncture, to which treatment by acupuncture is directed.

9. "Nothing was un-caused, but nothing was caused mechanically. The organic system in the prompter's book governed the whole. And the characters in the eternal dramatic cycle were, as has been said, in existential dependence upon the totality of the system" [86:283].

10. There has been a tendency to contrast East Asian thinking with Western thinking, the former is "holistic" and the latter not "holistic". This is a gross simplification of the situation. Unschuld presented evidence that many facets of TEAM are "ontological" rather than holistic, which parallels the trend seen in Western medicine, find the offending bug, virus, wind etc and get rid of it [126, 127]. Kuriyama has also presented evidence that it is not so easy to generalise that TEAM is holistic [55]. Thus the statement that TEAM is holistic is wrong [6, 12, 126, 127]. This does not mean that there are not holistic facets or aspects in TEAM [12, 127]. TEAM developed as a compilation of diverse ideas and methods, often contradictory and from different philosophical backgrounds. It has been called "polyparadigmatic" [39] in an effort to capture this diversity of philosophical approaches [124:4-8]. Thus it is equally incorrect to say in absolute terms that TEAM is not holistic. The situation is more complex. There are features in TEAM that are holistic and some that are not holistic. If one wants to investigate these approaches it will be necessary to have a background model that is capable of embracing both aspects [25]. Using only language and models that derive exclusively from non-holistic, reductionist views and ap-

proaches, it will be difficult if not impossible to ever describe the holistic features of a set of ideas or system [25, 76]. This point is important when we discuss the scientific investigation of qi and the jingmai (see chapter eight, [10]). Because of these confusions and this complexity, it may be more appropriate to stop using the term "holistic" as it is not applicable in any simple manner to, for example TEAM.

11. In a brief discussion of the different uses by which the term "jing" [經] has been used in acupuncture and the Shanghanlun Sivin cites a passage from the Suwen and concludes "Various sets of concepts that describe the parts of the body or the phases of a vital process, in other words, do not describe different things. They are ways of looking at different aspects of the body or process, which remains one. When the results of the two different analyses differ, the discrepancy does not lie in the reality described, but in the aspects chosen to characterize it. Each analysis is true for the aspects analyzed. Each is one way (sometimes of several ways) to understand the whole. This is not an 'either/or' mentality at work" [111:80-81].

12. Unschuld states it thus "The unique feature of the Chinese situation-and this should receive more attention from historians and philosophers of science-is the continuous tendency towards a syncretism of all ideas that exist (within accepted limits). Somehow a way was always found in China to reconcile opposing views and to build bridges." [124:57].

13. Of this Unschuld is very clear: "A specific pattern might be useful for handling a certain issue or situation successfully, and it might be contradicted by another pattern of knowledge that had also proven to be useful for handling the same (or another) issue. Both patterns –and this seems to have been the dominant attitude in Chinese history– were therefore legitimized. The 'either/or' approach that springs to a mind trained in the Western tradition appears to have been posed with much less persistence in traditional Chinese medicine" [125:7].

14. The same can be said of the term qi [氣] and how its meaning has evolved over time, Lo summarises this quite succinctly: "As qi is applied to the phenomena of the inner body, it goes through significant transformations. But rather than its new meaning replacing the old, the range of meanings grows inclusively – a process that is continuous to the present day" [67].

15. Here the word "signification" is a translation of the term "yi" [意] which will be discussed further below. Scheid and Bensky build up evidence for a dialectic of how yi and method "fa" [法] have been used as a conceptual underpinning in Chinese medicine [105].

16. Zhang discusses this tendency to "invoke a variety of cultural and philosophical assumptions" when we use English words like "body" or "emotion" [138:54-5].

17. The first chapter of the Suwen begins with a question from the Yellow Emperor and Qibo's response: "I have heard that the people of high antiquity, in [the sequence of] spring and autumn, all exceeded one hundred years. But in their movements and activities

there was no weakening. As for the people of today, after only half of a hundred years, the movements and activities of all of them weaken. Is this because the times are different? Or is it that the people have lost shis [ability]? Qi Bo responded: the people of high antiquity, those who knew the way, they modeled [their behavior] on yin and yang and they complied with the arts and calculations, [Their] eating and drinking was moderate. [Their] rising and resting had regularity. They did not tax [themselves] with meaningless work. Hence, they were able to keep physical appearance and spirit together…" after which he goes on to begin outlining how to address this problem [129:30-31].

18. Unschuld has argued that while not exclusively true of the models of TEAM, these represent general tendencies [126, 127]. The non-holistic tendencies in TEAM that Unschuld describes relate more to attempts at describing disease processes and pathology rather than the physiological systems and their interplay [5, 12] and are thus less relevant for our discussions here.

19. Puett has an excellent and thorough discussion of these themes in his book "To Become a God" [94].

20. In the context of the Confucian tradition it is more commonly translated as "virtue" while in the Daoist it is more common to find it as "inner power", "potency" [1:101-107].

21. See also the discussions in Lewis [62:29-32].

22. Reference to qi manifests in the early literatures in a variety of forms. Most often as simply "qi", but in some contexts, combined terms such as "jingqi" are used. The precise differences between these are not always clear. We will see below that in certain texts attempts were made to more clearly delineate between for example "qi" and "jing", where in the early self-cultivation literature, jing is a more concentrated and refined form of qi, intermediate between the shen, spirit and qi. By the medical literatures of the Huangdi Neijing, the nature and relationships of for example, qi, jing and shen are different again. We will see examples of these different and parallel uses below.

23. He also goes on to explain the parallel use of these ideas with existing medical practices, concluding "various groups used qi to explain 'invisible' concepts such as action at a distance or disease processes" [19:145].

24. The term "responds", is "ying" [應]. This, along with its extended correlate "ganying" [感應], resonance, is an important concept that captures the invisible mutual influence of things. Similar things influence each other in the same way that strings on musical instruments influence each other [86:282]. We will return to this below as it is important for an understanding of how qi was thought about.

25. See the discussion of ganying below.

26. It is not entirely clear what Mencius means here. Certainly he was discussing something of the relationship between the mind (here the "zhi") and qi. But this passage

appears to contradict other passages in other classics. For example the Zhuangzi says "As for qi, it is that which being empty, awaits things. Only the way accumulates in emptiness. Emptiness is the purification of the mind/heart" [1:90]. On the zhi and qi in Zhuangzi Allan comments "what is actually moved by the will is the qi of the heart/mind" [1:91]. Probably the Mencius was expressing different ideas about qi and the mind than others like Zhuangzi.

27. Hanson describes it thus "The qi unites the sage's dao, the sage's actions and the dao of the whole world. The sage's actions become perfect and natural responses to the total situation. Qi is the life I bring to my action. It is the force that carries that action into effect, and into practical significance. I control it and am controlled by it... Morality is not only in my mind but in qi" [37:175].

28. Allan translates a passage from the Mencius about how the cultivation of de changes the appearance of the body: "What a gentleman takes as his nature are humaneness, a sense of right and wrong, and wisdom; they are rooted in his mind/heart. They appear in his face's serenity, give form to his back and extend to his four limbs" [1:135].

29. "Xunzian self-cultivation thus changes the very physiological make-up of the self. Once the blood and qi have been harmonized with morality, the practitioner no longer has to compel himself to accord with ritual forms or other traditional norms –they are now such an integral part of the self that they are realized in the same spontaneous and joyous fashion that uncultivated people feel in satisfying the animal desires" [115:247].

30. Interestingly this hierarchy of qi-jing-shen is different than later descriptions. In later textual and practical traditions such as in the medical and "Daoist" practice traditions, jing is seen as being the root with qi arising out of that as the functional manifestation and shen as the higher forms of that manifestation. We have not explored the reasons for this discrepancy but can suggest that with the development of a medical model in the Neijing corpus where the physician needed to be able to divide and subdivide what had been previously seen as a unified/single form of qi [9, 18, 98, 128] it was necessary not only to divide everything into different functional named parts by function [18, 128] but also by location. In doing this jing came to be associated with the kidneys and reproduction, and these are the lowest organs in the body and thus become the root. Thus while shen retains its place at the top of the hierarchy, jing replaces qi at the bottom. As the medical literature became more and more detailed and further and further removed from its origins, this trend in thinking would solidify further, eventually becoming the "fundamental substances" of TCM in modern China [111].

31. Some have interpreted this passage as describing the more refined form of qi "shen" rather than simply "qi" [Dianne Sommers personal communication]. While it is possible to read the passage thus, we feel that it does not distract from the meaning and understanding we give for the following reasons. First, in the Neiye, qi-jing-shen are essentially the same but in different stages of concentration or purity. Second, it is common to find in the early medical texts the term "shenqi" [神氣] used to refer to a kind of basic "vitality" [59:118] which can be rendered in English in different ways [69:88]. An example of this generic use of the term "shenqi" is that the "qi" which is said in Lingshu chapter one to enter and

exit the acupoints is the "shenqi" [69:88, 73:14, 111:51]. Third, Lingshu chapter three states that "the spirit [神] is the zhengqi [正氣] [16], which itself is a form of generic qi that pervades the whole body. Finally, there is evidence that early medical authors were influenced by concepts in the Neiye [15, 16, 38], discussions about needling and how to influence the qi with the needle refer to the role of the "yi" –rendered by Roth in this passage as "awareness" [see 16].

32. Ames and Hall render this passage quite differently "way making (dao) gives rise to continuity, continuity gives rise to difference, difference gives rise to plurality, and plurality gives rise to the manifold of everything that is happening (wanwu). Everything carries yin on its shoulders and yang in its arms, and blends these vital energies (qi) together to make them harmonious (he)" [2:142-3].

33. Allan discusses the nature of this mirror in relation to still water, undisturbed and reflective, a state that comes from stilling the mind [1:90].

34. There are parallels here to passages found in the Neiye regarding stillness and its importance in the cultivation traditions [100] –see below. There are also parallels to some of the discussions of needling techniques we find in the Neijing. It is through quiet inactive focus on the needle tip and attending to the mechanisms of transformation and change (which lie in emptiness) and the timings of movements that the qi responds correctly see chapters four and five below. The goal of doing this is to help create more order in the movements of qi in the body "if they become empty, then they are filled and that which fills them becomes ordered" [1:84].

35. See later chapters for further discussions of this, especially chapter four [8].

36. We will see in chapter four especially how the early medical text, the Lingshu [靈樞], describes that this practice is required for needling to be effective, although the quotations are more directly traceable to the Neiye [15].

37. We find specific references to the idea of how the spirit [神] protects the body in the early medical literature; chapter eight of the Nanjing [難經] (circa 100 CE) discusses how the the "moving qi between the kidneys" [腎間動氣] is "also called the spirit guarding against the evil [一名守邪之神]" [125:130].

38. Yang takes this quote from Watson's earlier translation. Allan has a differently nuanced translation of the same passage "May I ask about the purification of the mind/heart? Confucius said, "when you unify your will (zhi), you do not listen (i.e. understand) with the ears, but listen with the mind/heart. When you do not listen with the mind/heart but listen with the qi, listening will stop at the ear and the mind/heart stop at what tallies with it. As for qi, it is that which being empty awaits things. Only the way accumulates in emptiness. Emptiness is the purification of the mind/heart" [1:90]. We cite this passage again in a discussion of the mind, xin. What Watson and Yang call "fasting of the mind", Allan renders as "purification of the heart/mind".

39. Yang has an interesting and extensive discussion of this last point [136:95-105], referring to a "common sense" and the state of "synesthesia", the blurring of perceptions so that one sees with one's ears, hears with one's eyes, etc. Yang draws attention to the documentation of how artists or religious adepts often manifest this ability through innate talent or cultivation [136:97].

40. The passage above from the Chunqiu Fanlu seems to imply that having emotions are normal and not a problem, which seems to contradict this passage from Zhuangzi. This is essentially correct, but makes sense when one realizes that in the Confucian influenced Chunqiu Fanlu, one follows the rituals and applies more external factors or allows those external rituals to regulate these, while for the Zhuangzi the experience of emotions is that they cause internal disruption, thus in order to stop the disturbance of one's qi one should follow internal processes rather than external processes –meaning to be as one without feelings.

41. Sterckx also discusses other texts that imply similar interpretations bringing the compound term "xueqi" [血氣] "blood and qi into focus [119:74-75]. Harper mentions that the term xueqi seems to first occur in the Lunyu, no earlier than the early fourth century BC [38:77]. Creatures that contain xueqi, both blood and qi (such as humans, certain larger animals), tend to have similar minds and intelligence "while acknowledging external physical differences between humans and animals based on the organization and refinement of the basic stuff that makes up all living creatures, more often possession of 'blood and qi' is said to unite them" [119:74]. For some, as is evidenced in the Liezi (third century CE), these similarities makes each susceptible to the moral authority of the sage.

42. The term Major translates as "spacetime" is [宇宙] yuzhou, "space and time" [75:294]. Le Blanc calls this the "space-time complex" [59:202]. It is unclear how or whether Major and Le Blanc were inadvertently influenced by Einstein's notions of space and time, but there is certainly a linguistic parallel.

43. "Self cultivation can thus refer to an immense domain, embracing daily instructions on eating, sleeping, breathing, or having sex, gymnastics and hygienic exercises (such as daoyin 'stretching and coiling') meditative practices, cosmological discourse and moral inspection" [34:465].

44. See the next chapter "The jingmai –a summary of their development" for more details.

45. For example, the Shiwen describes how spirit should be drawn into the body: "As for the way of inhaling qi, one must direct it to the extremities. Essence will be born and not cut off. Above and below all is essence. Cold and warmth are peacefully born. Breathing must be deep and long-lasting. The new qi is easy to hold fast to. Stale qi is old, new qi is long-lived. He who is good at controlling qi makes the stale qi dissipate nightly and the new qi collect in the morning so as to penetrate the nine apertures and fill the six cavities" [94:209]. In order to make the spirit long-lived the text describes the following: "If you wish to make the spirit long-lived, you must use the skin's patterns to breathe. When it comes to controlling the essence of qi, one exits death and enters life. Happy and joyous,

one uses this to fill the form. This is called concentrating the essence. Controlling the qi has an alignment. The task lies in accumulating essence. When essence flourishes, it invariably leaks. The essence that exits must be supplemented. As for when to supplement what has leaked: do it during sleep" [94:210].

46. Lingshu chapters ten and fifteen introduce the model of qi continuously circulating in the jingmai which was then adopted as a core model in the Nanjing [125:78-79].

47. This passage is matched by several others from different texts. The Shiwen and Tianxia Zhidaotan both from the Mawangdui contain parallel passages about sexual practices that cause the eyes and ears to become "perceptive and bright", the voice's sound "brilliant" the skin and hide to "glow", the spine to become "strong" and so on leading to engendering the "spirit illumination" [see 98:391 + 427]. Similar descriptions of the state of the body due to the cultivation of qi to develop shen can be found in the Neiye and later texts such as the Huainanzi [100:76-77].

48. See chapter four for detailed discussions.

49. For full translation see [38:425-438].

50. The term qi [氣] was found 1881 times in a search of the online Suwen database http://ctext.org/huangdi-neijing/suwen, and 1147 times in a search of the same website Lingshu database http://ctext.org/huangdi-neijing/ling-shu-jing.

51. At first there would have only been "qi" but in order to start classifying it new compound terms would need to arise, in addition to naming qi according to where it was and what it was doing, a number of very general forms of qi that are like a kind of "unitary qi" can be identified [58:42] such as yuanqi [元氣 ], zhengqi [正氣], and so on [7, 58:42-43, 98:58].

52. One of the more thorough analyses of these associations can be found in Chiu's PhD thesis from 1986 [18].

53. For example Suwen chapter five says fear injures the kidney [78:43] while Suwen chapter twenty one says fear can be associated with the liver [128:234].

54. In a terse discussion, Nanjing 33 raises the interesting question as to the similarity of the gan (liver zang) with the physical liver organ itself and the fei (lung zang) with the physical lung organ itself. The text suggests they are not the same since the zang maintain certain key relationships (via five phase, ten stem relationships) with other zang, while the physical organs removed from the body do not [77:59-60, 125:361-366]. It is the functionalities of the zang that characterize their nature not their physical qualities.

55. Such as the wuyun liuqi model found in Wang Bing's edition of the Suwen [128:393].

56. The reader is referred to various sources for more information [18, 45, 73, 111, 113, 125], such as Unschuld [128] and his Huangdi Neijing Suwen translation [129].

57. Here it is useful to cite Harper discussing the development of vessel theory in the Neijing from the Mawangdui texts "The manuscript texts graphically confirm the hypothesis that the Huangdi neijing is a summation of written medical knowledge edited so as to reframe older recorded teachings in terms of theoretical innovations" [38:89].

58. The term "form" is "xing" [形] commonly used as a general reference to the physical body.

59. Although we are drawing the distinction between cognitive and affective functions of the mind, we explicitly recognize the limitations of this. Daoist thinking is said to be "resolutely resistant" to this distinction [2:26]. We draw the distinction precisely because the various literatures explicitly discuss or hint at different effects of cognitive and affective manifestations of the mind. Essentially cognitive manifestations are thought to help order or move the qi while affective result from or trigger disorder and disturbance of the qi.

60. More accurately the heart and aorta.

61. It is interesting to point out that emotional self-mastery appears to be an important feature of other traditions, for example in Buddhism as exemplified in the Tibetan Buddhist tradition it seems to be crucial [20].

62. The Yinshu [引書] of the Zhangjiashan collection describes breathing techniques to normalise yin and yang qi and therefore control anger and joy: "If they (nobility) are joyful then the yang qi is in excess. If they are angry then the yin qi is in excess. On account of this, if those that follow the way are joyful then they quickly exhale (warm breathe), and if they become angry they increasingly puff out (moist breath), in order to harmonise it" [67].

63. Having said all that, the question remains whether these various authors intended that all emotional expressions would be disturbing to one's qi. The typical medical interpretation of this is that it is excessive or unregulated expression of an emotion that disturbs the qi. While a valid interpretation, the actual Neijing literature only states, for example "anger injures the liver" not that "too much anger" injures the liver. Perhaps this can be understood with reference to Allan's image of the heart-mind (see discussion below) as a pool of water, stirred up by emotion. The more intense the emotion, the more the water is stirred up and the less the ability of the heart-mind (which governs everything in the body) to perform its proper tasks. Perceptions of the outside world become distorted (we might say seen through an emotional lens that distorts the view) and various aspects of qi movement/physiology normally under the governance of the heart-mind become increasingly disturbed. The ideal state is to retain a calm heart-mind, to keep the surface of the pool still, hence the need to keep the emotions calm and controlled.

64. The contrast between the affective states of the xin, the emotions as disturbing and the regulating functions of the higher mental states (shen, yi, zhi) etc can be seen simply as a contrast of how the emotions are not physiological per se, they are the result of inner/outer factors while the higher mental states are more a part of the internal physiology, which undisturbed is self-regulating.

65. Throughout history in the medical literature we find examples of how authors instruct their readers to calm their minds and focus quietly on the task at hand, showing that this kind of focus has been involved in the practice of medicine from the earliest times. Sun Simiao (Beiji Qianjin Yaofang [備急千金要方] 650 CE) says "In the great physicians therapeutic practice, he must make his mind serene and his will firm, so that he desires nothing and demands nothing" [104:40], Yang Jizhou (Zhenjiu Dacheng [鍼灸大成] 1601 CE) says "In the mind (xin) of the physician there should be no desires, only a receptive and accepting attitude, then the mind can become spirit (shen). The mind of the physician and the mind of the patient should be level, in harmony, following the movements of the needle." [78:38]. Cheng Guopeng (Yixue Xinwu [醫學心悟] 1732) says "I admonished [my students in the following manner]. Awakening of the mind [refers] to the mechanism of reaching higher levels. Explaining through words is important for those studying at lower levels... Then when the mind becomes like a clear mirror, the brush can draw spring flowers [i.e. healing formulas] that rescue the people" [104:165].

66. This translation comes from Lewis who translates zhi as "intent", yi as "ideas" and jing-shen as "essential spirit energies". The fact that different scholars translate the same terms with different English words is confusing. This issue is elaborated below see especially boxes 2 and 3. The important point for our argument is that the yi and zhi when balanced help maintain a healthier internal, physiological environment.

67. Zhang continues "Again, yi, zhi, si, lu and zhi are not different things but descriptions of different phases of the same continuous process of heart-mind" [138:41]. Sivin renders the same Lingshu passage as "what the mind recalls is called thought (yi). What thought retains is called intent (zhi). Change of what is retained, in accordance with intent, is called ssu (si). Yearning for something distant in accordance with ssu is called concern (lu). Making decisions with regards to things on the basis of concern is called wisdom (zhi)" [111:287].

68. We assume an intended understanding of the stillness the results in clarity as referring to a moving or flowing but unstirred water, while the stillness that stagnates is one that has no additional movement. This intention can be seen in the Lushi Chunqiu's discussion of the importance of movement to keep the hinge of a door from rusting up "The reason the water in the stream remains vital, yet stationary water doesn't, and the hinge doesn't age yet the rest of the door does, is because they are moving. The relationship between the form and the chi (qi) is the same. If the form doesn't move, the jing doesn't stream. If the jing doesn't stream the qi becomes stagnant" [77:33].

69. Shen is also understood in the Neijing to refer to several different concepts, including the zheng qi [正氣], see chapter five for details.

70. "What Wenhui learns is that true mastery and skill, in life as well as in cooking, involve a knack, not a formula. The ideal is to "follow things as they are" and therefore never confront obstacles, just as water follows around a rock in the stream. The spirit or daemonic

(shen) to which Cook Ding refers can be seen as the "autopilot" that guides us in the absence of conscious intention... As A Graham says "people who really know what they are doing, such as cooks, carpenters, swimmers, boatmen, cicada-catchers, do not go in much for analysing, posing alternatives and reasoning from first principles, they no longer even bear in mind any rules they were taught as apprentices; they attend to the total situation and respond" [26:212].

71. Zhang expresses a more modern understanding of shen as "vitality as manifested through functional activities of mind and body" [138:6]. Kuriyama expresses an understanding of shen thus : "In everyday language shen referred most often to gods and divinities, but in medicine the term gestured toward the ineffable yet palpable difference between a stony cadaver and a breathing, responsive human being - the spirit of a person, the divine essence of life" [55:107].

72. Historically various theories and models of "shen", "qi" and "jing" can be found so that it becomes difficult making definitive statements about what they are. A common model is to see the three concepts as intimately interwoven, with shen being a more refined form of qi and jing being an essential concentration of qi: "The argument here rests on the claim that the universe is composed of qi, and that change is a product of alterations and transformations of this qi. Shen, the most highly refined form of qi, is able to understand the proper movements of the universe, and, since humans have this form of qi within themselves as well, they ultimately can attain the same comprehension through their own efforts" [94:115]. When qi is concentrated "it is jing; when it is dispersed it is qi. If jing is the nurturing aspect of this energy, qi is the configurational aspect of the same energy. They come together as jingqi [精氣] which is the basis of all forms of vitality" [138:57]. Zhang further captures their relationships "If jing and qi are the basics of life, then shen is the manifestation of that life" [138:58].

73. "Paying careful attention to the passage of the spirit in and around the body is a fundamental concern of the medical literature of Han times" [69:88].

74. The passage further describes the acupoints as being "neither in the skin nor the flesh, neither in the muscles nor the bones" (i.e. are not anatomically based) [73:14]. Sivin renders this passage as "'At the articulations within the body there are 365 points of communication... 'articulations' refers to where the divine ch'i (sic) travels freely and moves outward and inward, not to skin, flesh, sinews, and bones'. A modern Westerner expects these points of communication, where the physician's needles can affect the circulation, to be places in tissue, but here we find them related instead to processes" [111:51]. Lo goes on to explain how this distinction helps us grasp the difference between "crude and skilled practitioners", the latter pay attention to the shen (rather than the anatomical structures) [69:88-89].

75. "The loss of this substance or substances (i.e. the hun and po) led to mental disturbance or decline, rather than death. Moreover, they could continue to adhere to the body and function as mental powers even after death. They were in turn linked to other substances, the essential energies (jing) and spirit energies (shen), in a hierarchy of ascending refinement. The human body emerged from the fusion of all these energies as

well as the coarser energies that formed its physical structures" [62:55]. Paraphrasing Brashier, Lo suggests that the hun and po are "linked to medical states on anxiety and illness" [69:83].

76. Given one of the interpretations of yi as "attention" and one of the interpretations of zhi as "will" it is hard to ignore William James's insightful comments on these two: will is the effort of attention "The essential achievement of the will in short, when it is most 'voluntary", is to attend to a difficult object and hold it fast before the mind… effort of attention is thus the essential phenomenon of will" [118:37-38].

77. For the translation of the term yi as "judgment", see the enlightening discussion of Furth [29:144-5].

78. Larre and Rochat de la Vallee say of the "yi": "the heart recognizes if the vibration coming to it is true, that is, if its nature is such that the heart can compose with it... The heart, aware of itself, accepts or rejects what is being presented to it... Because it is vacant and calm, the empty and serene heart receives all the thoughts that germinate there like mushrooms...This recognition by the heart brings on the appearance of what we call 'intent' yi. Intent is a focal point, a concentration affected by the heart. This concentration allows form to occur: that which was presented to the heart is now represented by the outlines of a form: word, discussions, acts, work, conduct" [56:52-53].

79. "Therefore this vital energy cannot be halted by force, yet can be secured by inner power (de). Cannot be summoned by speech, yet can be welcomed by the awareness (yi)" [100:48], Rickett translates the same passage as: "Thus, this vital force –Never to be restrained by physical strength, it may be brought to rest by spiritual power (de) Never to be summoned by one's call, it may be made welcome by one's power of awareness (yi)." [96:39-40]. Yi is thus seen as an important mental function in relation to how one influences qi.

80. Chace and Bensky summarise it thus: "one's capacity for efficacy resides in effortless activity and the influence of one's consciousness resides in quiescence" [16].

81. Larre and Rochat de la Vallee tellingly state it thus: "Will, zhi is a movement initiated in the heart, but nothing appears, nothing comes out of the heart; the act has not yet begun: the will is the antecedent of all precise feeling, of all constructed thought... One's orientation, already apparent in intent (yi), is affirmed and becomes directive. But we must guard against intellectualizing the will. Its beginnings are before thought, before reflection, before meditation. However, there is nothing thoughtless about it. It is impulse, the natural and vital impulse in me, the injection of the vital life forces" [56:54-55].

82. "The will (zhi) is the governor of the qi. Qi is what fills the limbs. Wherein the will arrives is wherein the qi lodges. Thus it is said, 'hold fast to your will and do not violate your qi'... When the will is stopped up, then it makes qi move, when qi is blocked up, it makes the will move" [1:91].

83. An interesting parallel to this quiescent awareness is the observation in consciousness research that often intense concentration doesn't make the effect happen, rather soft willing or "gentle wishing" is more successful in making it happen [81:182].

84. See the discussions in Lingshu chapter one in the chapter by Chace and Bensky where the yi is clearly stated to be important in how one influences the qi during needling [16].

85. Chace and Bensky render the same passage a little differently "as for doctors talking about intention, the interstices and pores have extremely subtle divisions so to follow the qi requires skill. When inserting needles and the stone (probes) between them, being a hair off means failure. The knack exists in the connection between the heart-mind and hand. It can be understood but it cannot be spoken of" [16].

86. Of this Scheid and Bensky state: "physicians move towards healing power by the way of their yi – the ability to enter into the totality of a clinical situation, view it from different angles simultaneously, match it with ideas already present in the mind, compare and contrast them, weigh up possibilities for action and then, and only then, do exactly what is appropriate" [105:35].

87. For the term "gan" Larre and Rochat de la Vallee translate "reactions" [56:10].

88. Fox has a very nice statement about "ying": "just as text and reader constitute a reciprocally responsive whole, the same can be said of all human experience." As a result, suggests Zhuangzi, **the most effective mode of human experience is to 'fit' (shi) into any given situation in such a way as to allow ourselves to respond (ying) effortlessly and spontaneously, just like the hinge** (emphasis added). This kind of unobtrusive experience is what we might call 'wuwei'" [26:220].

89. The term "tuilei" [推類] is used to capture this kind of thinking. Sterckx describes it as an "epistemological method associated with five-phase and yinyang thinking, in general it refers to a process in which visible realities in the natural world are identified and categorized in order to 'push' or extrapolate this explanatory logic to realms beyond the visible" [119:80].

90. However Le Blanc quoting Major "the relentless cataloguing of categories of five-element and other correlations by Warring States and Han cosmologists points to a further doctrine that perhaps could be regarded as a genuine creation of the Tsou Yen school: ch'i (qi) and the concept of resonance" [59:143] implies a more common association of five phase correlations and ganying.

91. Major states it thus "Things within a correlative category (whether a simple or complex one) interact (even over long distances, and without any mechanical connection) on the 'like responds to like' principle not only because they emit imperceptible 'vibrations' through the medium of qi, but because they are made of the same kind of qi" [75:30].

92. This shift in the Huainanzi was a direct challenge to the emperor's "monopolization of sacred knowledge and authority" [130:187]. Puett and Wang discuss these changes at

length [94, 130:185-187]. What is relevant for us here is that both interpretations saw "tianren ganying", the resonance between heaven and man as being important and placed qi at the center of those models [130:187].

93. Slingerland continues: "the heart/mind of the perfected person –once emptied through psychic fasting– is completely open and responsive to things. The mirror-response is thus the behavioural correlate to cognitive emptiness or clarity" [115:192].

94. In his explanatory notes to the translation of this passage from the Wuxing, Csikszentmihalyi comments "The presence of a person of virtue is what allows the resonance of tian's way. The commentary equates the ability to balance hard and pliant in managing the affairs with goodness (and hence with the worthies), and the ability to effect a wuwei type of rule with sagacity (and hence with the sages)" [19:326].

95. The Huainanzi describes how the sage is able to connect to tianji inside the body [78:85].

96. Chace and Bensky render this passage as: "Ah, to know the incipience, how divine (shen)... Incipience is the most minute aspect of movement" [16].

97. This relates how being able to grasp the quiet spaces between things one can exert the most influence on those things. The arrival of qi is a subtle phenomenon in acupuncture needling –said to be like the "wind blowing away the clouds to reveal the blue sky" [68]. The superior physician attends to the ji in order to do this correctly and with maximum efficacy –for more discussion of this see Chace and Bensky and Birch in this volume.

98. If taken literally we feel that this is rather an overstatement, it could be more precise to say that the xin (mind), shen (spirit) or yi (attention/awareness) are pivotal in how things happen, meaning that they can act like a pivot so that they have the function of the ji. It can also be thought that these are what make the person efficacious in using ji correctly.

99. They state this in various ways: "Said another way, these processual events are porous, flowing into each other in the ongoing transformations we call experience" [2:15] and "life broadly construed is entertained through and only through these same phenomena that constitute our experience" [2:18].

100. "The arousal of qi in one's nature by external things causes one to react in a way that expresses emotion" [19:145].

101. Lo describes it thus: "every foodstuff, like every drug, had a sapor associated with the pentic system, a qi, a relative potency, and was associated with healing different parts of the body" [70:164].

102. The link between qi and wei (flavours) are not consistently used in the traditions of herbal medicine, thus this statement does not always clearly hold, see the chapter on herbal medicine [99].

103. Kuriyama additionally quotes Lingshu chapter four "the illness can first be seen in the face (se), even though it may not appear in the body. It seems to be there, but not there; it seems to exist, yet not exist, it seems to be visible, and yet invisible. No one can describe it" [55:179].

104. Graham comments on these effects: "Music, then, like ceremony, acts directly on man's tastes, it can modify his natural inclinations for the better. Sounds and movement act on the vitalizing fluids, the ch'i (qi) by 'arousal' and 'response' (ying)" [31:260]. It is also interesting to note the widespread use of sounds, bells, drums, chanting in shamanic practices by which the shaman can influence his followers.

105. The "obtaining of qi" is the "deqi" [得氣], seen by most modern Chinese practitioners to be the same as "qizhi", however some modern Japanese practitioners see them as different "In contrast to obtaining Qi (deqi), which is felt by the patient, the arrival of Qi (qizhi) is something that the practitioner feels" [109:181] as do some modern Chinese practitioners [137], "After inserting the needle, the next step is to get qi (得氣 deqi). Note that here the sensation of 'getting qi' is one that is felt by the patient. There is also the concept of 'arrival of qi' (氣至 qizhi) that involves a sensation felt by the practitioner" [131:533]. It should be apparent below in the chapter on acupuncture [8] and the chapter by Chace and Bensky [16] that the early literature implies that it is the practitioner that must "feel" the qi with needling.

CHAPTER TWO

# THE JINGMAI

## A summary of their development and nature

Stephen Birch, Manuel Rodríguez Cuadras, Miguel Angel Cabrer Mir

**余聞人之合於天道也內有五藏以應五音五色五時五味五位也外有六府以應六律六律建陰陽諸經..此五藏六府之所以應天道夫十二經脈者人之所以生病之所以成人之所以治病之所以起學之所始工之所止也**

I have heard that humankind is in accord with the way of heaven, thus they have five viscera internally and these correspond to the five notes, five colors, five flavors, five seasons and five directions. They also have six bowels externally which correspond to the six pitch pipes. These are analogous to the yin and yang channels... Thus these five viscera and six bowels correspond to the way of heaven. The twelve channels are responsible for life in humans and the development of illness. They concern the treatment and the origin of a person's illness. They must be studied by the beginner and yet they provide the skilled with limitations [they cannot exceed].

Lingshu chapter 11 [58:14]

**經脈者行血氣通陰陽以榮於身者也**

The Conduit vessels pass the blood and the influences, penetrating the yin and yang [sections of the organism], in order to provide nourishment to the body.

Nanjing chapter 23 [68:285-286]

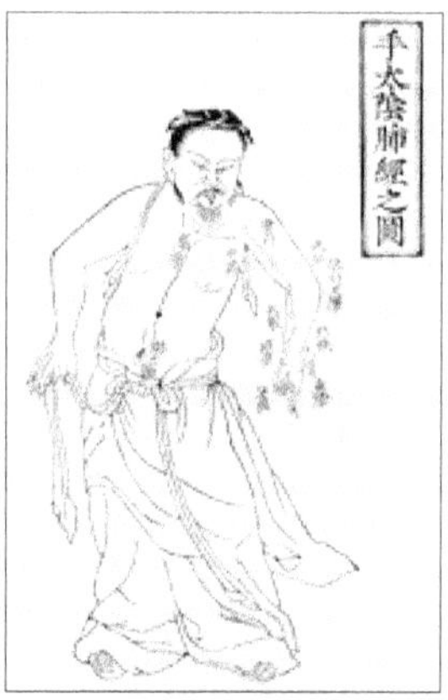


**手太陰肺經**
Arm taiyin-lung channel

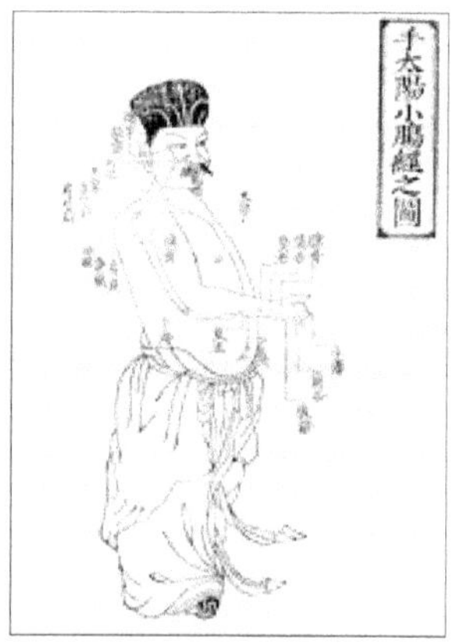


**手太陽小肠經**
Arm taiyang-small intestine channel

## Introduction

The development of the mai [脈] as a physiological system and the later development of the concept of the jingmai [經脈] as a more elaborated physiological system dates from the period of the late Warring States into the first portions of the Han dynasty (250-150 BCE). This theme has been explored by a number of authors, key among them Daly [17], Harper [20], Hsu [22, 23], Lo [35, 36, 37, 38, 40, 41, 42], Lo, Li [43], Lu and Needham [44], Unschuld [69]. Since the topic has been well addressed elsewhere, we will only summarise salient points here, propose some perhaps new ideas and explore how they were adopted or influential in the various traditions covered in this book. Chapter four, "Qi, jingmai and acupuncture" [6] will explore related ideas more fully. The basic purpose of the current chapter is to lay the foundation for those later discussions.

The term mai is found in the Guoyu [國語] of the fourth to fifth century BCE with reference to earthquakes "If the astrologer watches the earth at the right time, the yang is under stress and violently swells up, the qi [氣] of the earth trembles, on the morning of the first day of spring... the earth breaks out along the mai [脈]" [42]. Such convergence of ideas linking the mai and qi together in the context of an abnormal flow presages later developments in medical thinking where the terms become interrelated with reference to pain experiences, observations of location of blood vessels and palpable pulses and the physiology of the body; astronomical and meteorological observations and the terminology used for those helped set the stage for and permeated the language and concepts of physiology that emerged over the next centuries in China [41, 42, 43].

In the Chinese literature dating from the fourth century BCE the concept of the "body" started emerging [31:14]. We find it emerging in two distinct streams, in relation to "virtue" ("de" [德]) and "ritual order" through texts such as the Mencius [孟子], Zuozhuan [左傳] and Wuxing [五行] [16:59, 31:14] and in relation to self-cultivation practices in the text the Neiye [內業] [31:14] and early Han Mawangdui [馬王堆] and Zhangjiashan [張家山] texts [41, 43].[1]

The major medical corpus of the Huangdi Neijing texts have been dated at quite different times by different authors writing about them, but it has been possible to narrow down the dates of the earliest forms of these texts to somewhere mid to late second century BCE because of recent historical evidence and archaeological findings. In recent decades a number of tombs have been opened revealing many texts including a number of pre-Neijing medical texts. The most important tombs for us are those of the Mawangdui [馬王堆] from

168 BCE and the Zhangjiashan [張家山] from the mid second century BCE. These medical texts are thought to date from the late third early second centuries BCE. In them are thought to be the first descriptions of the mai in relation to physiology, and a number of these texts discuss qi within the "mai" [20:84][2] where the "mai" were both simple physiological systems and targets of treatment principally with cauterization (probably including moxibustion). Donald Harper has published a full translation of the primary texts [20]. Others have done detailed analyses of these texts [e.g. 17, 34]. It is thus unnecessary to dwell in detail upon these texts here since they have been described well by these authors. In addition to these early Han texts there are also the case records of Chunyu Yi recorded in the Shiji (circa 90 BCE), dating from around 154 BCE, analyses of this corpus are also available [22, 23, 24]. In this section we will summarise the important innovations and findings from these various historical texts regarding the "mai". The reader is especially referred to Harper [20], Daly [17], Lo [41] and Lo and Li [43].

## The mai

The term "mai" [脈] is translated as "vessel", "channel" or "pulse" [40] depending on context and the translator. Harper examines references and cross-references in the first etymological dictionary the Shuowen Jiezi [說文解字], circa 90 CE [20:83]. He then discusses how the common character component "pai" [𠂢] is linked to terms that are associated with water flows and channels in the earth and then describes it as reasonable to see how when the term "mai" [脈] was first adopted "there existed a conceptual correlation between the body and earth, and blood vessels and streams" [20:83]. The etymology of the term is discussed further below in the examination of the connections of the jingmai to their related internal organs.

It would have been known early on that "blood" is an important thing for life. With an injury or during animal slaughter, when it flows out of the living body it results in death. It would also have been known that it can be found in vessels inside the body; it is highly improbable that at least butchers, cooks, hunters and soldiers wouldn't have known this. The association with blood and these vessels would have resulted in an early use of terms to refer to these blood vessels. We would naturally expect the term "mai" to have first been used with reference to these important anatomical structures; a number of scholars describe how this is the original referent for the term "mai" [20:82, 27:41]. The first mention of blood vessels appears to be in the Zuozhuan description of a distraught horse (mid fourth century BCE) [20:82, 27:41, 64:74]. The use of the term "mai" as "blood vessel" can be found in the Neijing corpus in discussions of anatomical structures in the numerous discussions of the contrasts and correspondences of body tissues such as the skin, flesh, vessels, bones.[3]

Naturally as one touches living animals and people one notices that there are visible and non-visible vessels inside the body that can be felt to "move" "dong" [動]. These movements are regular and rhythmic. As we find later in the Greek medicine of Galen (second century CE) [27], these moving vessels or "pulses" can be palpated and used as indicators of the condition of the person or animal being palpated. In a parallel manner, we have reference to palpation of these vessels as early as 168 BCE in the Maifa text from the Mawangdui findings [20] and 154 BCE in the recorded cases of Chunyu Yi [22]. These "moving vessels" "dongmai" [動脈] are seen in a parallel way to the blood vessels palpated in Western medical traditions and hence the name "pulse" has come to be associated with them, though this can be conceptually misleading and confusing [27]. Kuriyama gives examples from the Neijing and earlier Zhangjiashan treatises that make clear rendering of the term "mai" as (blood) "vessel" or "pulse" difficult, arguing instead that the "duality in English renderings is an artifact of translation" [27:48]. It seems likely that palpation of these "vessels" as an indicator of the condition of the person palpated would come to be associated with the known anatomical structures that convey the blood within the body.[4] All of these are "mai".

Then, as the early models of the body start to be formulated in the late Warring States period, and physiological-functional structures were being sought and described, it seems reasonable that at least during some stage of this process these "mai" would have been discussed as they were already known to convey vital stuff that keeps one alive[5] (the blood) and can be palpated at "moving" places to give an indication of the state of the body. The "mai" as physiological-functional systems would thus emerge as a prelude to more detailed structures and systems and would then be incorporated in more elaborated forms in those systems. Hence the "mai" become conveyors of vital stuff associated with physiology. As we have seen in the previous chapter, during the late Warring states period, the term "qi" [氣] started to be used more and more to refer to important stuff in relation to for example, the mind, the emotions, virtue, self-cultivation, the weather, and through concurrently developing cosmological models and correlative thinking it came to become a central concept in thinking about the body. Thus it is natural that eventually this important evolving concept with all of its multiple implications and roles would come to be increasingly associated with the "mai" thus further extending the nature and thinking about the "mai". The first mention of the idea that "qi flows along with blood through the vessels inside the body" occurs in first half of the third century BCE [64:74.][6]

These associations and developments would have naturally involved incorporating older references, terms and concepts and merging them with newly evolving ideas, terms and concepts[7] as the model evolved and became more systematic.[8] As the relationships between blood and qi emerge, discussions of the compound term xueqi [血氣] (blood-qi or blood and qi) in relation to living animals can be found in the early literature [64:74]. Sivin cites the first usage of the term "xueqi" to be in the Analects of Confucius [60:46] where he translates the term as "physical vitality" or "physical powers". While there might be an inclination to see "xueqi" as referring to the blood and qi, many argue against this: Kuriyama argues, they are "essentially the same. Doctors did, to be sure, occasionally spotlight distinctions. Blood had form, for instance, while qi was formless... blood and qi were complementary facets of a unique vitality, its yin and yang manifestation" [27:229; see also 60:51-52]. Sterckx traces this inseparability of the two into the later Han: "According to Wang Chong, human beings live by the agency of refined qi (jingqi) which is made possible by the blood vessels. He further defines blood as the "jingqi during one's life period" and describes "blood and qi"(xueqi) as the seat of one's jingshen, hereby again associating the development of spiritual energy with the presence of a physiological substrate of blood vapor" [64:75]. This association helps us understand why Lingshu chapter eighteen states "the blood (xue) is the shenqi" [49:98]. The blood and qi together are vital to living things which are animated by "shen" [神] –often translated as "spirit", hence their close association. Kuriyama points to this natural type of association in other traditional systems, such as that of the Greeks with blood and pneuma, but there a polarization of the two gradually increased [27:229].

The story of the "mai" can be seen in relation to these developments in thinking and changes in society in China. What concerns us primarily is the role of "mai" as a system of physiological structures that preceded the innovation of the jingmai concept. The role of mai as "blood vessels" and "pulses" are peripheral to this story but will appear periodically in order to help embed developments into a broader background.

## Documented developments of the "mai"

The Mawangdui cache of texts buried in 168 BCE date from around 200 BCE to 170 BCE. They include not only medical texts but works on philosophy, ethics, history, astrology, divination etc. [20:4]. The medical texts included both treatises on health preservation and expansion from the yangsheng [養生] tradition, and texts on disease, diagnosis and treatment.[9] Of the medical texts, the most relevant to us are: The "Zubi shiyi mai jiujing" [足臂十一脈灸經], the "Yinyang shiyi mai jiujing" [陰陽十一脈灸經], the "Maifa" [經法] and the "Yinyang mai sihou" [陰陽脈死候]. There are two versions of the "Yinyang shiyi mai jiujing" in the cache. The Zhangjiashan cache of texts possibly buried in 186 BCE is a smaller cache of texts thought to date from 202-186 BCE. Of most relevance among them is the "Maishu" [脈書], which is a treatise that Harper describes in six parts, three of which are versions of the Mawangdui texts, the "Yinyang shiyi mai jiujing", "Maifa" and the "Yinyang mai sihou". The variants of the same texts allow for confirmation of the content and dating of them as there was naturally damage to some of the stored texts. Of the gymnastic and self-cultivation texts the "Daoyin tu" [導引圖] and the "Heyinyang" [和陰陽] of the Mawangdui and the "Yinshu" [引書] of the Zhangjiashan also provide input into how the mai were conceived and developed. In addition to these newly uncovered texts the case records of Chunyu Yi [淳于意] (circa 154 BCE), recorded in the Shji [史記] (circa 90 BCE) provide further information regarding how the concept of the "mai" was being used in the period before the Huangdi Neijing texts. Finally, a laquer figurine the "Shuang baoshan" figurine was unearthed in Mianyang dating from no later than 118 BCE [21, 37] that contains lines on it that appear to mirror some written descriptions of the mai.

Each of the above have been researched and described in detail, thus we will refer the reader to relevant sources[10] and simply summarize the primary findings that are relevant for a short history of how the "mai" developed into the more complex "jingmai".

## "Zubi shiyi mai jiujing" [足臂十一脈灸經]

The "Cauterization canon of the eleven vessels of the foot and forearm" uses the character "wen" [温] to refer to the "mai". It describes the trajectories of six leg vessels –three yin and three yang and five arm vessels– three yang and two yin. There is no mention of the concepts of qi or xue (blood). The eleven vessels lead from the extremities to the center of the body. For each of the eleven mai associated symptoms are described. Treatment is given by burning moxibustion on the relevant vessel, but with no specification of where along its trajectory.[11]

## "Yinyang shiyi mai jiujing" [陰陽十一脈灸經]

The "Cauterization cannon of the eleven yin and yang vessels" appears in three versions, two from the Mawangdui and one in the Maishu of the Zhangjiashan. Each text is of a different length, the most detailed being in the Zhangjiashan. Like the "Zubi shiyi mai jiujing" this text describes eleven vessels, classified the same way. There is one reference to the concept of qi in relation to one of the vessels and likewise one to the concept of blood [17:68]. The text gives more detail of the illnesses and describes how "dong" [動] movement or agitation of the mai lead to illness. The mai were described as controlling "zhu" [主] the illness which must be treated "zhi" [治]. Treatments are given in much less detail than in the previous text, application of moxa is only described for one vessel. Presumably this is an example of how to treat the other vessels.

## "Maifa" [經法]

The "Model of the vessels" does not describe the trajectories of the eleven vessels, rather it focuses on methods of palpation or pulse taking along the mai. It describes the qualities of the pulses and their significance. It gives a detailed understanding of qi and its movement thus making statements about the relations between qi and the mai. It describes if qi is moving in the wrong manner where to moxa or pierce with a stone needle. While it establishes a clear relationship between qi and the mai, it does not describe a flow of qi in the mai as such. In one discussion it mentions how cauterization (not necessarily with moxibustion)[12] can be used to influence the qi in the mai.[13] In the case of a vessel with excess qi in it causing the qi to ascend and not descend, applying cauterization on the waist was intended to make the qi descend (towards the warmth of the applied heat)[14], see discussions in Harper [20:91].

## "Yinyang mai sihou" [陰陽脈死候]

The "Death signs of the yin and yang vessels" is more theoretically detailed than the previous texts. It describes how the three yang mai are associated with tianqi [天氣] the qi of heaven and that they are said to control external affairs and life. The three yin mai[15] are associated with diqi [地氣], the qi of earth, and that they are said to control internal bodily affairs and death.[16] The text also describes how the mai need to be filled or emptied "suggesting either renewal of their contents, or a continual healthy state of flux" [17:72].[17] Blood and qi are described as having an intimate relationship. The Zhangjiashan version of the text is said to have been clearly influenced by the yangsheng tradition [17:72] thus hinting at the role of the yangsheng tradition in the development of the mai and jingmai.

## **"Daoyin tu"** ***and*** **"Yinshu" [導引圖] [引書]**

The Daoyin tu of the Mawangdui findings seems to describe movements, stretches and exercises for health. The Yinshu of the Zhangjiashan describes these also in relation to breathing exercises and massage. The two together are seen by Lo as an alternative "physical therapy" for treating pain, (alternative to the use of cauterization [moxa] on the eleven mai from the "Zubi shiyimai jiujing" and the "Yinyang shiyimai jiujing"), using movement and breath [41:390]. While not focused on the mai per se, they are "concerned with alleviating pain and discomfort... related to a body organized around mai" [41:391].

## *Mianyang figurine*

This ceramic figure has ten vertical lines drawn on it that appear to be related to the mai. Detailed analysis has shown that three seem to closely match descriptions of the mai, five appear somewhat similar while two of the ten do not at all correspond [17:75].[18] Lo has also suggested that the lines on the figurine are related to yangsheng exercises [21, 43] from the Daoyin (Mawangdui) or Yinshu (Zhangjiashan) texts [17:75]. After a detailed analysis of the figurine Lo states that we can think of the lines on the figurine "as a visual aid to guide medical intervention," but "whether intervention is styled in relation to a model of breath cultivation, to contemporary theories of pathological physiology or simply patterns of symptoms is as yet unclear" [41:388]. After further analysis she describes how the lines on the figurine seem related to superficial arterio-venous pathways and likely places where pulses can be palpated [41:390], they may also be related to the sensory systems of the eyes, ears etc [41:403] and are likely to be related to an idealized movement of qi in breath cultivation practices [41:404].

## *The case records of Chunyu Yi*

Chunyu Yi's twenty five case records are found in the Shiji from around 90 BCE. The cases have been dated to between 164-153 BCE [22:52]. They show how an experienced clinician was using ideas that existed in his time in the treatment of patients. The cases focus more on diagnosis, etiology and treatment, especially by herbal medicine. His focus was less on the practice of acupuncture.[19] His cases describe a model of how qi [氣], the mai [脈] and bing [病], disease were seen to be related [22]. He details relationships between the mai and the internal viscera, something missing in the Mawangdui and Zhangjiashan texts but clearly present in the Neijing corpus. He has extensive discussion of examination of the mai, which could be palpation of the pulses and/or palpation of the mai themselves [22:73-74], he stated how when he treated patients "I invariably press their vessels first and then treat them" [20:94]. In his writings examination of the mai leads to an understanding of the condition of the internal viscera and an understanding of the (condition of) qi in the body.[20] His writings reflect an "understanding of vessel theory different from the Huangdi Neijing, but definitely more elaborate than the Mawangdui texts" [20:39]. It appears that his writings may lie somewhere between the Mawangdui and Zhangjiashan texts and the Neijing texts and are the first to start introducing relationships between the condition of the mai and the internal organs, with a clear emphasis on the emotional state of the patient as well [24].

Vivienne Lo argues cogently that examination of the trajectories of the mai in texts such as the Maishu and the Yinshu evidences a link between the location of pain symptoms, movements of qi and the locations of the mai. She argues that the trajectories and descriptions of the mai may have been influenced by experiences and descriptions of pain, for which they were treated [35]: "So consistently is the link between the symptoms and channels made that the sites of pain and discomfort cited in the second list virtually mirror the description of the channel itself. They are close enough to suggest that the phenomenon of pain and disturbance was largely responsible for determining the spatial dimensions of the channel itself." Given the focus we saw in the last chapter that concepts such as qi and the mai would have developed not from purely descriptive anatomical considerations, but rather from practical considerations such as how to help someone in pain [8], it makes considerable sense that such links are found in an examination of the texts. This trend will have influenced the later developments of jingmai as well.

It is generally agreed that the writings found in the Mawangdui and Zhangjiashan manuscripts coupled with the Chunyu Yi case studies have been influential in the development of concepts and methods that are found in the Huangdi Neijing corpus [17, 20, 22, 23, 24, 36, 37, 41, 43, 69]. The details of those influences are not all obvious and as Harper warns,[21] it is premature to try making definitive statements about publications in the period leading up to the publication of the Neijing texts [20:39].[22] However, with regards the development of the concept of the "mai" and its transition into the Neijing concept of the "jingmai" it does seem clear that these earlier publications set the stage and that we are able to look at some of the important stages of this evolution.[23]

## The jingmai

The development from discussion of the "mai" in the pre-Neijing texts to discussion of the "jingmai" in the Neijing texts marks a turning point in medical thinking.[24] With the jingmai we see many influences being drawn together into a comprehensive model of physiology, health and disease in the form of the "theory of systematic correspondence" [67, 68]. A passage from chapter twenty-five of the Suwen "exemplifies such a correlative account of the body:

> Heaven and earth blend qi (and the result) is called man. If man is able to remain responsive (ying [應]) to the four seasons, heaven and earth are father and mother to him, as when he who shoulders the burden of dominion over the myriad things is called Son of Heaven. In the sky there are yin and yang; human beings have their twelve major mai-channels. The sky has its hot and cold weather, human beings have their depletions (xu) and repletions (shi). He who can model (jing [經]) himself on the transformations of sky and earth, yin and yang, will not fail to be attuned to the four seasons. He who can know the pattern (li [理]) underlying the (motions) of the twelve mai-channels (jingmai) will not be surpassed in wisdom even by a sage [17:8, from 60:58].

This passage captures in part the role of the theory of systematic correspondence by which the jingmai are explicitly related to heaven and earth, yin and yang, through which they help import order into the body (see discussions in the previous chapter), but it does not describe the more extended application of the theory of systematic correspondence to the body through the jingmai. There is already correspondence to yin-yang in the naming of the "mai". With the development of the jingmai we see the application of the additional correspondences to the wuxing [五行], the five phases and to the internal organ systems. The system of five phases had, by the time of the Huangdi Neijing become an important tool. The jingmai's correspondences to both yin-yang and the five-phases allows for the further import of order into the body when the jingmai are used in treatment, many systems inside the body were seen to fit within the five-phase correspondence system, thus implying a kind of targeted ordering of systems within the body was now possible (see further discussions in chapter four [6]).

The term "jingmai" has been translated to English as "meridian", "channel", "conduit-vessel", "sinarteria"[25] each term reflecting the understanding and conceptual framework of the person using it. The etymology of the term jing [經] shows that it refers to or is like the vertical threads (the "warp") in a fabric [60:80, 69:169-170]. In weaving, these vertical threads form the basis upon which the pattern of the fabric is woven with the horizontal threads (the woof). Thus in a sense the warp forms the foundation for the structure.[26] The various translations of the term "jing" invoke an understanding of the jing as something that orders or brings regularity to things: Levi translates the term as "regularity" [30:689] while Sivin says that the term "implies regularity" [60:80], Puett translates the term as "aligning" [54:2], Daly in the last quote used the term "model" as in modelling oneself on. [17:8], Rochat de la Vallee [56:12] and Unschuld [69:17] translate jing as "norms" such as the "norms in heaven", while Cook translates it as "constant" [15:259] and Lewis as "guiding principle" [31:30].[27] Perhaps the incorporation of the term jing into the compound term "jingmai" was intended to imply a further ordering of the body, which is why Lingshu chapter ten, the pivotal jingmai text tells us [經脈者... 調虛實] "the jingmai... regulate vacuity and repletion" [70:427, 73:556]. A conceptual basis of this is argued for by Unschuld as a parallel to the ordering of society that was experienced during the early Han dynasty [67][28] and the healing or governing, zhi [治] [17:122], that is applied to restore natural order. It is thus possible to see the term "jingmai" as having a meaning like "ordering vessels", or "vessels that (bring) order" to the structure, the body.[30] They would thus be implicitly and explicitly about restoring and maintaining order or regulating the body. Since the mai contained qi and blood, which were seen as fundamental for human life, a natural focus as medicine developed in the early Han went to correcting disturbances of the mai. This way of thinking is further expressed through the utilisation of the six yin-yang categorisations of the "jing". We see a partial application of this six-fold categorisation in the Mawangdui texts [17, 20], but the full categorisation is not found till the Neijing texts where twelve jingmai are described (instead of the eleven of one of the Mawangdui texts) –see Table 1. The six-fold categorization of six jing used in premedical texts as a six fold yin-yang cosmological categorization, being used for example to refer to the movements through yin and yang during the course of the year [60:80-83].[31]But the six-fold yin-yang categorization of the six-jing that we find in the Neijing are "not, in other words, a single concept in the Inner Canon, but a variety of sixfold schemata related in various ways to the circulation tracts (jingmai) by way of yin-yang theory" [60:82].[32] Sivin states that the "main purpose of the six warps (jing), in other words, is to describe the order and symmetries of normal energy distribution through the body" [60:82].[33] Daly argues that the incorporation of the term "jing" to create the novel term "jingmai" not only links the mai to more cosmological theories, but adds a temporal dimension [17:73]. The textual descriptions of the mai in the Mawangdui and Zhangjiashan texts describe the spatial dimensions of the mai, by incorporating more philosophical and cosmological dimensions the Neijing's term "jingmai" expand the understanding of the mai considerably to reflect a much richer vision of the changing body, its vessels and its environment [17:73].[34]

The systematic correspondence of the twelve jingmai to the wuxing [五行] five-phases introduces further the idea of increasing the order of things inside the body. The jingmai may already be about helping create alignment in the body, they help create and maintain order. Through their five-phase correspondences not only is it possible to target specific structures and systems within the body but it becomes possible to help import order from the environment (heaven and earth) which outside of human affairs is in more ordered and natural states.

In addition to and as part of these expanded visions of the body Harper [20:45-54] and especially Li Jianmen [40] argue that at the centre of these changes lie the "art of calculations" or "art of numbers" shushu [數術]. The calculations and arts had a broad applicability in Chinese society important for example for the correct timing of rituals that were to aid in the summoning of certain powers or effects on behalf of the person performing the ritual [42]. This has a long history in China, helpful in the negotiations between heaven and the ruler to ensure correct outcomes, in astrology, calendars and their making, yinyang and five phase correlations, it also includes a collection of occult literatures including divination, demonology, incantation [20:45, 52]. The development of the "jingmai" brought together multiple strands of thinking and acting, allowing much expanded conceptualization schemes for understanding the body in health and disease, in its interactions with the environment and a greatly expanded range of treatment options.

Table 1 summarises the various mai that can be found from Mawangdui texts, the lacquer figure found in a site in Mianyang and in the Lingshu.

**Table 1: Historical Precursors of the twelve jingmai –channels***

| **Zubi shiyimai jiujing (mai)** | **Yinyang shiyimai jiujing (mai)** | **Mianyang laquer figure** | **Lingshu chapter 10 (jingmai)** |
|---|---|---|---|
| arm tai yin | arm tai yin | arm tai yin | arm tai yin-lung |
| arm yang ming | tooth | arm yang ming | arm yang ming-large intestine |
| leg yang ming | leg yang ming | leg yang ming | leg yang ming-stomach |
| leg tai yin | leg tai yin | - | leg tai yin-spleen |
| arm shao yin | arm shao yin | arm shao yin | arm shao yin-heart |
| arm tai yang | shoulder | arm tai yang | arm tai yang-small intestine |
| leg tai yang | leg tai yang | leg tai yang | leg tai yang-bladder |
| leg shao yin | leg shao yin | - | leg shao yin-kidney |
| - | - | arm jue yin | arm jue yin-pericardium |
| arm shao yang | ear | arm shao yang | arm shao yang-triple burner |
| leg shao yang | leg shao yang | leg shao yang | leg shao yang-gallbladder |
| leg jue yin | leg jue yin | - | leg jue yin-liver |

It is not too much of a speculation to suggest that the utilization of the term jing in "jingmai" brings with it another interesting implication. The mai were already described as running vertically in the body in the pre-Neijing texts such as the "Zubi shiyi mai jiujing" [足臂十一脈灸經] [20:86]. In the Neijing the jingmai also run vertically in the body, which matches the concepts of the jing as the warp or vertical threads in a woven fabric. But since the mai were seen as being of the body and thus of earth, and the jing as being related to broader models of nature, and thus of heaven, perhaps the term "jingmai" is also intended to capture the idea that the human being is a product of the interactions of heaven and earth.[35] There are many discussions of how humans are the product of the interaction of heaven and earth, the jingmai could thus be seen as a way of conceiving how the qi of heaven and earth interact through the body to help order and structure the body according to the more universal rules of yin and yang.[36] "In medical texts, like the "Yinyang mai sihou" [陰陽脈死候], yang vessels circulate tian's qi, while yin vessels circulate earthly qi" [16:156 and see 20:219], in other words in at least one of the Mawangdui

*(After Engelhardt [18] and Daly [17])

texts, we find an explicit articulation of a similar concept, the yang mai contain the qi of heaven while the yin mai contain the qi of earth. Thus we find in the passage above from Suwen chapter twenty-five the statements about how heaven and earth "blend qi" to create the human being, and the obviously important role of the jingmai in grasping both the nature of and disorders of the human being; "a regulated flow of qi, the vital substance of life, was as basic to physical health as it was to the harmony of heaven and earth, and the channels through which it flowed were as carefully mapped as the waterways of the empire" [36:31]. The jingmai had become an important part of the physiology of the body, Lingshu chapter forty-seven states it thus: "The function of the tract-channel network system (jingmai) is to promote a normal passage of the blood and the qi, so that the vital essentials derived from man's food can nourish the yin and yang, sustain the muscles, sinews and bones, and lubricate the joints" [44:28-29]. Huang Fumi in his Zhenjiu Jiayijing states "The twelve channels are responsible for life in humans and the development of illness. They concern the treatment of a person's (illness) and the origins of illness" [74: 95]. In the modern period Wang in a discussion of the clinical importance of the twelve channels quotes Lingshu chapter ten [經脈者所以能決死生, 處百病調虛實不可不通]"The channels are determiners of life and death. They treat the hundred types of disease by regulating excess and deficiency. They cannot be allowed to not be open!" [70:427].

Diagnosis and treatment consequently focus on understanding and correcting the disorders of the jingmai. This is a model of medical practice that exhibits major developments in the Neijing and reaches a kind of pinnacle in the later Nanjing where clearer and more systematic descriptions of health and disease are given [68] that utilise systematic diagnosis and treatment of the twelve jingmai by correcting qi disturbances of xu [虛] (vacuity) and shi [實] (repletion) to regulate the body. This theme will be explored in chapter four in the examination of how different models of acupuncture practice have evolved that employ the concepts of qi and the jingmai differently.

## Qi movements in the mai-jingmai

While qi was described in relation to the mai and jingmai, the descriptions of its movements in the pre-Neijing and Neijing texts were varied. Lo argues that in the pre-Neijing texts the movement of qi is not limited to the mai alone.[37] Further, there are passages that suggest varied opinions or ideas about how and in what direction qi moves in the mai. The "Maishu" [脈書] of the

"Zhangjiashan" [張家山] texts describes: "The vessels are something the sage prizes. As for vapor, it benefits the lower part (of the body), and harms the upper part; it follows warmth and departs from coolness.[38] Thus the sage has a cold head and warm feet.[39] To treat ailments, take away the surplus and increase what is insufficient" [20:81]. Harper suggests that with the vertical alignment of the mai in the pre-Neijing texts the Yinshu [引書] and the Maifa [經法] which have clear discussions of movement of qi in each that this movement was not in an interconnected circuit but was instead probably from head to feet citing the passage "the sage has a cold head and warm feet" [20:86]. Harper describes a parallel discussion of downward moving qi on a twelve sided jade block dating from the late fourth early third century BCE [20:125, see also 37]. The jade block is inscribed with phrases that describe breathing techniques to help develop qi. The text is translated as

> Swallow, then it travels; travelling, it extends; extending, it descends; descending, it stabilizes; stabilizing, it solidifies; solidifying, it sprouts; sprouting, it grows; growing, it returns; returning, it is heaven. Heaven –its root is above; earth –its root is below. Follow the pattern and live, go against it and die [20:126].

Thus, in what seems to have been an important description of qi movements in relation to breathing, we find a downward movement, that while not limited to the mai, certainly sets precedence for ideas about qi movements in the body. Lo also explores the role of breathe as a treatment method to guide the qi for relief of pain, citing descriptions in the Yinshu, suggesting that the movements of qi were certainly at least in part guided by breathing techniques and that these may have influenced descriptions of the mai [35].

In the pre-Neijing texts of the Mawangdui there are also clear descriptions of a kind of centripetal movement in the mai, where, rather than a circulation, there is a movement towards the centre of the body (see Table 2). In none of the pre-Neijing texts do we find description of a circulation or circuit for qi movement within the mai [17, 20].

The Neijing itself is a compilation of many ideas from different times. Within the Neijing there are clearly older and later portions [26, 69, see also discussions of the passage about needling from Lingshu one translated and discussed by Chace and Bensky [11] in chapter five] and the text exhibits different competing influences and parallel developments [69]. There is evidence that the pre-Neijing texts of the Mawangdui and Zhangjiashan provided influences for the development of different ideas and models. So it should not be surprising that when we read the Neijing descriptions of the jingmai and

**Table 2: Pathways/Directions of the mai and jingmai[i]**

| | Zubi shiyimai jiujing* | Yinyang shiyimai jiujing* | Lingshu 17 Nanjing 23 | Lingshu 10** |
|---|---|---|---|---|
| Arm yin | hand > chest | hand > chest (or shoulder) | hand > chest | chest > hand |
| Arm yang | hand > head | hand > head (except taiyang head > hand) | hand > head | hand > head |
| Leg yin | foot > thigh or abdomen | foot > abdomen (except taiyin abdomen > foot) | foot > chest | foot > chest |
| Leg yang | foot > head | foot > thigh, head | foot > head | head > foot |

qi movements that we find a number of different descriptions that appear to be contradictory,[40] which later settle out as a commonly accepted circulatory system model with a standard description of qi flow.

For example chapter seventeen of the Lingshu and even chapter twenty-three of the Nanjing describe very similar centripetal movements of qi in the jingmai probably influenced by texts such as those found in the Mawangdui site [20, 68:298] (see Table 2). However the more widely accepted model is one of a continuous circulation through the jingmai in a specific sequence. Citing Suwen thirty-nine which states "The flow in the conduit vessels (jing-mai) does not stop. It circulates without break", Unschuld states that we have the first reference to a circulation in the jingmai, but, as he points out, the Suwen does not specify what is flowing in the jingmai [69:175]. It is in Lingshu chapter fifteen, where a continuous qi circulation is proposed that we start to get clarification of what is flowing in the jingmai. This was further reinforced as the basic model upon which diagnosis and treatment is to be focused starting in Nanjing chapter one.[41] Lingshu chapter fifteen and Nan-jing chapter one detailed this in relation to the circulation of a subset of qi, the "ying qi" [營氣] nutritive qi which is said to be localised in the jingmai

i.(After Unschuld [68:298])

* while the vessels contain qi and move, there is no mention of a circulation between them.

** the channels explicitly circulate the yingqi [營氣] nutritive qi, in a continuous circuit, as described in Lingshu fifteen and Nanjing one: lung > large intestine > stomach > spleen > heart > small intestine > bladder > kidney > pericardium > triple burner > gallbladder > liver > lung and so on.

and continuously circulating through the twelve channels, where it is propelled by the breath [44:29-31, 68:65-79] and closely related to astronomical cycles [35].[42] This model additionally included the contrast of the yingqi with the weiqi [衛氣] protective qi;[43] Lingshu eighteen tells us how the yingqi circulates within the jingmai while the weiqi circulates outside the jingmai, and how "They circulate without a break. [After] fifty [passages they have] another great meeting" [69:176].

This model rose to a position of great influence within the field of acupuncture following the Nanjing's systematic elaboration of the model within the framework of yinyang, five phase theories. While the Suwen and Lingshu had descriptions of this approach, they were not so systematic due to the nature of those texts as compilations of many ideas which were at times contradictory. The Nanjing is generally seen as being more systematic and Unschuld identifies this as a kind of pinnacle in the development of the "Theory of Systematic Correspondences" [67, 68, 69]. This model of qi circulation thus became for many that practice acupuncture the target of diagnosis and treatment. Pulse diagnosis, palpation of the radial arteries, became the principle method for understanding the state of this circulation[44] and for identifying where and how it might have gone wrong.[45] The principle target of treatment became the correction of this circulation using fine needles to influence the qi in the channels focusing on the use of bu [補] supplementation/tonification technique where xu [虛] vacuity/depletion/deficiency is found and xie [寫] draining technique where shi [實] repletion/excess is found. Thus as we look to how the qi and jingmai concepts influenced the practice of acupuncture we will find traditions that have tried to adhere more closely to this model. But, we will also find other traditions of practice that evolved different approaches using as justification other ideas and passages from the early medical literature.

In textbox 1 we have proposed a way of thinking about the seemingly contradictory passages about the jingmai and movement of qi in them from Lingshu fifteen, Nanjing one and Lingshu seventeen, Nanjing twenty-three. We have tried to account for a number of evolving concepts in relation to how an understanding of physiology developed and how the natural influences of heaven and earth may have been seen.

Since the qi is said to be propelled through the jingmai by the breath, it is natural to ask what about before birth? Lingshu chapter ten addresses this question in a cursory manner "[After labour when the] gu [grains] come into the stomach, the vessel-meridian pathways are [all] connected, the blood and qi [begin to] move" [49:154].[46] This text is generally understood to imply that the flow of qi and blood within the jingmai start after birth –which makes

**Box 1 – speculations on heaven-earth influences on the jingmai**

We can speculate on the possible role of different influences in how the different models of flow of qi in the mai and jingmai arose. When the arms are raised above the head, the yang jingmai are all see to run downwards, half from finger tips to the head half from the head to the toes, while the yin jingmai are all seen to run upwards, half from the toes to the torso and half from the torso to the finger tips. In the model we have suggested where the compound term jingmai may have been intended to describe the flow of energy from heaven and earth in a mutual movement to create the human being, we see an interesting possibility. In this standing posture heaven's energies would flow downward in the same manner as the yang jingmai while earth's energies would flow upwards like the yin jingmai. This two way flow of energies could also help explain why the twelve jingmai are paired as, for example arm taiyang and leg taiyang or leg taiyin and arm taiyin. The pairing gives a kind of continuity of the flow. This also fits to the idea from Suwen sixty-eight "Above tianshu (tianshu, ST-25 is an acupoint level with and to either side of the navel –a natural axis between upper and lower body halves) is controlled by heaven qi, below tianshu is controlled by earth qi" [49:72]. Taking this logic a step further, it is not unreasonable to see the development of the circulation model as a kind of synthesis of these mutual movements. Further, the centripetal flow of the mai in the pre-Neijing texts and of some Neijing (Lingshu 17), Nanjing (Nanjing 23) passages may have been related to the idea that the mai/jingmai on the arms are more yang and related to heaven's downward flow while the mai/jingmai on the legs are more yin and related to earth's upward flow (in this standing posture with arms raised above the head). That the description of these different flows appear contradictory does not imply anything wrong. As we discussed in chapter one, 'either-or' type thinking was not usual in historical Chinese texts, apparent contradictory statements normally co-existed without problem [8]. Besides the centripetal descriptions may relate more to how the body is influenced by or resonating with some of the energies of heaven and earth, while the circulation flow, which runs through the internal organs, may relate more to the body's normal circulation which is a synthesis of bodily, functional, heavenly and earthly influences. What circulates is the product of normal physiology and its interactions with the energies of heaven and earth. What runs centripetally are additional, non-physiological influences from heaven and earth, which would naturally act to align, order or regulate the body. We see further evidence for this simple distinction with the shu-transport xue or acupoints system on the arms and legs, which describe an analogous water flow running from fingers to elbows and toes to knees. This system of acupoints is very important in acupuncture, they are used to help regulate the body; these same acupoints appear later in the biorhythmic literatures as influential treatment points based on cyclical actions of heaven (the ten stems) and earth (the twelve branches) in the ziwuliuzhu system of the najiafa [32], see chapter four [6].

sense since the theory of the Lingshu and later texts such as the Nanjing is that qi flow is propelled by breathing,[47] and the production of the yingqi said to circulate in the jingmai is from the stomach.[48] One obvious implication of this is that the jingmai are probably not in a mature state before and for a period after birth since they appear not to have functioned before then. This has led some to speculate that in babies and small children the jingmai and its system of acupoints are in a different state than in adults and that thus treatment needs to be different [5]. We have not found much discussion of this theme and thus will not pursue it further here.

## Qi flow –the hydrological analogy

There is considerable evidence that the descriptions of movements of qi in the jingmai were based on a water flow analogy [17, 20, 39, 69] which had become generally influential in Chinese thinking [1, 62]. The flow of water is unidirectional (like the later models of the jingmai), when water does not flow it can cause problems. This latter idea has found various expressions: The Maishu text of the Zhangjiashan manuscripts perhaps of the second century BCE states: "Now, the reason why flowing water does not become putrid and the doorway pivot is not devoured by bugs is because they move. By moving, you fill the limbs and empty the depots. When the five depots are empty, the jade body will benefit" [20:144]. The relevance of this becomes perhaps clearer with an earlier reference from the Lushi Chunqiu [吕氏春秋] (circa mid third century BCE) "The reason why flowing water does not become putrid and the doorway pivot is not devoured by bugs is because they move. The form and vapor (qi) are also thus. If the form does not move, the essence does not flow. If the essence does not flow, the vapor clogs" [20:145]. With these pre-existing analogous ideas it seems natural that movements in the jingmai should be seen related to a hydrological analogy [17]. Other evidence for this can be seen in the descriptions of the mechanics and timing of actions in needling techniques aimed at influencing the qi in particular ways. While the descriptions we find were not intended as descriptions of how qi flows, we can, using an understanding of water flow and wave movements, interpret these descriptions using a hydrological analogy.

We have already seen that the Lingshu and Nanjing both propose that qi is propelled in the jingmai by the breath, but these descriptions do not allow a clear imaging of the flow. We have already mentioned (see endnote 28) that Lingshu chapter twelve draws the analogy between the twelve jingmai of the body and the twelve great rivers of China [44:23, 49:134, 67:82]. Mirroring a passage in Lingshu seventeen,[49] Nanjing thirty-seven has an explicit discussion using the flow of water analogy for the flow of qi in the jingmai "The passage of the influences (qi) is like the flow of water, it never comes to rest" [68:388] while Huang Fumi in his Zhenjiu Jiayijing [鍼灸甲乙經] makes a similar analogy "Qi never fails to circulate. It circulates forever like the flow of water or the sun and moon" [74:103]. Thus we see water flow analogies for the jingmai and flow of qi. There are other passages that more indirectly imply this or at least can be interpreted in light of this analogy.

In several places in the Neijing and Nanjing subtle aspects of needling are discussed that mention how the practitioner must feel or divine the movements of the qi.[50] Some of these passages allude to the "coming and goings" of the qi[51] and how the timing of needle insertion,[52] needle removal[53] or other actions[54] must follow these. Often the texts and later commentaries describe these as being difficult tasks that only the superior physician or one who knows what they are doing can do.[55] We thus find clear discussions about how the qi comes and goes, like an ebb and flow which can be understood through an extension of the hydrological analogy. It is possible that the imagery is like a wave breaking and running up the beach, one feels it arrive and then withdraw. But this seems improbable since it would imply that before the wave arrives and after it leaves there is no qi. It seems more reasonable to see this in a different hydrological analogy as like the waves that move across the surface of water. The jingmai itself is the river which has a certain flow and movement of water within it, across its surface are waves that can be felt to come and go in the sense of rising and falling. Understanding what is meant by the "qizhi" [氣至] the "arrival of qi" which is essential for the needling to be effective,[56] is touched on in chapters four and five, but it is unlikely it refers to the notion of going from the state of "no qi" to that of "having qi", rather of going to an increased state of qi with the needling. We feel it reasonable to interpret the various discussions of the "coming and going" of qi in these passages on needling as like the rising and falling levels of water as a wave passes through. This interpretation is reinforced by discussions of how one should approach the acupoint and prepare it so as to encourage the qi to arrive;[57] the act of touching creates a change in qi movements that can be taken advantage of just as touching the surface of water can create changes that promote this wave like motion and which can then be detected and responded to with appropriately timed actions.

Here in this chapter we have discussed the flow of qi in the jingmai. Chapter four will return to discussions of the different types of qi flow in the body [6], including the weiqi [衛氣] protective qi,[58] that occur within, outside of and in relation to the jingmai. Also, the description of needling techniques found in the Nanjing imply a conceptual model that appears to link weiqi and yingqi in a different way.[59] But since this model is linked to the needling techniques of the Nanjing, the contrast of these with the images of needling technique found in the Neijing can also be found in chapter four [6]. In the appendix to this chapter we return to the theme of qi circulation in the jingmai, where we discuss questions about this circulatory model.

## The jing and mai a comparison of various jing and mai structures

The transition of mai as vessels that contain and conduct blood and qi into a system of interconnected jingmai that provide a continuous circulation of qi through the interconnected network appears to have arisen concurrently with descriptions of the luomai [絡脈], the "connecting" or "network" vessels. The first treatise to describe the twelve jingmai, Lingshu ten also describes the fifteen luomai. The jingmai run vertically in the body and the luomai horizontally.[60] While other branches and trajectories of the luomai are given, the primary role seems to be to interconnect the jingmai so that a continuous circulation of qi can occur. For example the qi that flows through the hand taiyin (lung) jingmai flows to the hand yangming (large intestine) jingmai via a luomai that passes from the hand taiyin jingmai to the hand yangming jingmai. The system of the luomai thus interconnect the twelve jingmai at the extremities on the arms and legs. At the very end of the primary treatise on the jingmai and luomai, in Lingshu chapter ten it says [人經不同脈亦所別也]. This literally says "Jingmai are not the same, luomai are also (not the same)". This has been understood and interpreted in quite different ways,[61] but it seems to imply that the jingmai may not have been thought of as being the same in different people, or at the very least that the jingmai exhibit individual differences between people. If the primary treatise on the jingmai ends with a statement about this implicit variability of the jingmai, it is understandable why later authors such as Huang Fumi might want to try to standardise things by codifying the descriptions more systematically and clearly.

Descriptions of jing and mai in the Neijing do not stop with the systematisation of the jingmai and luomai, other categories of jing and mai are given. Some of these do not appear to have developed or been used beyond their description in the Neijing (eg the "jingshui"), some exhibit on and off developments and uses (eg the "jingjin" and "jingbie") while others exhibit later development and elaboration (eg the "qijingbamai"), see Table 3 for a listing.

**Table 3: various systems of jing and mai**

| **Jing and mai structures** | **Relevant Neijing chapters** | **Examples of modern uses** |
|---|---|---|
| 12 Jingmai – 12 channel vessels [經脈] | Lingshu 10 | a |
| 15 Luomai – 15 network vessels [絡脈] | Lingshu 10 | b |
| 12 Jingbie – 12 channel divergences [經別] | Lingshu 11 | c |
| 12 Jingjin – 12 channel sinews [經筋] | Lingshu 13 | d |
| 12 Jingshui – 12 water channels [經水] | Lingshu 12 | e |
| 8 Qijingbamai – 8 extraordinary vessels [奇經八脈] | Suwen 44, 60; Lingshu 2, 10, 11, 17, 21, 33, 38, 62, 65 | f |
| Numerous sunluomai – 'grandchild' luo vessels[62] [孫絡脈] | Lingshu 17 | |

a. Many traditions: *Chinese* –[3, 13, 70]; *Japanese* –[19, 25, 46, 59]; *European* –[63].
b. [25, 70].
c. [25, 58].
d. [46].
e. Except as theoretical constructs we are unaware of any practical applications.
f. Using the Zhenjiu Daquan tradition with the eight acupoints (for history see [48]): [3, 13, 46, 50, 63, 70].
Using a Lishizhen based approach [12] of needling pathway points [25].

It is interesting to note that in this elaboration of channels and vessels, some are named as mai –"vessels" (jingmai, luomai, sunluomai, qijingbamai) while others are named as jing –"channels" (jingbie, jingjin, jingshui). What is intended by this distinction in naming? In the historical literature descriptions of the jingmai include the idea of qi circulation. The luomai and sunluomai as adjuncts to this circulation are also considered to include circulating qi. But in none of the historical texts examined has a circulation of qi been described for the jingbie, jingjin, or qijingbamai.[63] Thus on the basis of this we can suppose that all of these mai and jing contain qi in some form, but only the jingmai/luomai have a circulation of qi. It is also unclear what kind of qi is contained in each of these different mai/jing. The absence of clear statements about this is curious since the Neijing tries to make clear statements about and distinctions within the body and its physiology. For example, why do the system of jingbie still, to this day, remain obscure with regards what they are supposed to contain and what their function is? With the system of qijingbamai, we see an evolution of the system, as it gradually became more and more articulated with the fullest accounts appearing in the Ming dynasty.[64]

## The jingmai-luomai-sunluomai as protective boundaries

The Neijing has several discussions of how environmental "xieqi" [邪氣] evil qi (such as wind, damp, cold) enter the body [69:171-173]. Two of these descriptions (Suwen sixty-three and thirty-one) describe these penetrations in relation to the channel system. Suwen chapter sixty-three gives the following interesting account of how xieqi from the environment penetrates into the body. It does so in stages and at each stage if the body's healthy qi cannot drive it back out, it then penetrates deeper. The jingmai, luomai and sunluomai play important roles in these defensive layers: first it comes to the skin and body hair level:

> It stays there [for a while] and does not leave. Then it enters [further] and lodges in the tertiary vessels (sunluomai). It stays there [for a while] and does not leave. Then it enters [further] and lodges in the network vessels (luomai). It stays there [for a while] and does not leave. Then it enters [further] and lodges in the conduit vessels (jingmai). It links up with the five depots (zang) internally and spreads into the intestines and stomach [69:171].

While the "weiqi", "protective qi" is supposed to help protect the body from these environmental influences, the qi circulatory system of the jingmai-luomai itself also appears to play this protective role. Presumably the increasingly deeper penetration of the xieqi described in this Suwen passage is not automatic but is the result of the inability of the body to drive it out. Many translators render the Suwen passage a little differently by adding the term "if" in front of each expression "it stays there", "if it stays there [for a while] and does not leave... then it enters [further]" [see for example 73:293]. This interpretation implies that somehow the sunluomai, luomai and jingmai are involved in efforts to drive out or expel the invading xieqi. How this is accomplished is not clearly stated, but it has led some modern practitioners to see the qi circulating channel system (jingmai-luomai-sunluomai) as being a kind of protective layer for the body [66:59 + 81]. This passage from Suwen sixty-three also implies that the luomai were seen as being more superficial than the jingmai, an idea also found in Lingshu ten in a discussion of the differences between the jingmai and luomai. The jingmai are not visible while the luomai are frequently visible, especially when in a full state,[65] the condition of the jingmai is determined by feeling the radial pulses, while the luomai being more superficial are visible [73:570]. The descriptions of the luomai found in the Lingshu and some of the treatments of them by bloodletting [71:409] have led some commentators to suggest that they are related to the blood vessels visible at the surface of the body.

## Jingmai –organ connections

As medical traditions emerged out of the late Warring States –early Han dynasty period, it was necessary to have a developed physiological understanding of the body that allowed physicians to grasp something about the nature of what was occurring and be able to make practical decisions about what to do about it. This required that a refinement of the concept of qi be made, specifically that it be subdivided into numerous subsets and labeled according to where it was and what it was doing. Thus the concept of qi evolved from a unified undifferentiated concept[66] into a multi differentiated concept [4, 14, 29, 55].[67] The concepts of the jingmai –channels and their corresponding zang-fu– organ systems seem to have developed in part at least as a response to this practical need. While in the pre-Neijing texts from Mawangdui and Zhangjiashan there are some references associating the mai to some internal organs, this was by no means thorough, systematic or complete.[68] As one of the primary goals during the medical developments of the Neijing was to create a more thorough and systematic knowledge of physiology, we can also suggest the transition of the mai to jingmai in the Neijing was in part an effort to capture and provide a basis for such elaborated discussions. In her arguments about the role of touch in the development of early medical literature [23], Hsu demonstrates that in his cases from the Shiji [史記] Chunyu Yi [淳于意] (circa 154 BCE) not only directly perceived qi in the mai through touch but also that "the tactile exploration of the mai leads to the recognition of qi coming from the viscera" [23:22]. In other words in some of the early medical literature we find theory and practical applications developing suggestive of a connection between the mai palpated at the body surface and the qi of the internal organs.[69]

Hsu also suggests that in the Neijing we find an increasing recognition of the connection between the emotions and corresponding organs and that perhaps the palpation of the mai described in the earlier Maifa and by Chunyu Yi allowed access to information about the condition of related organs via the qi-emotion relationships [23:24-25]. Since emotions were also associated with disordered movements of qi –see discussions in the previous chapter [8], the jingmai may be seen as providing a further link between disturbances of the qi flowing in the jingmai and their associations to the internal organs. This may have been another factor related to the transition from mai to jingmai and the more elaborated connections of jingmai with the internal organs.

It is also possible to see this interlinking between the internal physiology of the body and its functional structures, the organs, with the outside and surface of the body through the use of the name "jingmai". Harper analyses the etymological evidence for the origin of "mai" from the Shuowen Jiezi. The term "mai" [脈] in the Shuowen Jiezi is glossed as "water angling and flowing separately" and is related to a cognate "yong" [永] which is often used interchangeably with "mai" and is glossed in the Shuowen Jiezi as "water which is long, it depicts the long extension of the network of subterranean channels" [20:83]. In the last definition "subterranean channels" is the term "jing" [巠] which is the right half of the character for jing [經]. In this analysis, not only does the term "mai" imply a flow of water and through its cognate, a deeper flow of water channels, but within this we find the right hand half of the term "jing" [經]. The use of the fused term jingmai [經脈] thus could be seen to capture the extended image in physiology of the surface vessels connecting to the internal physiological systems of the organs (zang-fu). Perhaps further evidence of this can be seen in how the first use of the term jingmai is found in the Neijing texts coinciding with the appearance of the elaborated and systematic literature on the zang-fu and the systematic interlinking of the jingmai with corresponding organs. Table 4 lists the jingmai –organ correspondences. However the links between the jingmai and internal organs developed, there is a systematic description of these links found in the Neijing corpus.

## Jingmai and the xue [穴] acupoints

In the early medical literature of the Huangdi Neijing we not only find the first mention and description of the system of jingmai, their associated structures such as the luomai, and a continuous circulation of qi, but it is here that we find first mention of discrete locations on the jingmai as targets of treatment, the "xue" [穴] or acupoints.[70] Citing various numbers probably based on shushu, calculations and arts, Suwen chapter nine describes how the person has three hundred and sixty-five acupoints [see 73:57] while the actual number of named acupoints in the Nejing was far less than that and even today has not reached this idealized

**Table 4: Jingmai –zangfu correlations**

| jingmai | Zang | Fu | jingmai |
|---|---|---|---|
| arm taiyin | fei [肺] lung | dachang [大肠] large intestine | arm yangming |
| leg taiyin | pi [脾] spleen | wei [胃] stomach | leg yangming |
| arm shaoyin | xin [心] heart | xiaochang [小肠] small intestine | arm taiyang |
| leg shaoyin | shen [肾] kidney | pangguang [膀胱] bladder | leg taiyang |
| arm jueyin | xinbao [心包] | sanjiao [三焦] triple burner | arm shaoyang |
| leg jueyin | gan [肝] liver | dan [胆] gallbladder | leg shaoyang |

number of three hundred and sixty-five –see chapter four for more details. The passage does not use the term "xue" or "acupoint" but is understood to refer to them since a parallel passage in Suwen fifty-eight explicitly mentions the three hundred and sixty-five acupoints and their relationship to the year [69:166]. The importance of this passage from Suwen fifty-eight is that it not only provides corroborative evidence for the interpretation of the shushu numerological (calculations and arts) descriptions in Suwen nine, but associates the acupoints explicitly to the system of minute branch vessels, the sunluo: "The 365 holes of the meeting points of the tertiary network [vessels], they, too, correspond to a year" [69:166]. This is an important association which gives novel insights into the nature of the acupoints. This is discussed further in chapter four [6].

It is important to recognise that descriptions of the acupoints come only after the earlier vessels or mai had been upgraded to the more complete system of "jingmai".[71] Thus there is likely to be an important relationship between the nature of the acupoints, the jingmai, qi and needling. In fact the acupoints were defined by nature as being related to the movements of qi rather than anatomical structures.[72] This theme is discussed further in chapter four, the chapter on acupuncture, qi and the jingmai as the acupoints become relevant in the practice of acupuncture.

## Conclusion

In this chapter we have traced the development of the "jingmai" from earlier conceptions of "mai" as (blood) vessels, to "mai" as a kind of primitive physiological system, to "mai" as trajectories or locations in which are found qi and blood (xue [血]) which are responsible for one's health and physiology, and are targets of treatment by moxa or lancing. Next we looked at "jingmai" as trajectories in which the qi (and blood) flow, connecting to the internal organ systems and to each other in a continuous circulation with treatment predominantly by use of metal needles. We briefly examined qi movements within the jingmai. The jingmai are deeply embedded in the theory of systematic correspondence and its attending theories, cosmologies and influenced by other convergent traditions such as the yangsheng theories and techniques. At each stage of development we have seen how efforts to capture physiology became more comprehensive, eventually evolving to places from which one can influence the body's internal workings and eventually as a primary target of diagnosis and treatment. Connections to related organs, the acupoints that lie on the jingmai and the variety of "jing" and "mai" were briefly examined as developments out of emergent jingmai theory. The jingmai represent an extension of the mai concept to a circulatory system that not only regulates and maintains a healthier inner state or functions but also serves to protect from outside influences. Throughout this sequence of changes we have also seen that the concept of qi has played a central and later pivotal role for understanding these different aspects and stages. The novel development of the concept of the jingmai in the Neijing texts can be traced to numerous converging influences with multiple implied and explicit intentions. A full accounting of the development of the jingmai is not yet possible.

## Appendix one

Lingshu chapter fifteen describes the circulation of qi in the twelve jingmai in a continuous circuit as follows:

> As the heavens turn around 28 lodges [宿], each lodge is 36 divisions; the human qi moves one revolution of one thousand and eight divisions, and the sun moves through twenty-eight lodges. The human circulation tracts (jingmai), upper, lower, left, right anterior and posterior amount to 28, and they encircle the body, sixteen zhang and two chi long (37 metres), in order to correspond to the 28 lodges, and to 100 clepsydra divisions, dividing day and night. Thus with one human exhalation,

> there are two movements [of the pulse] in the channels and qi moves three "cun" inches; with one inhalation, there are two movements [of the pulse] in the channels and the qi moves three "cun" inches... with thirteen thousand five hundred breaths, the qi moves fifty ying (circuits) in the body in 100 clepsydra (water clock) divisions, and the sun moves through twenty eight lodges; as the water in the clepsydra empties, it has traveled throughout [the body]... [42].

Here we see the circulation of qi related to the twenty-eight astronomical divisions [宿] lodges or mansions through which the sun is seen to move one cycle in the course of one day (due to the rotation of the earth). The qi moves in relation to the pulse movements and breath. The total length of the system of jingmai (sixteen zhang and three chi) is traversed by the qi fifty times a day during the course of thirteen thousand five hundred breaths. Vivienne Lo clearly shows the relationships between the jingmai, qi movements within them and astronomical, astrological systems [42]. Cause-effect relationships between the jingmai, qi movements, the twenty-eight lodges and the breath are not linear in an ordinary Western sense of relationships. The system of qi movements in the jingmai was conceived to begin with in part due to the complex relationships of many things [35, 40, 42]. What do these numerical relationships refer to? Clearly these numbers are not intended to take into account "normal" breathing and daily activities, they are a kind of numerological ideal based on the ever present systems of shushu [數術] [40, 42]. It seems likely that these relationships are more than an ideological description intended to convey an understanding of broader theories of physiology, rather they convey an experience of some sort. If so, then what? Since the description of qi circulation is one of making 50 rounds through the jingmai so that it moves a certain distance every day and is propelled by rhythmic breathing, then the numbers of breath may relate to some idealized pattern of breathing that enables the person practicing it to achieve an ideal physiological state. Given that in daily life breathing varies considerably during the day with different activities, it makes sense to see this breathing pattern as based on a kind of yangsheng breath cultivation practice as part of a meditation practice. When one cultivates one's breath so as to breathe in this way a kind of ideal condition of qi movement maybe established that aids the person practicing the techniques in terms of their own cultivation and health. It is helpful to recall what Lo says of breath cultivation techniques from the pre-Neijing texts: "Mawangdui breath cultivation texts confirm that the aim of breath cultivation is to move qi. So we can assume that the implicit object of breath cultivation in Yinshu is to resolve pain by means of different techniques to move qi through the body" [35]. In more recent publications Lo is more explicit about the notion of the earlier mai concepts; in a detailed analysis of the possible relationship of the Mianyang figurine to the mai discussed in other contexts, she states it may be "a model of perfect physiology, a plan for the movement of qi in breath cultivation, so well described in the Mawangdui and Zhangjiashan breath cultivation" [41:404]. Is the description of qi movements in the jingmai in relation to breath in Lingshu fifteen an extension of the notion that with the proper breathing techniques (of for example the Yinshu) one can get the qi to move so as to help correct health problems? If so, does this not then imply that naturally normal breathing has little or insufficient effect on qi movements so as to help correct health problems? If so, then this further supports the interpretation that the circulation of qi model in Lingshu fifteen does not refer to normal physiology, rather an idealized conceptual model of it. Perhaps the qi does not move as such in the jingmai during the course of a day, rather it can be made to flow when appropriate breathing or needling techniques are applied. Is the circulation of qi model in the Lingshu and Nanjing more based on the syncretistic inclusionist tendencies of East Asian historical thinking? Where the notion of the mai which contain blood that moves was extended to the broader concept of the "jingmai" so that by extension the jingmai must also have movement within them, and the thing that moves is the newly stressed concept or qi. Extending the model to reflect broader astrological and meteorological models gives the qi movements a circulatory nature. Of course, we cannot say for sure, but it makes sense to discuss this as it will have profound impact on any scientific investigation of the jingmai and qi. First, without a clear model or series of reasonable alternate interpretive models, any scientific "measurements" may be completely irrelevant. Second, it may be that circulation as such does not happen *unless* one applies an appropriate technique to the jingmai such as needling or a breathing technique. Third, even if no measurements of the jingmai ever reveal a "circulation" that matches the historical descriptions, it does not necessarily invalidate them, rather it confirms a non-ontological description of them.

## Bibliography

1- Allan S. *The Way of Water and Sprouts of Virtue*. Albany, State University of New York, 1997.
2- Ames RT, Hall DL. *A Philosophical Translation: Dao De Jing –making this life significant*, New York, Ballantine Books, 2003.
3- Anon. *Essentials of Chinese Acupuncture*. Beijing, Foreign Languages Press, 1980.
4- Birch S. Filling the whole in acupuncture. Part 1:1 What are we doing in the sup-

plementation needle technique? *European J Oriental Medicine*, 2009:6(2):25-35. Part 1:2, 2009:6(3):18-27.

5- Birch S. *Shonishin –Japanese Children's Needle Therapy*. Stuttgart, Thieme Medical Publishers, 2011.

6- Birch S. Chapter four: The Jingmai and qi –acupuncture perspectives. In this volume.

7- Birch S, Bovey M. Chapter eight: Qi, Jingmai –Scientific investigation of concepts based in traditional East Asian medicine: challenges to cross-paradigm research. In this volume.

8- Birch S, Cabrer Mir MA, Rodriguez M. Chapter one: Qi and the mind –explorations of the links between qi, the mind, mental and emotional states. In this volume.

9- Birch S, Felt R. *Understanding Acupuncture*, Edinburgh, Churchill Livingstone, 1999.

10- Chace C. On greeting a friend, an approach to needle technique. *Lantern*. 2006:3(3):4-7.

11- Chace C, Bensky D. Chapter five: An axis of efficacy –The range of meaning in chapter one of the Lingshu. In this volume.

12- Chace C, Shima M. *Exposition on the Eight Extraordinary Vessels*, Seattle, Eastland Press, 2010.

13- Cheng XN. *Chinese Acupuncture and Moxibustion*. Beijing, Foreign Languages Press, 1987.

14- Chiu ML. *Mind, body, and illness in a Chinese medical tradition*. Ph.D. thesis, Harvard University, 1986.

15- Cook CA. Ancestor worship during the Eastern Zhou. In J Langerwey, M Kalinowski (eds). *Early Chinese Religion*, Leiden, Brill, 2009, pages 237-279.

16- Csikszentmihalyi M. *Material Virtue: ethics and the body in early China*. Brill, Leiden, 2004.

17- Daly NP. *Hybridizing the human body: The hydrological development of acupuncture in early Imperial China*. Masters thesis, Department of East Asian Studies, McGill University, 1999.

18- Engelhardt U. Neue archaologische funde zur leitbahntheorie. *Chin Med*. 1998;13:93-100.

19- Fukushima K. *Meridian Therapy*, Tokyo, Toyo Hari Medical Association, 1991.

20- Harper D. *Early Chinese Medical Literature: the Mawangdui Medical Manuscripts*. London, Kegan Paul, 1998.

21- He ZC, Lo V. The Channels: A preliminary examination of a Lacquered Figurine from the Western Han Period. *Early China* 1996;21:81-124.

22- Hsu E. In Hsu E, (ed). Pulse diagnostics in the Western Han: how mai and qi determine bing. *Innovation in Chinese Medicine*, Cambridge, Cambridge University Press, 2001:51-91.

23- Hsu E. Tactility and the body in early Chinese medicine. *Science in Context*, 2005:18(1):7-34.

24- Hsu E. *Pulse Diagnosis in Early Chinese Medicine The telling touch*, Cambridge, Cambridge University Press, 2010.

25- Irie T. *Keiketsu Keikin Kikeiryoho*, Yokosuka, Ido no Nippon, 1982.

26- Keegan J. *The Huang-ti nei-ching: the Structure of the Compilation; the Significance of the Structure*, doctoral diss. Berkeley; University of California, 1988.
27- Kuriyama S. *The Expressiveness of the Body and the Divergence of Greek and Chinese Medicine*, New York, Zone Books 1999.
28- Larre C, Rochat de la Vallee. *Rooted in Spirit*, New York, Station Hill Press, 1995.
29- Larre C, Rochat de la Vallee E. *Essence, Spirit, Blood and Qi*, London, Monkey Press, 1999.
30- Levi J. The rite, the norm and the Dao: philosophy of sacrifice and transcendence of power in ancient China. In J Langerwey, M Kalinowski (eds). *Early Chinese Religion*, Leiden, Brill, 2009, pages 645-692.
31- Lewis ME. *The Construction of Space in Early China*. Albany, SUNY Press, 2006.
32- Liu BQ. *Optimum Time for Acupuncture*; Jinan, Shandong Science and Technology Press, 1988.
33- Lloyd G. The techniques of persuasion and the rhetoric of disorder in late Zhanguo and Western Han texts. In Nylan M, Loewe M (eds). *China's Early Empires –A Re-appraisal*, Cambridge, Cambridge University Press, 2010, pages 451-460.
34- Lo V. *The influence of yangsheng culture on early Chinese medical theory*. University of London, doctoral thesis 1998.
35- Lo V. Tracking the Pain: Jue and the Formation of a Theory of Circulating Qi through the Channels. *Sudhoffs Archiv*, 1999, pages 191-211.
36- Lo V. The influence of nurturing life culture on the development of Western Han acumoxa therapy. In Hsu E, (ed). *Innovation in Chinese Medicine*, Cambridge, Cambridge University Press, 2001:19-50.
37- Lo V. Spirit of Stone: Technical Considerations in the Treatment of the Jade Body. *Bulletin of the School of Oriental and African Studies*, University of London, 2002; 65:1:99-128
38- Lo V. Introduction. In Lu GD, Needham J. *Celestial Lancets*, London, Routledge Curzon, 2nd edition, 2002, pages xxv-li.
39- Lo V. Huangdi Hama jing 'The Yellow Emperor's Toad Manual' in a special edition of Asia Major, 2001;14(2):61-99, edited by Nathan Sivin: Essays Contributed in Honour of Michael Loewe [published in Spring, 2004]. See also http://www.ihp.sinica.edu.tw/~medicine/ashm/lectures/Lo.pdf.
40- Lo V. The territory between life and death. *Medical History*, 2003, 47: 250-258.
41- Lo V. Imagining Practice: Sense and Sensuality in Early Chinese Medical Illustration. In: Bray F, Dorofeeva-Lichtmann V, Métailié G, (eds). *The Warp and the Weft: Graphics and Text in the Production of Technical Knowledge in China*. Leiden, Brill; 2007, pages 383–424.
42- Lo V. Heavenly bodies in early China: astro-physiology in context. In A Akasoy, C Burnett and R Yoeli-Tlalim (eds), *Astro-medicine: astrology and medicine, East and West*, Florence: Micrologus Library, 2008, pages 143-187.
43- Lo V, Li JM. Manuscripts, received texts and the healing arts. In Nylan M, Loewe M (eds). *China's early empires – a re-appraisal*. Cambridge, Cambridge university press, 2010, pages 367-397.
44- Lu GD, Needham J. *Celestial Lancets*; Cambridge, Cambridge University Press, 1980.

45- Major JS. *Heaven and Earth in Early Han Thought.* Albany, State University of New York Press, 1993.
46- Manaka Y, Itaya K, Birch S. *Chasing the Dragon's Tail*, Brookline, Paradigm Publications, 1995.
47- Matsumoto K, Birch S. *Five Elements and Ten Stems*, Brookline, Paradigm Publications 1983.
48- Matsumoto K, Birch S. *Extraordinary Vessels*, Brookline, Paradigm Publications, 1986.
49- Matsumoto K, Birch S. *Hara Diagnosis Reflections on the Sea*; Brookline, Paradigm Publications, 1988.
50- Nagatomo T. *Nagatomo MP Shinkyu Kuowa Hachiju Hachisyu*, Kyoto, Shinkyu Shinkuokaisha 1976.
51- Nylan M. Classics without canonization: learning and authority in Qin and Han. In J Langerwey, M Kalinowski (eds). *Early Chinese Religion*, Leiden, Brill, 2009, pages 721-776.
52- Poo MC. Ritual and ritual texts in early China. In J Langerwey, M Kalinowski (eds). *Early Chinese Religion*, Leiden, Brill, 2009, pages 281-313.
53- Porkert M. *The Theoretical Foundations of Chinese Medicine.* Cambridge, MIT Press, 1974.
54- Puett MJ. *To Become a God: cosmology, sacrifice, and self-divination in early China.* Cambridge, Harvard University Asia Center, 2002.
55- Rochat de la Vallée E. *A Study of Qi in Classical Texts*, London, Monkey Press, 2006.
56- Rochat de la Vallée E. *Wu Xing the Five Elements in Classical Chinese Texts*, London, Monkey Press, 2009.
57- Rodriguez M. Chapter six: Qi, jingmai, yaoyi –a study of their relationships. In this volume.
58- Shima M, Chace C. *Channel Divergences: Deeper Pathways of the Web*, Boulder, Blue Poppy Press, 2000.
59- Shudo D. *Introduction to Meridian Therapy*, Seattle, Eastland Press, 1990.
60- Sivin N. *Traditional Medicine in Contemporary China*, Ann Arbor, Centre for Chinese Studies, University of Michigan, 1987.
61- Sivin N. State, cosmos and body in the last three centuries BC. *Harvard J. Asiatic Studies.* 1995:55(1):5-37.
62- Slingerland E. *Effortless Action*, Oxford, Oxford University Press, 2003.
63- Soulie de Morant G. *Chinese Acupuncture.* Brookline, Paradigm Publications, 1994.
64- Sterckx R. *The Animal and the Daemon in Early China*, Albany, State University of New York, 2002.
65- Sunu K, Lee Y. *The Canon of Acupuncture: Huang Ti Nei Ching Ling Shu*, Seoul, Korea Acupuncture Society, 1985.
66- Toyohari Association. *Toyohari East Asian Needle Therapy: the study and practice of Toyohari.* European Branch of the Toyohari Association, Amsterdam 2010.
67- Unschuld PU. *Medicine in China: A History of Ideas*, Berkeley, University of California Press, 1985.

68- Unschuld PU. *Nan Ching: The Classic of Difficult Issues*, Berkeley, University of California Press, 1986.
69- Unschuld PU. *Huang Di Nei Jing Su Wen –nature, knowledge, imagery in an ancient Chinese medical text.* Berkeley, University of California Press, 2003.
70- Wang JY. *Applied Channel Theory in Chinese Medicine.* Seattle, Eastland Press, 2008.
71- Wiseman N, Feng Y. *A Practical Dictionary of Chinese Medicine*, Brookline, Paradigm Publications, 1997.
72- Wu JN. *The Spiritual Pivot*, Honolulu, University of Hawaii Press, 1993.
73- Wu NL, Wu AQ. *Yellow Emperor's Canon Internal Medicine*, Beijing, China Science and Technology Press, 1997.
74- Yang SZ, Chace C. *The Systematic Classic of Acupuncture and Moxibustion*, Boulder, Blue Poppy Press, 1994.

## Endnotes

1. In a parallel discussion Slingerland states "As we have seen, the rise of theories concerning the biological self and subsequent focus on the individual called for a reformulation of Confucius" vision in a way that would respond to the new state of the art in self cultivation technology, which in turn required addressing the specific functions of the heart/mind and the qi" [62:134].

2. References to "qi" in the "mai" are found in several of the Mawangdui texts [20:84] and Zhangjiashan texts [37], see also the summary discussions by Daly [17] of the Mawangdui and Zhangjiashan texts. Though some of the references are to the term "xueqi"[血氣], which can be seen as "blood-qi" or as "blood and qi".

3. See for example Suwen chapters five, nine, ten which describe how the mai, the vessels relate to the heart [69:119], Suwen chapters twenty-three and forty-four how the "heart rules the vessels" [69:133, 143], while Suwen sixty-one describes how the heart "stores the qi of the... vessels" [69:153].

4. After the Han dynasty an extensive literature on pulse diagnosis, "mai" began with the publication of the Nanjing (circa 100 CE) and especially following Wangshu He's "Maijing" [脈經] late third century CE. The term "mai" is thus often seen today as associated with this corpus of literature and the practice of pulse diagnosis.

5. In the Analects Confucius cautions about three things that the young, mature and elderly person must guard against to protect their qi and blood, thus clearly indicating that "Blood and qi were thus associated from the beginning with core aspects of a person's being" [27:103]. Given the influence of Confucian thinking on the early medical literature [67], it is not surprising that we see the focus on the conveyors of the blood and qi –the mai– in relation to core physiology.

6. There is a dispute about the dating of the Guanzi passage that likens water flow through the earth to blood and qi flow in the body's vessels [20:83]

7. Such as the earlier use of the term mai in the combined astronomical-meteorological contexts that we saw above with reference to earthquakes [42].

8. Unschuld describes this tendency in Chinese thinking quite clearly "The unique feature of the Chinese situation-and this should receive more attention from historians and philosophers of science-is the continuous tendency towards a syncretism of all ideas that exist (within accepted limits). Somehow a way was always found in China to reconcile opposing views and to build bridges" [67:57]; this theme is discussed in the previous chapter [8].

9. Including an early text on herbal medicine, the "Wushier Bingfang" [五十二病方], "Recipes for fifty-two ailments."

10. Harper [20] gives a full translation of the available texts with extended commentaries and explanations. Daly [17] explores the use of hydrological analogies as a way of understanding the development of the "mai", pages 67 and following give a good summary of the content of the texts. Hsu [22] gives a good summary of the Chunyu Yi case records exploring how palpation was used in the early medical literature [23] and has a more recent full annotated translation [24]. Lo explores the Mianyang figurine [21] and the development of the mai [35, 41, 43].

11. The "acupoints" that we find in the Neijing corpus are not found in the Mawangdui or Zhangjiashan texts describing the mai. It is now generally accepted that the mai vessels pre-date the development of the acupoints [27:43-44]. We return briefly to this below and Birch addresses it in more detail in chapter four [6].

12. See discussions in Harper [20:91 and 95-96].

13. Another Mawangdui text the sexual cultivation text "Tianxia Zhidaotan" [天下至道談] also describes how moxa (or more accurately cauterization) can be used to influence the qi in a positive way [20:429, 36:41].

14. This notion that the qi moves towards the warmth or heat is found in the Maishu of the Zhangjiashan, see the discussion in the section "Qi movements in the mai –jingmai" below and in Harper [20:81 and 86]. It is important for other reasons, see chapter four [6] and chapter eight [7].

15. The text names three yang mai and three yin mai, this parallels the naming of the twelve jingmai in the Neijing according to the three yin-yang classification –see table 1. This thus hints at the notion that the text is referring to twelve mai rather than the eleven of the other texts, which is attested to by Daly [17:78]. This represents another sign of the stepwise development of the concept of the jingmai out of the early discussions of the mai.

16. The idea of the yangmai being related to the qi of heaven and the control of external affairs seems to us to carry the idea from earlier traditions of how one tries to cultivate de [德] or virtue which comes from heaven – a theme discussed in the previous chapter [8]. The characterisation of how the yin mai are related to the qi of earth and the control of internal bodily affairs fits with this same model. In the heaven-earth pairing, heaven is yang (hence related to the yang mai) and earth is yin (hence related to the yin mai).The cultivation of de is important in both Confucian and Daoist texts, through its cultivation one can positively influence other people and therefore this is an important attribute of the sage and the political leader. The control of one's external affairs is greatly influenced by one's virtue, and virtue comes from heaven. This theme is discussed in the previous chapter and is clearly repeated in the later Huangdi Neijing Lingshu (chapter eight): "Heaven within me is virtue (de). Earth within me is the breaths (qi). Virtue flows down, the breaths expand, and there is life." [28:16]. The living body was seen as a construct of qi, imbued with virtue from heaven.

17. This appears to be a precursor for the bu [補] supplementation and xie [寫], draining methods of correcting xu [虛] vacuity and shi [實] repletion respectively in the Neijing. See chapter four for more discussion of needling techniques in early medical texts [6].

18. If they are related it is further evidence for the influence of the yangsheng tradition on the development of the mai and jingmai. Lo presents evidence from another Mawangdui text, the "Heyinyang" [和陰陽] the "Conjoining yin and yang", a text on sexual cultivation [36]. She shows clear influences of this yangsheng tradition in the language of named acupoints and description of techniques in the Neijing [36]. This theme is examined further in chapter four [6].

19. Fourteen cases are treated with drug therapy, two with cauterization and two with acupuncture [20:94], and appears to have had a model for deciding when to use drug therapy and when acupuncture or cauterization "he explicitly cautions against using them when "according to the model one should not perform acupuncture and cauterization" [20:94-95].

20. Hsu presents evidence that Chunyu Yi was directly perceiving qi in his examination of the vessels [23], there are references to feeling the qi coming from for example the liver, kidneys etc as he examined the mai [22:75], this issue was touched on in the previous chapter in the examination of the nature of qi in relation to consciousness [8]. Chunyu Yi also discussed deqi [得氣] in his examination of the vessels [22:75]. Hsu suggests a possible interpretation relative to the "dong" [動] or movement, agitation or impulsion in the mai and its feeling as a kind of qi, so that Chunyu Yi's use of the term "deqi" can be seen as something like getting the qi as the feeling of what is wrong with x "The doctor's statement that he got liver qi would thus amount to saying that there was a potential for (pathological) change in the liver" [22:77]. The term "deqi" is explored further in chapter four "The jingmai and qi –acupuncture perspectives" [6].

21. If only because further archaeological findings may reveal quite new evidence and perspectives.

22. After detailed analysis of the mai Lo concludes "it is impossible to find a unitary concept of mai, one that is represented equally in the excavated texts and in the Shuangbaoshan figurine…it may be safer to assume that the term mai is flexible and has popular, technical and specialised usages all of which come to bear on one another at different times" [41:393-4].

23. Harper has a very good discussion of different lines of evidence that link the earlier discussions of mai and the Neijing discussions of the jingmai, presenting various perspectives and arguments for and against [20:77-90].

24. We can propose other potential explanations as the search for a more elaborated physiological description shifted from the mai to jingmai and their corresponding zangfu. Since the early focus was about describing things in practical terms, potential actions rather than ontological structures (see discussions in the previous chapter in the section "philosophical perspectives"), the mai were those things to which you can direct treatment and improve the internal functioning systems; thus in a way the mai represent those systems and were thus viewed as physiological systems. The development of mai to jingmai, congruent with starting to use metal needles targeted to acupoints further evolved the mai as a representational physiology system to a more abstracted action oriented functional system. Since they are connected to the functional structures (zangfu etc) in a continuously connected system, regulation of that system automatically regulates the connected (internal) functional structures, hence the jingmai are more explicitly seen as having regulatory influences rather than being a representational physiological system and it is thus natural that there be a concordant physiological system elaborated such as we find with the detailed descriptions of the zangfu organ systems.

25. "Meridian" [59], "channel" [71], "conduit-vessel" [69], "sinarteria" [53].

26. The term jing [巠] is glossed in the first etymological dictionary from China (circa 90 CE), the Shuowen Jiezi [說文解字] as "subterranean channel" [20:83], which both matches the implications discussed here and the water analogy implications discussed below.

27. Lewis also says "The character jing [經] is used in early texts to indicate the division of a city by a grid of streets and the market by stalls. It had the broader meaning of 'to put in order' or 'rule' and came to be applied to the canonical texts that provided order in the world" [31:248]. Nylan explains the term jing thus: "In pre-Han and Han literature, *jing* conveys four main meanings besides that of 'a classic text': (1) a 'constant' (*chang* 常) that is regular and predictable; (2) the 'main thread' or 'warp' in a fabric… (3) 'to manage', 'to arrange' or 'to rule'; and (4) 'to pass through.' Early writers kept all these meanings in mind when they theorized about authoritative texts. Supposedly, the *jing* represented reliable distillations of the 'constant rules' and 'main models' employed through the ages by recognized experts when they wielded specific arts or techniques... in their areas of special competence… What mattered was how effective the arts and techniques proved to be in practical application" [51].

28. Unschuld makes an extended argument about how the development of the waterways in China brought with it a new order to society, a system of communication (and hence control) [67]. This is further supported by the parallel arguments about the appropriation of water analogies both throughout early Chinese thinking [1] and in direct relation to the mai [17] and jingmai (specifically discussed in parallel to the great rivers of China in Lingshu chapter twelve [44:23, 49:134, 67:82]).

29. Unschuld translates the term zhi [治] as 1) to rule, 2) to cure, 3) to treat, 4) to regulate [68:736], Rochat de la Vallee as to "govern", "rule" or "treat" [56:10], Lloyd as to "order" [33:451].

30. Rochat de la Vallee, personal communication, 2011.

31. Hsu states this as "These concepts testify to a certain cosmological speculation not found in other Mawangdui medical texts such as" the Wushier Bingfang [五十二病方] [23].

32. It is also useful to look at Nanjing chapter seven which explicitly describes the three yin-three yang governing of qi according to the seasons and certain numbers of days throughout the year [68:122]. Presumably the Nanjing author saw the use of the term "jing" in "jingmai" as employing these relationships.

33. This usage is quite different than the six warps usage from the Shanghanlun [傷寒論], which is instead concerned with the transmission of cold pathogen in stages into the body [60:82-84] also see chapter six below [57].

34. Daly states that they add "a temporal dimension to medical theories and altering the field of space, opening the possibility for modes and qualities of movements previously unimaginable" [17:73]. The expanded vision of the body in the more elaborated theories of systematic correspondence, allows for a much richer approach to understanding the diagnosis and treatment of the patient.

35. See for example the Daodejing, Huainanzi [2, 45]. The fact that the earliest descriptions of qi circulation in the jingmai (Lingshu chapter fifteen) and the systems of acupoints associated with the jingmai (Suwen nine) relate these things to specific astronomical-astrological phenomena are specific examples of how the influences of heaven and earth on humans. Following Suwen chapter three the Taisu [太素] (circa 610 CE) states "since ancient times (it has been understood that) penetration by (the qi of) heaven is the basis for life which depends on (the universal qi of) yin and yang. The qi (of everything) in the midst of heaven and earth and the six directions, from the nine provinces and nine body orifices to the five visceral systems and the twelve joints is penetrated by the qi of heaven" [61:15].

36. Harper appears to support this "The transition from the old idea of blood vessels to a physiological theory whose main purpose was to explain the movement of vapor in the

body directed attention away from the blood-vascular system per se and towards an idealized system which enmeshed with correlative cosmology" [20:83-84].

37. "On the evidence of the excavated texts alone (pre-Neijing texts) there is very little to suggest that qi in the body is present only in the channels, let alone that it travels in a particular direction in those channels" [36:30].

38. On the basis of this sentence the qi "follows warmth and departs from coolness" we can propose a way of understanding why moxibustion was applied on the mai for treatment. By burning moxibustion on the mai, it might tend to attract the qi away from the symptom area (qi follows warmth) thereby reducing the relative amount of qi where the symptom is located, and thus reduce the symptom. This model works well especially if the symptom were seen to involve inflammation or infection, i.e. presence of warmth. This passage is also relevant for the scientific understanding of qi and its investigations; here "qi" is seen to flow from cool to warm, which is contrary to the usual way of thinking of "energy" in the second law of thermodynamics (where "energy" flows from warm/heat to cool"), thus implying that "qi" cannot be easily if at all equated with the "energy" that physicists talk of, see chapter eight which discusses the scientific investigation of the jingmai and qi [7] for further discussions.

39. Lo translates this sentence instead as "the sages cool the head and warm the feet" arguing that the text seems to be about treatment principles [36: 29].

40. Not only would the compilers and authors of the Neijing have been collecting the different opinions and ideas from experts but they would not have been much involved in trying to resolve differences of opinion, which as a trend in Chinese culture were tolerated and by and large allowed to co-exist - see chapter one in this volume [8] and especially [67:57].

41. As usual, the details of this are more complex, see the discussion in [69:175-176].

42. We discuss this astronomical aspect in appendix one below.

43. See chapter four, "The jingmai and qi - acupuncture perspectives" for further discussion of the weiqi [6].

44. The first treatise to describe the jingmai in detail, Lingshu chapter ten states that the condition of the jingmai is determined by feeling the radial pulses "commonly, one cannot see the channel, its condition of sthenia (repletion) and asthenia (vacuity) can only be determined by feeling the cunkou (radial) pulse" [73:570]. This sets the stage for the later focus on the use of pulse diagnosis for grasping the condition of the channels.

45. Unschuld cogently argues that palpation of the radial pulses was taken up by the Nanjing as the principle method for understanding the condition of qi in the body [68]. The argument ties together a number of developing themes. The "mai" (as palpable vessels on the body surface) came (in the Mawangdui and Zhangjiashan texts) to be asso-

ciated with the "mai" as precursors of the "jingmai", associated with blood and qi and a kind of primitive physiological understanding. As the "jingmai" became elaborated in the Neijing and the model of them as composing a continuous interlinked circuit for circulation of qi developed, it was natural that it would be proposed that to understand the condition of the whole circuit one could palpate a key point along that circuit, in this case the pulses at the wrist, at LU-9, the "great meeting" place of the pulses. In this model, palpation of the radial pulses naturally becomes a primary target for diagnosis in order to understand the condition of the jingmai system, and the condition of qi throughout the body.

46. Wu and Wu translate the same passage as: "When the five-cereal enters the stomach, it produces the refined substances which causes the unimpediment of the vessels and the unceasing operations of the blood and energy" [73:556]. While rendered differently, it expresses a similar idea: the qi starts moving after food enters the stomach.

47. Lingshu fifteen and Nanjing one.

48. Lingshu eighteen describes this [49:97-98].

49. Chace and Shima translate the passage as "At no time does the qi not circulate. It is like the flow of water, like the ceaseless movements of the sun and moon" [12:178].

50. The passages either mention qi explicitly or mention other concepts such as "shen" [神], spirit or "ji" [機], dynamic which are interpreted to refer to the qi, see chapter four for more explicit discussions of needling and chapter five for annotated translation and commentaries of relevant passages.

51. Lingshu one states "To understand its goings and comings, emphasize its periodicity" (Chace, Bensky, chapter five in this volume [11]). Lingshu nine describes how one should "divine the comings and goings of the spirit" [10].

52. Nanjing eighty tells us "as soon as one [notices] with one's left hand that the influences appear, one inserts the needle" [68:646].

53. Nanjing eighty states "When the needle is inserted and when it is apparent that the influences have left completely, then one withdraws the needle" [68:646].

54. Suwen twenty-seven states "When the qi has arrived, this is exactly the moment for which one has to be on the alert" [69:283].

55. See the passage from Lingshu one translated and discussed in chapter five below, see also Nanjing seventy-eight [68:635].

56. This concept is clearly stated in Lingshu chapter one providing the background for application of needling techniques.

57. Nanjing seventy-eight gives a clear descriptions, see [68:635].

58. The weiqi, protective qi, was basically said to run rapidly across the surface of the body to help protect the body from potentially invading xieqi, thus offering a kind of protective boundary for the body. But the descriptions of the early texts give varied accounts (see chapter four for further discussion [6]).

59. Unschuld describes how the terms yingqi and weiqi "were used with different meanings by different authors of the Suwen texts, of the Lingshu and of subsequent commentaries" [69:163]. It is thus not surprising that different models of how needling affects qi can be found.

60. This model has persisted into modern times. Li Shizhen in his text Qijing Bamaikao (1577) repeats this idea thus: "People have channel vessels and network vessels throughout their body. Those that travel longitudinally are called channels (jing), while those that branch off are called networks (luo)." [12].

61. For example Matsumoto, Birch render the first sentence "because each person's meridian is not the same" [47:153]. Wu and Wu see the two sentences in relation to different conditions of the jingmai and luomai "As the conditions of the channels in different persons are different, the conditions of the collaterals are different also" [73:574]. Sunu and Lee see the two sentences as referring to the different lengths of the jingmai and different sizes of people "It is because the length of the meridians or the locations of the starting points of the connecting meridians are different from person to person as the human bodies are different from one another in their fatness and leanness" [65:166]. Wu approximates the last interpretation "People and channels both have their variations, so the luo linking vessels have their differences and separations as well" [72:65]. The first and last translations imply that the jingmai are not consistent between people.

62. Several authors have noted the parallel between the jingmai, their branches, the luomai and their many small branches the sunluomai and the arteries arterioles capillaries [44:16-19, 49:141-142]. Lu and Needham cite Wangbing from the eight century (who seems to be citing Lingshu chapter seventeen): "the tracts and channels (jingmai) are inside the body and the branches which connect them horizontally are the luo. And the luo again have further branches which are called the sun" [44:18]. Suwen fifty-eight suggests a "meeting" between the sunluo and the three hundred and sixty-five acupoints through which qi moves "The 365 holes of the meeting points (acupoints) of the tertiary network [vessels] (sunluo), they too correspond to a year... They serve as passage[ways] of the camp (ying) and protective (wei) [qi]" [69:166]. This passage suggests not only that the sunluo are involved in the circulation of qi, but that the acupoints lie at intersections with the sunluo –see below and especially chapter four for further discussions of this.

63. Some modern Western authors have proposed a circulation of some kind in the qijingbamai, but as documented elsewhere [9:74-76] this appears to be based on mistranslation.

64. Li Shizhen, the first medical author to write a treatise on the qijingbamai, the Qijing Baimaikao [奇經八脈考] said of them "[Discussions of] the eight vessels scattered throughout the masses of [medical] texts, are sketchy and incomplete" [12:94]. For a discussion of the development of the qijingbamai [奇經八脈] see Matsumoto, Birch [48]. At the time of the Neijing (early Han) the descriptions of the qijingbamai are of not well articulated trajectories (even with apparent contradictions) with varied symptoms associated with them and no clear treatments given. In the Nanjing (later Han) the theories and trajectories become more systematised, but are still absent clear treatment ideas. Fully articulated trajectories of the pathways of the eight qijingbamai start to emerge especially with the Shisi Jingfahui of 1341, but still with different trajectory sequences given by different texts after this [48:25-67]. The tradition that associates the eight qijingbamai with eight paired acupoints for treatment did not emerge until the Zhenjiu Daquan of 1437 described them (probably based on an earlier pairing of the eight acupoints in the Zhenjing Zhinan of 1289 [48:5-7] independent of the qijingbamai). Treatment via the four pairs of eight points developed further in the Zhenjiu Juying (1529) and especially the Zhenjiu Dacheng (1601) with increasingly long lists of symptoms to guide their selection, but with almost no theory given [48:69-137]. There is also a different and less well known tradition that emerged through the work of Li Shizhen in his Qijing Bamaikao (1578) [12]. Li Shizhen appears to have developed a completely different understanding and use of the qijingbamai, not at all using the eight treatment points indicated in the bulk of traditional literature from the fifteenth century onwards. Li Shizhen's model of the qijingbamai used a combination of neidan [內丹] or internal alchemy practices with herbal medicine and acupuncture, his text "Qijing Bamaikao" represents a radical departure from other medical texts of the time discussing the qijingbamai. Clearly by comparison to the jingmai, the qijingbamai were in more "embryonic" stages of description at the time that the jingmai were being elaborated in the Han dynasty, the qijingbamai came to mature clinically only much later [48].

65. See [73:570 and 574, and 47:153].

66. Of this Rochat de la Vallee writes "Another point developed in the medical texts is that all qi expressed through the five zang or through yin yang, is just one qi existing in a unity" [55:58]. Larre and Rochat de la Vallee discuss this with the following quote from Lingshu thirty "Huangdi: I know that a human possesses jing, qi, jin, ye, xue and mai. At the deepest understanding they are all one qi, but they are differentiated by six names. I want to know what the meaning of each of them is" [29:42]. The Lingshu chapter states that qi is one of the six qi, identifying a specific subset by location and function.

67. Rochat de la Vallee lists several types or named forms of qi that are equivalent to this unitary qi: zongqi [宗氣] "ancestral qi", zhenqi [真氣] "true qi", zhengqi [正氣] "correct qi" and yuanqi [元氣] "original qi" [55:58-59], to which Birch [4] adds the shengqi [生氣], "vital qi", the yuanqi [原氣] "source qi" and the weiqi [胃氣] or "stomach qi" (at least as referred in the Neijing and Nanjing as that which reflects in the pulses, see Unschuld [69:157]). Given the way the terms "shen" [神 ] "spirit" [see for example Nanjing eight –(68:130) "the spirit guarding against evil"] and "shenqi" [神氣] "spirit-qi" [see for

example Lingshu one –(36:31), the acupoints as places "where the qi of the shen travels in and out"] are used it makes these terms also good candidates as referents to this "unitary qi", Sivin states that "shenqi" is "the normal vitality of the body" [61:14]. While various traditions make distinctions between these terms, they are all whole body or unitary forms of qi. See also Birch, Cabrer Mir and Rodríguez in this volume for further discussion [8].

68. Harper discusses this [20:87].

69. Here we need to distinguish between different uses of the term "mai". In one the term refers to all the blood vessels. In the second to the specific mai of the Mawangdui that contain the qi, and are the precursors for the jingmai system. In the third the term mai refers to the vessels that are palpated in pulse diagnosis, especially on the radial arteries at the wrists. The use of the term mai in this passage refers to the Mawangdui's concept of the mai (as jingmai precursors). The palpation may include pulsating vessels (as in pulse diagnosis) but will include the whole length of the mai trajectory, whether pulsating vessels are felt or not.

70. While the first mention of the acupoints is found in the Neijing texts, not many of the later named acupoints are found in the Neijing texts [39]. It is in the post Han text of Huang Fumi, the "Zhenjiu Jiayijing" (circa 282 CE) that we find the first systematic naming and descriptions of the acupoints where many more are named than are found in the Neijing [39, 44] - see chapter four for more details [6].

71. This is important when we examine the scientific exploration of the jingmai in chapter eight [7].

72. "At the articulations within the body there are 365 points of communication... articulations" refers to where the divine ch'i (sic) travels freely and moves outward and inward, not to skin, flesh, sinews, and bones" [60:51].

CHAPTER THREE

# HOW TO BECOME A SHANG YI OR "SUPERIOR PHYSICIAN"

## An exploration of the influence of the practitioner in early China

Dianne Sommers

## Introduction

The physician in early China was a craftsman who worked with particular instruments and techniques like needles, cauterisation or moxibustion, herbs and incantations. To become a skilled practitioner he started as an apprentice to grasp the theoretical basis and master the practical techniques, in a discipline that would show quite a varied picture. There were diverging strategies on diagnosis and treatment and a lively scene that was involved in keeping the body fit and healthy as long as possible. Simultaneously another movement was going on, one that had the aim to unify all the different theories –including medicine– in one big master plan, one that would encompass all existing phenomena in the universe.

To set the scene, the situation in the period that led to the basic medical writings of the Han era (206 BCE-220 CE) will be described. The general notion of the "Superior Person" as the man who had acquired qualities of excellence through extensive study and training will be discussed. The second part of the paper explores the role of the practitioner in the early years of Chinese Medicine. Who was the physician in that era and what skill was expected from him? What do the classical texts say about the bearings and training of the physician? The last section is concerned with the "Superior Physician" or shang yi [上醫], who occasionally appears in the classical medical texts. What does this predicate mean in the context of its time and how can we understand this? What is expected of a physician in order to fulfil such a qualification?

In modern medicine the starting point is that practitioners who perform the treatment –as long as they all administer the techniques in exactly the same way– do not influence the results. In research the personality of the therapist is of no concern because every trained practitioner is considered to deliver the same product. The question I will research is if the physician as a person has an influence and impact on treatment results. Does it matter *who* administers treatment if the applied techniques are the same? In early China they certainly believed it did. Why did they think that and what were their arguments?

Although we can never view the ideas of the early practitioners with the eyes of their time and culture, we can clarify a lot of the circumstances that were at stake for the practice at that time. To see how *our* Chinese medicine practiced today (which still follows the basic tenets of that era) differs from the traditional way the role of the practitioner was viewed. The ancients claimed that the character of the practitioner formed an important aspect in the given treatment, which provides us with issues for reflection and maybe also some inspiration to see different ways and possibilities.

## Time sketch

In 221 BCE the Warring States came to an end when Qin Shi Huangdi (256-210 BCE) unified the former feudal states in one empire. The Qin emperor did not defeat his enemies because of superior technology, but because he found new ways to organize the state. In the establishment of his bureaucratic organisation that was based on merit, he followed the advice of his Legalist ministers who supported the abolition of all special rights and privileges of the nobility. Instead, he applied laws that would treat all subjects impartially. They thought that only if the laws would be systematically applied, the essential evil nature of man could be controlled. This formed an adequate preparation for a new kind of government far more efficient than the aristocratic dominion of the Warring States. The new type of government created a powerful and strong country that was able to succeed where the other states failed [9:97].

The Qin emperor had a short reign that lasted only eleven years. After his death in 210 BCE many of the former states rebelled once again. The rebel that defeated all his rivals was the founder of the new dynasty that would stay in charge for more than four hundred years. The new Han emperor took over the bureaucratic government system of the Qin emperor, but with a different perspective. Instead of the strict and sometimes harsh measures of the legalistic and militaristic government, the Han focussed more on idealized stories of mythological and historical figures from ancient times to take as examples for high moral behaviour.

In the second century BCE the Confucian scholar Dong Zhongshu [董仲舒] was responsible for transforming the diversity of more regional ideas and thoughts into a state synthesis. In his doctrine of the natural order of the universe a new worldview was born in which ethical ideas, five phases and yin-yang theories are interwoven. The notion of qi [氣] formed the bridge between philosophy, science and state politics. The basis of his cosmological framework already lay in the late Warring States period. While in the real world everything was rapidly changing and in the old state structures were breaking apart, the synthesis was an attempt to establish a new underlying order.

In the vocabulary of the new synthesis the cosmic process is described together with its analogues in the state and human body [32:5-6]. The links between cosmos, state and body had already been discussed in earlier times, but in the first century BCE it reached the systemized form that became part of all the other theories of the period. The emperor was the central actor in this network of resonant systems. The underpinnings for this system were found in "The Grand Plan" (Hong Fan [洪範]) a short text from the Book of Documents (Shujing [書經]), probably written around 300 BCE. Here the fundamental correspondences between Heaven and Earth, Five Phases, planetary connections and calendric calculations were written down. The text had a clear purpose in supporting the authority of the emperor, next to a secondary goal that was de facto an attempt to control his behaviour. By performing the right rituals the emperor would influence the whole network of correspondences in a positive way. A neglect of the rites or incorrect behaviour would create the opposite effect.

The state is also a cosmos in itself. In Springs and Autumn Annals of Mr. Lü (Lüshi Chunqiu [呂氏春秋]), completed in 241 BCE is said:

> The Way of Heaven is round; the Way of Earth is square. The sage kings took this as their model, basing it on [the distinction between] above and below. How do we explain the roundness of Heaven? The essential qi alternately moves up and down, completing a circle and beginning again, delayed by nothing; that is why we speak of the way of Heaven as round. How do we explain the squareness of Earth? The ten thousand things are distinct in category and shape. Each has its separate responsibility [as an official does], and cannot carry out that of another: that is why one speaks of the way of the Earth as square. When the ruler grasps the round and his ministers keep the square, so that round and square are not interchanged, the state prospers.
>
> The One is most exalted of all. No one knows its source. No one knows its incipient form. No one knows its beginning. No one knows its end. Still, the myriad things take it as their progenitor. The sage kings took it as their model in order to perfect their natures, to settle their vital forces and to form their commands.
>
> A command issues from the ruler's mouth. Those in official positions receive it and carry it out, never resting day or night. It moves unimpeded all the way down. It permeates the people's hearts and propagates the four quarters [of the realm]. Completing the circle, it reverts to the place of the ruler. That is the round Way"
> (Lüshi chunqiu jiao shi 3:5. [1:239]).

This expresses that when in the state the universal Way (dao) [道][1] is followed, the tasks of the emperor and officials are clearly separated. The duty of the ruler is to act according to the ritual and to cultivate the Way, so that his deeds are in harmony with the cosmos and therefore powerful. In this way, the sage emperor, his officials and the rest of the empire establish a microcosm, where everything has its place and both spontaneous and orderly actions shape the correct norm.

The factor that ties cosmos, state and body together and enables an organic resonance between them is the universal qi. The sage emperor forms the central axis, whose power is mediating all the processes in the three realms. Medicine fits the cosmological picture like a glove because the body –just like the state– is a cosmos in itself. Humans are made out of qi from Heaven and Earth and therefore inseparable from the Heavenly and Earthly rhythms. In the Basic Questions of the Yellow Emperor's Inner Classic (Huangdi Neijing Suwen) [黃帝内經素問], hereafter Suwen[2] is stated in chapter twenty-five (adapted from Suwen seventy-one) [34:419]:

> 天復地載，萬物悉備，莫貴於人。人以天地之氣生，四時之法成。
> Covered by Heaven and carried by Earth,
> The ten thousand creatures have all become completely perfected
> None has a nobler position than man.
> Man comes to life through the qi of Heaven and Earth;
> He matures in accordance with the laws of the four seasons.

In moving away from the earlier occult practices, the Han cosmologists and medical writers used the concept of qi resonating between the three areas to build their theories. These concepts mirror the ideals of the state elite with the image of an emperor who is not concerned with politics but who forms nothing but the embodiment linking man and cosmos. The qi of the cosmos is the same qi that fills the body. The correspondences between man and the universe are extensively elaborated in the Lingshu [15]:

> 歲有三百六十五日，人有三百六十節。地有高山，人有肩膝。
> 地有深谷，人有腋膕。地有十二經水，人有十二經脈。
> In the year there are 365 days; humans have 365 joints.
> On the earth there are high mountains; humans have shoulders and knees.
> On the earth there are deep valleys; humans have armpits and hollows.
> On the earth there are twelve cardinal watercourses; humans have twelve cardinal circulation tracts...[3]

Likewise are the correspondences between body and state. In Suwen chapter eight the hierarchy of the twelve internal organs is shown as departments of the state [16]:

心者，君主之官也，神明出焉。
肺者，相傳之官，治節出焉。
肝者，將軍之官，謀慮出焉。
The heart (xin 心) fills the office of master and sovereign.
Spirit brightness (shenming 神明) stems from it.
The lungs fill the office of minister and governor.
Order and moderation stem from it.
The liver fills the office as general.
Planning and deliberation stem from it...

What was said about the state also holds true for the human body, which means that when the ruler (i.e. the heart) is wise and his behaviour is according to the Way, all under him are safe and the body will flourish. In sickness, the resonances between the different realms are disturbed. To find out which cycles or phases are involved in a disease is an important diagnostic task, just as making a prognosis and designing a suitable treatment to rectify the illness.

## Being the best you can be: The image of the Superior Person

The image of the Superior Person is found throughout Chinese thinking and already played an important role in early texts. It was considered perfectly normal for every human being to strive to become a superior man, perhaps superior to his fellow man, but surely superior to his own past and present self. The aim to excel was approved and accepted throughout Chinese society, man could always become better than he was before. It was a conviction that became an art of living and acted as a powerful transformative force for various groups in the whole nation.

In Confucian circles[4] a range of terms was used to describe the various dimensions of accomplishment. At the basic level there is the "petty" person (xiaoren) [小人], more concerned with his own benefit and trivial business. He simply copies what is already there, rather than adding something constructive to society or the situation. Stages that refer to some kind of achievement include a person with special interpersonal qualities (renzhe) [仁者], an exemplary man with outstanding social and political affinities (junzi) [君子] or the supreme level of the universal sage (shengren) [聖人] who represents the highest degree. Some regard these different categories as stages of a process, others see them more as descriptions that emphasize the focus of their efforts [8:158].

The different classifications have shared attributes like a commitment for learning, cultivation and refinement. For the adept it provided meaning, value and purpose that added to personal and political influence. In the cultivation process effective communication plays an important role. In this, language is the aspect that shapes and embraces the world: "the exemplary person (junzi) is what he says, and where he is exemplary, the world is as he speaks it" [8:161]. Because of its influence, language presents both a danger and an opportunity. The importance of living up to one's word or trustworthiness (xin) [信] and integrity (cheng) [誠] for human society is clearly illustrated by Mencius (Mengzi) [孟子], 372–289 BCE:

> If a man serving in a subordinate position fails to win the confidence of his superiors, he cannot hope to govern the people. There is a way for him to win the confidence of his superiors: if friends do not trust him, he will not gain the confidence of his superiors. There is a way for him to win the trust of his friends: if in serving his parents he fails to please them, he will not win the trust of his friends. There is a way for him to please his parents: if upon looking within he finds that he has not been true to himself, he will not please his parents. There is a way for him to become true to himself: if he does not understand goodness he cannot be true to himself. It is for this reason that being true is the Way of Heaven, and to reflect upon this is the Way of man. There has never been a man totally true to himself who has not affected others, just as there has never been a man not true to himself who has been able to affect anyone at all.[5]

This excerpt shows that the Confucian idea of becoming a Superior Person always bears a social and ethical dimension. It also reveals the absence of a distinction between private and public, which is so prevalent in western thought. In this context personal cultivation is not seen as a private affair and therefore it is always connected with the social environment.

Likewise the Daoist texts had their expressions for various states of realisation. In the Laozi [老子] and Zhuangzi [莊子] terms are found like the genuine man (zhenren) [真人], spirit man (shenren) [神人], great man (daren) [大人] and the whole or complete man (quanren) [全人]. As in the Confucian texts these terms should not be understood as "fixed or final categories" as their meaning changes in different contexts and circumstances. For the realisation of what is seen as the Daoist fulfilment of the Superior Person, the notions of genuineness (zhen) [真] and what is so-of-itself (ziran) [自然] articulate the pureness and naturalness of human existence. In a rather piquant conversation in the Zhuangzi, Confucius is brought on stage in a chat with an old fisherman [7:251-252]:

> Confucius said solemnly "Let me ask what you mean by 'genuine'".
> The genuine is the most quintessential, the most sincere. What fails to be quintessential and sincere cannot move others. Thus, forced tears however sorrowful fail to sadden, forced rages however formidable do not strike awe, forced affection however much you smile will not be returned. Genuine sorrow saddens without uttering a sound, genuine rage strikes awe before it bursts out, genuine affection is returned before you smile. The man who is inwardly genuine moves the external with his spirit. This is why we value the genuine.

The text continues with the "Zhuangzian" view on social interaction. The argument here is not that anything is wrong with conventions in themselves –after all they do have their function and role– but rather it concerns the bond with which one sticks to rites and rules, at the expense of the release of one's own inner genuineness [7:251-252]:

> When it is applied to relations between men, in service within the family the son is filial and the father compassionate, in service within the state the minister is loyal and the lord just, in a wine-feast you enjoy, in mourning you grieve. What matters in being loyal and just is that you do fulfil the charge, in a wine-feast that you do enjoy, in a mourning that you do grieve, in serving your parents that you do please them. To the glory of fulfilling the charge you can pick your own route; in serving parents, if you do please them they won't raise difficulties in how you did it; in the wine-feast, if you do enjoy you won't be finicky about the cups; in mourning, if you do grieve no one quibbles about the rite. The rites are what the custom of the times has established. The genuine is the means by which we draw upon Heaven, it is so-of-itself and irreplaceable. Therefore the sage, taking Heaven as his model, values the genuine and is untrammelled by custom. The fool does the opposite; incapable of taking Heaven as his model he frets about man, ignorant of how to value the genuine he timidly lets himself be altered by custom, and so is an unsatisfied man. What a pity you were steeped so soon in man's artificialities, and are so late in hearing the greatest Way!

The notion of genuineness is also connected with the term "brightness" or "clarity" (ming) [明], as an expression of the quality of understanding. Commentators explain it as "to make manifest", by which it becomes clear how things are related and how these relationships pattern the world. The highest form of clarity is the ability to see "how things really are", called the "divine" insight or "spirit brightness" (shenming) [神明].

Both Confucians and Daoists have placed specific accents in their definitions of the Superior Person, but found a common vocabulary in two types of personal transformation that can be seen as results of the cultivation process. The changes reveal a direct remodelling of one's individual perspective and a reshaping of the attitude towards the world. A first group of modifications showed "extension, development, widening, deepening", qualities referring to an opening up to a broader and different perspective, to an insight in patterns that were obscure before and an enhancement of mastery and skill. The second type of transformation that was shared by both Confucians and Daoists included better "integration, blending, unification and merging" which created opportunities for establishing harmony, empathy and care.

The way these characteristics were expressed and communicated would be quite different. In general the worldly manifestation for the Confucians would take place through language and ritual, resulting in the development of virtues (de) [德] like humanity and propriety. For Daoists the transformations would happen in accord with natural processes, expressed in the enhancement of intrinsic power (and for which they also used the term de [德]) and which coincided with a more intuitive human virtue.

## The medical practitioner

Before the Han era the treatment of disease could be in the hands of a shaman (wu) [巫], recipe master (fangshi) [方士] or physician (yi) [毉 or 醫]. Shamans were usually more associated with prayer healing practices through maledictions or incantations. The recipe masters, as their name already suggests were involved with drugs, herbal medicine but also diverse occult practices. Those known as the physicians used various therapeutic strategies with needles (ci) [刺] or (zhen) [針/箴], stones (shi) [石][6], lancets (zhan) [鑱] and cauterization (moxibustion jiu) [灸] techniques. Although this might seem to offer a clear contrast, the differences between the groups were certainly not distinct [17:359]. Some of the practitioners lived in shrines and would use a personal combination of strategies with needles, stones or herbal remedies, practicing divination and expelling demons [22:404-406]. They could work with physical movements (daoyin) [引導], contemplative discipline and macrobiotic techniques for nurturing the spirit (xiushen) [修身] and methods for conserving the qi in the quest for long life (changshou) [長壽] or to transcend death (yangming) [永命] [11:112-119].

Records testify of rituals to nurture the personal power (de) of the practitioner, which could accumulate over generations within a lineage of healers. A novice would act in accordance of a process called "modelling" (xing ) [型][7] which was a long way of following the lineal pattern, to secure the physical embodiment of ancestral power and to blend his personal aspects with the pattern of his lineage. The transition from apprentice to master took place in a musical ceremony to ritually "open the heart" and "grasp the power" from the ancestral predecessor.

Usually shamans and recipe masters did not stay long at one particular spot but travelled from place to place, wherever they could find support for food, clothing and a roof over their heads. In special cases they could be working together with state officials, lineage elders with special expertise or diviners. In general the physicians tended to be the most educated practitioners. Late in the Warring States specialization became more common; surgeons *avant la lettre* who were skilled with lancets treated external wounds, excised dead flesh and lanced boils, dieticians prescribed food according to the time of the year and "seasonal doctors" worked with acute problems like headaches in spring, itchy skin diseases in summer, fever and chills in autumn and coughing in winter [4:11].

Most practitioners of medicine also involved themselves in self-cultivation and nourishing life (yangsheng) [養生] practices, which were considered a form of healing. The nourishing practice concerns the physical body (xing) [形], inner nature (xing) [性], the heart (xin) [心], spirit (shen) [神] and –last but not least– improving one's understanding (zhi) [知]. Their attention was not only for sick people but also for those seeking longer or even eternal life [4:14].

Exercises for moving the qi often used props (staffs, jade disks or items that had special associations with healing) and sometimes also music and dance. Uniquely designed movements were meant to cure specific symptoms or illnesses. Their associations linked the early dances to mythical ancestors and seem to have played an important role in the different forms of healing (exorcism, purification, strength building, transcendence) [3:255]. Other techniques might include breathing exercises, dietetics, sexual cultivation (intra-chamber, fangzhong [房中]) and the use of "calculation arts" (shushu) [數術].[8]

The physicians of the Han dynasty (206 BCE–220 CE) built on these earlier medical practices and used them as a solid foundation for the new medicine based on qi, yin and yang, and the five phases (wuxing). As described earlier, the body of medical knowledge gradually transformed into a more unified theory that fit the encompassing cosmological system.

What forms a surprising and major break with the earlier medical writings is the way disease and the effects of treatment are explained. The novelty of this development that soon became the norm in the Han era is often overlooked. According to this theory illness arises from pathological conditions of qi in the vessels (mai) and internal organs (zangfu), caused by naturalistic phenomena such as wind, cold, dampness, etc. That illness could be caused by excessive qi from outside was already an old idea[9], but now in the Neijing these pathogenic substances became the main reason for disturbances that would manifest themselves on a deeper level, rather than some external form of qi. The new medicine replaced the older aetiology of demons and evil spirits with pathogenic agents of a more naturalistic origin. The thought that ghosts and spirits would be able to cause disease in the human body was explained away as "a shadowed spirit of a mind in doubt" [20:1148].

Although a different medical theory became dominant, new archaeological evidence demonstrates that a great deal of the old healing practices sustained [10: 217]. This means that at the official theoretical level the ideology of the cosmological model prevailed, but underneath a wide variety of healing techniques and remedies continued and "survived" the systematization [13:76-77]. Outside the official theoretical framework the widespread exorcist therapeutic practices continued.

The Neijing is seen as a proponent of the new aetiology. In the Neijing[10] the existence of demons as cause of disease and the efficacy of treatment with spells and incantations is dismissed and discounted [10:211]. Students in the Han era who wished to become physicians (yi) would officially have primarily encountered the naturalistic model as described in the Neijing, but would certainly have been aware of the specialist knowledge of the magical and demonological world. Traces of shamanism and a belief in the occult can occasionally be observed as in Lingshu chapter seventy-three, "On deploying ability" (Guan neng) [官能], where the qualities of the adept who wished to become a practitioner were explored [12:93]:

> He whose eyes are bright can be made to examine the colour. He whose ears are sharp can be made to listen to the sound. He who is nimble at discourse can be made to transmit the teachings. He who is slow and steady, whose hands are skilled and whose heart is discerning can be made to handle the needles and moxa so as to put blood and qi in order and adjust various contrary or concordant conditions; and to investigate yin and yang so as to integrate the various techniques. He whose joints are relaxed, whose muscles are pliant and whose heart is in harmony can be made to "guide and pull" (daoyin) and "circulate qi" (xingqi). He who berates others with speech that is cutting and poisonous can be made to spit on abscesses and eliminate ailments with incantations. He whose nails are harsh, whose hands are poisonous and who is prone to causing injury in the conduct of affairs can be made to

> massage accumulations and apply pressure to numbness. In each case, by obtaining his abilities the techniques then can be performed and his name then becomes illustrious. When the right man is not obtained, his achievement is incomplete and his teacher is without fame. Thus it is said "when the right man is obtained, then speak: do not transmit to the wrong man" which refers to this situation. He whose hands are poisonous can be tested by having him massage a turtle. Place the turtle under a vessel and have him massage from above, and it will die in fifty days. He whose hands are sweet restore it to life just like it was before.

It is clear that a student must have had manifold talents that we don't quite understand today. Also the candidate is expected to add some status to the teacher. Without the necessary skills both teacher and student will suffer: the teacher is left without fame and the student without achievement.

## Transmission

In the early Han period most physicians would pass on their knowledge orally [27:36] to students they selected, but it became much more common that the medical wisdom was written down in manuscripts. These texts were highly valuable and served to establish personal authority and prestige. Disciples should study them thoroughly [31:184-185]:

> The Thunder Duke inquired of the Yellow Lord: "Insignificant though I am, since you permitted me to receive your patrimony I have gone through the sixty bundles of wooden slips on which the Nine Needles is written, ardently applying myself to them from daybreak to dusk. The bindings of the older ones are broken, and the slips of the newer ones are grimy, but still I chant and memorize, never setting the book aside.

The transmission was the next step for the student and an important moment. In the same Lingshu chapter the ritual is described, that presumably accompanied the solemn ceremony of handing over the texts from teacher to student [31:184-185]:

> The Thunder Duke bowed repeatedly and then arose, saying "Please command me with respect to this." He purified himself for three days and then sought permission. "I venture to make a request. Insignificant though I am, I hope to take the oath today at the epochal time of yang." The Yellow Lord accompanied him into the room where he had done the purifications, and carried out the cutting of the arm and the smearing of the blood. The Yellow Lord himself recited this formula:

*Today at the epochal time of yang*
*We smear the blood, transmit the formulas.*
*He who dares defy these words.*
*Will surely suffer.*

The Thunder Duke bowed repeatedly and spoke: "Insignificant though I am, I receive it." The Yellow Lord grasped his hand with his left hand, and with his right conferred the book to him, saying: "Take care! Take care! I will now explain it to you.

The significance of the oath and the use of blood form an initiation that bonded teacher and disciple as father and son: it established their connection in the lineage. As the legitimate successor in the line of physicians he could use the text in his practice and transmit it to his future student. After the handing over another aspect the transmission began. In oral teachings the thoughts and ideas of the former masters of lineage would be explained to make sure that nothing of the ancient material was lost. Also these served as the necessary supplement for a correct interpretation of the written tradition. In a later phase also these instructions would be written down and added to the transmission, often accompanied by warnings against teaching them to "unworthy persons".

Some aspects of the transmission process are also described in the story of Chunyu Yi, a physician in the early Han who lived in the kingdom of Qi. In the Shiji[11] twenty-five of his medical case histories are recorded. At some point in his career he was accused of an unknown crime and was sent to the capital Chang'an for punishment by mutilation. His daughter however persuaded the emperor to abandon this idea, and he was put under house arrest. Imperial orders summoned him to defend his case and explain his medical practice and craftsmanship. In his answer he makes a clear point that his participation in a lineage, together with the texts that had been transmitted to him were both important aspects as proof for his technical qualifications as a doctor. From Chunyu Yi's written testimony it also becomes clear that diagnosis of the disease in those days was already done through a quite systematic use of observation and palpation of the patient. The treatment that was given was apparently based on what he perceived in his observation, most often combined with what he felt in the pulse and on the channels [14].

## Practical skills

The Neijing gives instructions on how to needle and how to improve practical skills of the practitioner. Diverse therapeutic aspects and methods, mostly concerning acupuncture, are explained in chapters that are scattered in the text. For example in Lingshu four Qibo teaches how to find the acupuncture points and how to needle them [15]:

> 黃帝曰。刺之有道乎。岐伯答曰。刺此者。必中氣穴。無中肉節。中氣穴則針游於巷。中肉 節則皮膚痛。補瀉反則病益篤。
> Huangdi inquired: is there a special method for needling the patient?
> Qibo answered: He who needles must hit the (centre of the) qi hole.
> Do not hit the flesh or joints.
> If you hit the qi hole, the (effects of the) needling will travel through the alleys.
> If you hit the flesh or joints, the skin will be painful.

The needling requires correct localization so that an effect on qi circulation will take place and that pain will be prevented. The correct application of techniques is of vital importance, otherwise it can cause a worsening in the condition and create chaos. The text continues [15]:

> 補瀉反則病益篤。中筋則筋緩。邪氣不出。與其真相搏。亂而不去。反還內著。用 針不審。以順為逆也。
> If you reverse tonifying or draining (if you apply tonification while you should have used draining and vice versa), the disease will become more severe.
> If you hit the tendons, then they become slow and the pathogenic qi will not come out.
> Rather it will grapple with the real (qi).
> There will be chaos and it will not leave,
> But on the contrary it will turn back to the inside and manifest itself.
> If using the needles does not happen in a careful way,
> Then going along will become contrariness.

## The Superior Physician

### Knowledge and lineage

A first and basic quality for somebody who would be called a "Superior Physician" is an outstanding medical knowledge. Biographies of famous doctors all mention hard study and reverence for the medical and philosophical texts often learned by heart. Their respect for the written words honoured the literary tradition in which they stood. The prestige of the texts was derived from the fact that the wisdom was directly transmitted

In the era that the Huangdi Neijing was written the education of the practitioner of medicine would have shown contrasting views. Its cosmology based medicine is all about qi: man is formed out of the qi from Heaven and Earth, has a metabolism that extracts qi from food and drink, a meridian system that circulates it through the body, comes in contact with pathogenic qi that carries diseases in the body and food, and can employ the qi qualities of herbs, needles and moxibustion techniques to harmonize the imbalance in the system. The Neijing uses categories as yin-yang and five phases to analyse the condition in naturalistic terms. All this provided a powerful and sophisticated explanatory model of the body corresponding with the cosmological framework at work at a universal scale.

This 'canonization' that was put down in the Neijing was in contrast with the diversity found in other medical manuscripts of the time [27:37], which show a pragmatic approach which was transmitted in a lineage of practitioners in combination with oral teachings. These included spirit healing, ancestral influences and demonical causes of disease far more varied than is pictured in the received canon.

through legendary sages from the far past who laid the foundation of the culture and gave it to the Chinese people. For medicine this was Huangdi, the Yellow Emperor who had revealed the secrets of the body. The herbalists had Shennong, who had tested all the plants and minerals on their healing qualities.

The lineage, formed by the chain of doctors that handed over their knowledge to a next generation, formed the continuity in which the wisdom was secured and how transmission took form. An unbroken line connected physicians and their students in a direct way with the original source. Scholars argued that this direct line was the only way to secure the correct understanding of the classic texts [25:205-206]. In his preface of the Pulse Classic (Maijing) [脈經] the physician Wang Shuhe (265-316 CE) wrote [35]:

> Through the ages few have been able to draw on the extensive meanings of the writings that survive. The secret implications of the old classics have been kept arcane rather than been broadcast. This has left scholars of later eras in the dark about their fundamental meaning, each with his own partial view, unduly confident of his abilities. The result is obvious: minor illnesses transformed into life threatening ones, and chronic problems dragging on until all hope of recovery is lost.

He points out that those who study "tread in the footsteps of the ancient worthies and can avoid causing premature deaths". The various teachings will lead them back to the founding revelations of medicine and only then it will guarantee of the efficacy of treatment.

## And beyond...

Basic knowledge and technical aspects of acupuncture formed the basic training that practitioners should have been able to learn without big difficulties. Several chapters of the Neijing describe two types of practitioners; one group of more ordinary, crude (cu) [粗] physicians and a category that carries the ambition for the highest form of treatment, the Superior (shang) [上] or even sage-like Practitioner. The information and instructions about the way for obtaining this status are scattered over the different chapters. Usually the passages are vague and it is clear that it had been essential that text study would be combined with oral instructions and practical guidance. Descriptions of their methods and ideas show affinity with techniques coming from self-cultivation traditions and divinatory and alchemical texts.

To be a Superior Physician required different sorts of qualities, related to enhancing one's influence on the patient's qi. Without doubt this can be seen as a crucial aspect in a medical practice where a special potency (de) could form the neutralizing force against still smouldering demonic powers, supernatural beings or other entities that could cause disease. The vocabulary that is used in the texts is not easily translated and needs the contextual spectrum that is discussed earlier in this paper.

## Shenming 神明 –Spirit brightness

Some aspects of the special qualities required for the Superior Physician are stated very clearly, others more vaguely. The first chapter of the Lingshu points out [15]:

> 小針之要。易陳而難入。
> The essentials of the fine needle are easy to explain, But it is difficult to understand the deeper aspects of it.

Apparently it is problematic to tell how the needle process exactly works. But another aspect that is meant here is that the practitioner cannot directly observe what is going on. The patterns of illness, the causes of disease and other aspects of a patient are not directly revealed for the physical senses, hence they are called "obscure". Suwen twenty-six explains [16]:

觀其冥冥者，言形氣榮衛之不形於外，而工獨知之。
As for "observing the obscure":
This means that the thriving and defensive (aspects) of the formed qi,
Is not visible on the outside,
But it is only the skilled practitioner who understands this.

The inability to perceive "what does not have a physical form" is exactly the reason why not all practitioners get the same results:

是故工之所以異也。然而不形見於外，故俱不能見也。
視之無形，嘗之無味，故謂冥冥，若神髣彿。
This is the reason why practitioners are different.
But it takes no visible form on the outside,
Therefore none of it can be seen.
He looks at it without it having a form, and tastes it without it having a flavour.
And therefore it is called obscure.
As if it were a spirit.

Where the crude do not really know what is going on, the Superior Practitioner can observe things that are not so obvious on the outside. This clarity can only come from the spirit by which the power of observation can extend to more hidden and internal aspects. In Lingshu one the practitioner is urged to attend to the spirit [15]:

粗守形上守神。
The crude guard the form (xing), the superior guard the spirit (shen).

## Ji 機 mechanism

The practice of the Superior Physician uses a highly refined skill that utilizes the concept ji to explain an essential element of the needle technique. Lingshu one continues [15]:

刺之微在遲速。粗守關上守機。
機之動不離其空 空中之機, 清靜而微。
其來不可逢。其往不可追。
The subtleties of needling lie in the speed:
The crude guard the passes (guan), the superior guard the mechanism (ji);
The movement of the mechanism is not separated from its empty centre,

The ji is in the empty centre; clear, quiet, yet subtle,
When it comes cannot be met, when it leaves it cannot be pursued.

The full passage from Lingshu one and several of its crucial concepts are analysed by Charles Chace and Dan Bensky in their chapter "An Axis of Efficacy" [2]. It makes clear that for the practitioner it is most important to understand what the term ji means. In their chapter they mention several aspects that help translating and interpreting it; as a mechanism or dynamic of qi (as an expression on how qi –or different forms of qi– are moving in the channels), as the firing mechanism of a crossbow, the crux or hinge of a thing, or as a trigger that engages something.

Other explanations of what ji (mechanism) might involve can be found by examining its use in astronomy, alchemy and divination. In Chinese astronomy the ji forms the pole around which celestial bodies revolve. When we extend this aspect to the field of medicine, ji could refer to the correct point on the body that is selected. It is the point of stillness that does not move itself, but around which movement of the whole system circles.

In alchemy ji is the exact moment when the adept starts his alchemical work and "begins the process in an open space containing nothing" [29:536]. In divination ji refers to the point of control in both temporal and spatial senses [26:120]. The aspect that involves the correct time and place is also an important issue in some styles of acupuncture treatment. For example the exact time when the treatment is given, at which moment a certain point is approached or when exactly the needle should be removed. The correct place concerns finding the exact topographical spot where the best conditions are found for the intended goal, the ideal location for the treatment or for the placement of the needle.

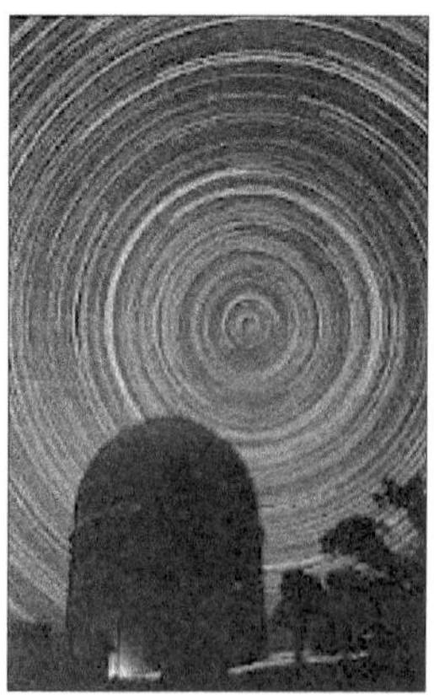

The Celestial Pole

The earlier mentioned shushu [數術] (calculation arts) were already an ancient skill but they rose to great heights together with the cosmological model. The great phenomena of the outside world, the movements of planets and stars are mirrored in the state and human body and their movements of qi. The calendar that linked both worlds used the twelve Earthly Branches and ten Heavenly Stems. They provided a key for predicting lucky or unlucky moments, the right time prescribing ritual or medical interventions or proscribing certain actions. This would provide the correct alignment of the human world with the patterns of Heaven and Earth [27:61]. In the state the emperor's first duty is to take care of this process and performing the leading role, in the human body it is the heart (xin) that is responsible [15].

The crude guard the passes (guan), the superior guard the dynamic (ji).

The crude work with the larger areas around the joints (jie) or passes (guan)[12] to find the points, but the Superior Physician has to attend to all the subtleties that are concerned with the mechanism (ji). The authors of the Neijing clearly state that it is not about finding the point somewhere in the physical structure of the body. Here palpation is taken a step further and asks for more subtle and refined skill. At the correct site (that is, where the ji can be activated) the practitioner may become aware of a specific feeling or a physical experience.

Lingshu three reiterates some aspects that already were said in the first chapter but adds some subtleties concerning the superior needle technique [15]:

粗守關者。守四肢而不知血氣正邪之往來也。
上守機者。知守氣也。機之 動不離其空[13] 中者。
"Crude" is who guards the passes (guan).
He guards the four limbs and does not know about the comings and goings of the straight and the oblique (pathogenic) of blood and qi.
"Superior" is who guards the dynamic (ji),
He knows how to guard the qi.
The movement of this mechanism never strays from its empty centre.

知氣之虛實。用針之徐疾也。空中之機。
清靜以微者。針以得氣。密意守氣勿 失也。
He knows about the fullness or emptiness,
And of the slowness or speed with which the needle is applied.

The mechanism of the empty centre is something clear, quiet and subtle.
The needle is used to obtain the qi.
Guard the qi with close attention: do not let it slip away!

## Yi 意 –attention, intention, concentration

That last line from this Lingshu three passage admonishes to give "close attention" to the process of working with qi. This is the concept yi [意] that most often is translated as concentration, attention or intention and is a next crucial aspect to explore. In some sources it is called "the Yellow Dame" (huangpo [黄婆] as it represents the communicative principle of the Yellow Centre that harmonizes yin and yang [24:88-89]. The two central organs of the body, the spleen and the heart, are associated with the concept. In Lingshu eight Huangdi and Qibo discuss the source of attention [15]:

所以任物者謂之心；心有所憶謂之意
That with which we fulfil our tasks we name the heart.
That what the heart holds (in its heart) we name attention.

Our attention (or intention) is what the heart selects and holds inside from the manifold impressions that we experience during our conscious lives. For example, if someone tells a story and we would ask several people to repeat what the story was about, each person's yi would pick out those specific elements it considered important. If a group of people would read a newspaper, every reader will remember different aspects of its content. It is the heart that chooses, and what we call "yi" are the images and ideas that are formed out the immense ocean of particulars and facts present in the outside world and of which only some are taken into consideration. The role of the spleen is an important assistant in the transformative process, as it provides the energy for selecting and transforming the images that are ingested. In alchemical texts the yi is seen as "the rider of qi", as the conductor who orchestrates the movement of qi in the body [6:1158].

Lingshu nine explains how yi or attention is used in the needling process [15]:

精神內守。而後可以行針。 專意一神。精氣之分。
毋聞人聲。以守其精。必一其神。令志在針。
Only when on the inside essence and spirit are safely guarded, can the needling start.
Pay special attention to the single-mindedness of the spirit, and the separation of essence and qi.

Do not listen to the talking of people, with this you guard the essence.
You must be at one with the spirit, this causes the will to go into the needle.

The physician Guo Yu [郭玉] lived during the reign of Emperor He [和帝] (89-105 CE) and was famous for his needling techniques. He was compassionate and caring for his patients, even for very poor people. But sometimes when he treated a noble person he could not cure him. To test Guo Yu, the emperor ordered a sick aristocrat to dress like a poor man and to ask for Guo Yu's treatment on the street. Guo Yu cured him with a single needle, and when the emperor asked him an explanation he replied [5:359-360]:

> The word "medicine" yi embodies the idea of "attention" yi. The regions of the skin are very finely divided. Following the flow of qi consummates skill. When inserting needles an error of a hair's breadth will mean failure. A kind of spirit connects the physician's heart with his hand, and that is something that I can know but cannot explain.
>
> Now when it comes to treating nobles, they look down on me from the heights of their distinguished place, and I am filled with anxiety that I might not please them. Curing nobles presents four difficulties. First, they do as they please and not as I advise. Second, they are not at all careful in caring for their own health. Third, their bones are frail, so they cannot bear strong medicine. Fourth, they love a life of ease and hate labour. Though the acupuncture needles demand precise measure, with them I am often in error. I am burdened with a heart full of trepidation, compounded by a will reduced in strength. Thus attention is not fully there. Consider what influence this has on treating the disorder! This is the reason I cannot bring about a cure.

The passage explains how the yi becomes seriously impeded when the heart is not at ease. In the theory of Chinese medicine the heart is in charge and responsible for these tasks that form the centre of life: intelligence, thinking, feeling, reasoning. When the heart is agitated, thinking will be influenced by it, experiences will be felt different. In the Masters of Huainan (Huainanzi) [淮南子], a text that was presented to Emperor Wu [武帝] in 139 BCE, is said (translation adapted from Major et al. [23:567]):

> 心有憂者，筐床衽席弗能安也，菰飯犓牛弗能甘也，琴瑟鳴竽弗能樂也。
> When the heart is agitated, though provided with a well-made bed and soft mats, you will not feel comfortable. Though provided with a meal of wild rice and succulent beef, you will not find the taste good. Though provided with the music of qin and se, and the piping of the flute, you will not find joy

## Xin 心 –The heart

Traditionally the heart, xin is designated as the ruler of man, more specifically as the organ that is responsible for both mental and emotional aspects. It is often translated as "heart-mind" because of its "mastering" activities like thinking (si) [思], loving (ai) [愛], grieving (bei) [悲] or intending (yi) [意]. As long as the heart is not overwhelmed by different sensitive and cognitive impulses and is able to maintain a quiet, empty and balanced centre the energy of Heaven can be guarded, securing a save place for the shen and ensuring long life in harmony.

Sometimes the heart is compared to a horse, which strays in all directions and must be tamed. To "empty the heart" (xu xin) [虛心] means to release oneself from the restlessness, desires and thoughts which come with everyday life [29:1102]. For a practitioner who wished to improve his skills it was a crucial aspect that his heart should not bothered by emotions (qing) [情]. In a famous quote Huizi asks Zhuangzi (Zhuangzi ch. 5, transl. adapted from [28:131]):

> "How can a man without his emotions still be called a man?" Zhuangzi responds, "Distinguishing 'right' and 'wrong' is what I mean with the emotions. What I mean by being without emotions is that man should not allow likes and dislikes to enter and thus harm himself. He should always accord with the spontaneous and not add to life."
>
> Huizi then asks him what that means, "adding to life". Zhuangzi replies:
>
> "The Way gave us appearance, and Heaven gave us form. Do not use likes and dislikes to enter and harm the self. Now, you are putting your spirit on the outside, and wearing out your essence."

"To empty the heart" or xu xin had to be carefully learned and practiced, required personal dedication, regular training and self-discipline. Some sources also mention purification practices and physical exercises for a correct ordering of the body and (heart-) mind [18: 48]. The Neiye [內業][14] speaks of "regulating the heart" (zhi xin) [治心]. The character zhi is the same as is used in medical texts for "governing" a physiological function or "curing or treating" a disease [21:938]:

> 我心治官乃治，我心安官乃安，治之者，心也。
> 安之者，心也。心以藏心，心之中又有心焉。
> When our heart is well regulated, our senses are well regulated too.
> When our heart is peaceful, our senses are peaceful too.
> What regulates them is our heart.
> What makes them peaceful is our heart.
> The heart contains a heart.
> Within the heart there is another heart.

"In the heart is another heart" forms a central point in the text. The heart with a void in its inner core: an empty space where the spirit[15] can reside. On the one hand the heart acts as the sovereign, responsible in fulfilling his tasks as ruler, but within that heart is another space where the dwelling shen can find a place to stay. This double function of the heart has been elaborated in later medical theory and is expressed as the sovereign fire and ministerial fire of the fire element [30:9-12]. The Neiye states that it is the heart that creates the basis for the great accomplishments [21:939]:

心全於中，形全於外，不逢天菑，不遇人害，謂之聖人。
人能正靜，皮膚裕寬，耳目聰明，筋伸而骨強，乃能戴大圜而履大方。
If the heart is complete on the inside,
the form is complete on the outside.
Calamities of Heaven will not harm you.
Human evil shall not visit you.
We call such a man a sage.
If you can hold on to correctness and quiescence.
Your skin will be relaxed and glow with health.
Your ears and eyes will be sharp and clear.
Your tendons taut, your bones strong.
Only then you are able to wear the Great Circle.
And to tread on the Great Square.

If the heart is kept at peace, it will bring health and harmony both inside and outside the body. It will strengthen the physical abilities to accomplish the challenges on the outside, symbolized in "carrying the Great Circle of Heaven" and "treading on the Great Square of Earth". The wisdom that attends to this condition brings a mastery of the self and the world around us.

## Conclusion

Reviewing the different characteristics of the Superior Physician it becomes clear that people wearing this predicate were able to apply a unique intervention on the human body. Their special qualities were attained through a process of dedicated cultivation, bringing about healing and harmony for himself and for his patients.

The qualities and skills described in the Neijing texts for the Superior Physician closely relate to the features that were mentioned earlier in this paper characterizing the Superior Man. The "widening and deepening possibilities" that formed the first group of transformations, unveil as the capacity to perceive different qualities of qi, seeing patterns in the body, knowing what goes on and what needs to be carried out at a certain moment in time. This insight is called shenming [神明] or "spirit brightness". Whereas the ordinary (or crude) practitioner dwells in oblivion, the enhanced perception of the superior physician enables him to make a better diagnosis and be more aware of what would be a good treatment. The other aspect in this category of "extension" is the mechanism ji [機], the ability to engage the qi in optimal time and space conditions. To know the right moment (exact timing) and the right circumstances (exact location) for engaging transformations provides an extended form of skill that allows for maximum therapeutic effect.

The second group of qualities that was seen as characterizing the Superior Man was couched in notions like "integration, blending, unification and merging". This can be seen in the Superior Physician as the ability to create a focus, giving strict attention to what is necessary to restore the patterns and what is called yi [意] (intention, attention or concentration), what gives qi its focus and direction. What brings all these features together also belongs to this second group of qualities. It is the heart, the great ruler and coordinator of all processes and the emperor of the nation, where all emotional, intellectual and mental aspects are being processed and where the decisions are made. The heart decides in all matters what it wants to keep and what it discards. The "emptying of the heart" (xuxin) [虛心] forms an important strategy in the ability of the heart to clear everything that should be swept aside. Through this conscious action the heart becomes the empty space where the emperor can rule his country with an untroubled and unbiased mind, to do the things that are best for the whole nation without prejudice.

In Suwen fifty-four Qibo gives several guidelines about needle technique. After explaining some more general instructions there follows an almost poetic description on the bearings of the practitioner by which he can control the spirit and guide the qi [16]:

> 如臨深淵者，不敢墮也。手如握虎者，欲其壯也。
> 神無營於眾物者，靜志觀病人，無左右視也。
> 義無邪下者，欲端以正也。必正其神者，欲瞻病人目，制其神，令氣易行也。
> As if standing on the edge of an abyss, not daring to go down.
> The hand, as if grasping a tiger, wanting it to be sturdy.
> The spirit, without being troubled by trivial things,
> Quiet and devoted to the observation of the patient, without looking left or right.
> Righteous, without being deflected downwards, wanting to correct it until it is straight.
> He must keep his spirit straight, desiring to look in the eyes of the patient,
> To control his spirit and make his qi move easily.

In a different language we could say:

The physician perfects his posture, stabilizes his hand and creates a total focus for his mission. In him are the best intentions to bring about the finest for his patient. Without being distracted, his focus is on bringing back the right patterns. For this his spirit is single-minded, and by looking in the patient's eyes he is able to control the spirit and qi. By settling his own spirit, he uses himself as an instrument to control the spirit of the patient. The correct posture, quiet intention and the determination of the practitioner enable the heavenly alignment to take place, through which the response of the spirit and essences of the body can take place.

In the Chinese name Lingshu [靈樞] the character shu [樞] meaning "axis" or "pivot" helps to explain this process. A pivot is a central shaft that allows for a connection between different aspects. In a human being the character shu refers to "opening and closing" between different areas, or, in other words to function as an intermediary through which different aspects and layers can interact.

In disease patterns (most typically where the normal restoration processes are disturbed) these life-giving and healing connections are disrupted. This is seen as the reason why natural healing (as the capacity of the healthy body) does not take place any more. Only when the communication between different levels has come back on line and the qi is able to pass through, the life-giving Heavenly force (ling) [靈] can access the body again. The ling is what comes down from Heaven and is received in the earthly body. Without this health cannot be restored, as it is Heaven's role to give the correct lines, to restore power to put the original pattern (li) [理] back in place. Only when this happens can construction take place, which is a matter of the Earth. Nothing can be built without the plan, which is provided by Heaven. In the same way, nothing can take form without the essential materials, for which Earth is responsible.

The Lingshu or Spiritual Axis is the name for the tool that reinstates the connection between Heaven and Earth. The axis is the acupuncture needle, allowing the repair of the disturbed connection and the restoration of the pattern. In the same way the Superior Practitioner is the treatment tool, now using his own body as the connecting pivot to engage the qi. This describes what could be called the Superior Way.

"Superior" in this context is not what we would call morally or ethically superior, nor is it about following the better protocols or having the best intentions, but it is about a sensitivity to perceive the unique aspects and qualities that are present in the actual situation, it is the capacity to recognize what is going on in both external and internal environment and to bring about what would be the best solution given these circumstances.

The different techniques that were described are sometimes called "mental training" in western terminology. It is misleading if the mental aspect is placed opposite the physical aspect; working with qi always involves both aspects. This can also be observed in talking about the eastern martial arts. It would also be misleading to call these "physical training" as the primary goal here is to bring about a state of mental peace and clarity. An important part of the practice is to learn not to be deceived by the direct visual or auditory experiences and to detect the opponent's qi. Our senses can lead us astray and show an illusion; someone who is big and tall can harbour a weak qi and something heard at a certain spot does not mean that the qi is there. Only with stillness in the heart things can be perceived as they really are.

In the medical texts of the Neijing the notion of the Superior Physician alludes to a vast spectrum of ideas and techniques, rooted in cosmological ideas and combined with all sorts of methods concerning inner cultivation in early China. Although the special powers or virtues (de) [德] that would be the result of this development are connected to the person, it is not something directly seen as "personal". Although patterns can be restored and healing can take place through the development of his individual talents, inner refinement and opening up of senses, we may also become aware that there is no "owner" of this power, only somebody who can and may use it. And the texts warn: do not let it slip away!

The Superior Person is the mediator connecting the portals of the different realms, the intermediary who is able to perceive the patterns of the microcosm of the patient and the bigger patterns of the macrocosm in order to bridge the gap that other people cannot cross. In this way he can influence the qi of the world and bring about harmony and healing in the patient.

本末，一體也；其兩愛之，一性也。
先本後末謂之君子，以末害本謂之小人。
君子與小人之性非異也，所在先後而已矣。
Roots and branches constitute a single body.
What both of them cherish is a single nature.
One who places the root first and the branches behind is called a Superior Man.
One who uses the branches to harm the root is called a petty man.
The natures of the Superior Man and the petty man are not different;
Rather, it is a question of their priorities.
(Huainanzi translation by Major et al. [23:832]).

## Acknowledgements

I am deeply grateful to many people who provided me the stimulating thoughts, environment and a supportive space to develop my ideas concerning this topic. Especially I wish to thank Burchard Mansvelt Beck for his kind support, precise comments and wise insights in reviewing this paper.

## Translation notes

Some Chinese characters (like qi) are never translated, others (like shen, ji or yi) are used both in Chinese and English, to express that their meaning hardly can be conveyed in one single translation. All translations, unless indicated differently, are by the author.

## Bibliography

1- De Bary T, Bloom I. *Sources of Chinese Tradition, from Earliest times to 1600*, Volume I, Sec. ed. New York: Columbia University Press, 1999.
2- Chace C, Bensky D. Chapter five: An axis of efficacy –The range of meaning in chapter one of the Lingshu. In this volume.
3- Cook CA. Ancestor worship during the Eastern Zhou. In: Lagerwey J, Kalinowski M. (eds.) *Early Chinese Religion: Part One: Shang through Han (1250 B.C. – 220 A.D.)*, Leiden: Brill, 2009 pages 237-279.
4- Cook CA. The Pre-Han Period. In: Hinrichs TJ, Barnes LL. (eds) *Chinese Medicine and Healing –An Illustrated History*. Cambridge Massachusetts: Harvard University Press 2013.
5- DeWoskin K. Three Biographies from the History of the Later Han. In: Minford J, Lau M. (eds.) *Classical Chinese Literature: An Anthology of Translations*. New York; Columbia University Press, 2000.
6- Esposito M. on yi. In: Pregadio F. (ed.). *The encyclopedia of Taoism, Volume II*. London and New York: Routledge, 2008.
7- Graham AC. *Chuang-Tzu –The Inner Chapters*. London, Harper Collins Publishers, 1991.
8- Hall DL, Ames RT. *Thinking from the Han –Self, Truth and Transcendence in Chinese and Western Culture*. Albany New York: State University of New York Press, 1998.
9- Hansen V. *The Open Empire –A History of China to 1600*. New York: Norton & Company, 2000.
10- Harper D. The Conception of Illness in Early Chinese Medicine, as Documented in Newly Discovered 3rd and 2nd Century BC Manuscripts, part I. *Sudhoffs Archiv*, Band 74, Heft 2. Stuttgart: Franz Steiner Verlag, 1990.

11- Harper D. *Early Chinese Medical Literature: The Mawangdui Medical Manuscripts.* Sir Henry Wellcome Asian Series. London and New York: Paul Kegan, 1998.
12- Harper D. Physicians and Diviners: The relation of divination to the medicine of the Huangdi Neijing (Inner canon of the Yellow Thearch). In: *Extrême-Occident* 1999, N°21, pp. 91-110.
13- Harper D. The Textual Form of Knowledge: Occult Miscellanies in Ancient and Medieval Manuscripts, Fourth Century BC to Tenth Century AD. In: Bretelle-Establet F, (ed). *Looking at it from Asia: The processes that Shaped the Sources of History of Science.* New York: Springer, 2010 pages. 37-80.
14- Hsu E. *Pulse Diagnosis in Early Chinese Medicine –The Telling Touch.* New York: Cambridge University Press, 2010.
15- *Huangdi Neijing Lingshu*: 1: 靈樞經Wenlin digital version 4.1.1. Wenlin Institute Inc. 2012. 2: Huangdi Neijing Lingshu jizhu (Collected commentaries) 黃帝內經靈樞 集注 Zhang Zhicong張志聰 (1672).
16- *Huangdi Neijing Suwen*; 1: Wenlin digital version 4.1.1. Wenlin Institute Inc. 2012. 2: CD complement to the annotated translation (Zheng Jinsheng, Zhang Tongjun, Tessenow H, Unschuld P.) Berkeley, Los Angeles: University of California Press, 2011. 3: Huangdi Neijing Suwen jizhu (collected commentaries) 黃帝內經素問集注Zhang Zhicong張志聰 (1672).
17- Kalinowski M. Diviners and Astrologers under the Eastern Zhou: Transmitted texts and Recent Archaeological Discoveries. In: Lagerwey J, Kalinowski M. (eds.) *Early Chinese Religion, Part One: Shang through Han (1250 BC-220 AD).* Leiden: Brill, 2009, pages 341-396.
18- Kirkland R. *Taoism –The Enduring Tradition.* New York and London: Routledge, 2004.
19- Lau DC. *Mencius*, revised ed. London: Penguin classics, 2003.
20- Li Jianmin, They shall expel Demons. In: Lagerwey J, Kalinowski M. (eds.) *Early Chinese Religion: Part One: Shang through Han (1250 B.C. – 220 A.D.)*, Vol.2. Leiden: Brill, 2009, pages 1103-1150.
21- Li Xiangfeng, *Neiye* in *Guanzi jiaozhu*, 3 vols. Beijing: Zhonghua Shuju, 2004.
22- Lin Fu-shi. The Image and Status of Shamans in Ancient China. In: Lagerwey J, Kalinowski M. (eds.) *Early Chinese Religion: Part One: Shang through Han (1250 B.C.-220 A.D.)*, Leiden: Brill, 2009 pages 397-458.
23- Liu An, Translation adapted from Major J, Queen S, Meyer A, Roth H. *The Huainanzi –A Guide to the Theory and Practice of Government in Early Han China.* New York: Columbia University Press, 2010.
24- Liu Yiming, translation in Cleary T. *The Inner Teachings of Taoism.* Boston and London: Shambala, 1986.
25- Lloyd G, Sivin N. *The Way and the Word – Science and Medicine in Early China and Greece.* New Haven: Yale University, 2002.
26- Lo V. Spirit of Stone: Technical considerations in the Treatment of the Jade Body. *Bulletin of the School of Oriental and African Studies*, University of London, 2002;65(1): 99 128.

27- Lo V. The Han Period. In: Eds. Hinrichs TJ, Barnes LL. *Chinese Medicine and Healing – An Illustrated History*. Cambridge Massachusetts: Harvard University Press 2013.
28- Puett MJ. *To Become a God: Cosmology, Sacrifice and Self-Divinization in Early China*. Cambridge MA: Harvard University Asia Center, 2008.
29- Robinet I. On ji. In: Pregadio F. (ed). *The encyclopedia of Taoism, Volume I.* London and New York: Routledge, 2008.
30- Rochat de la Vallée E. *The Double Aspect of the Heart*, Monkey Press, 2012.
31- Sivin N. Text and Experience in Classical Chinese Medicine. In: Bates D. (ed.) *Knowledge and the scholarly medical traditions*. Cambridge: Cambridge University Press, 1995A.
32- Sivin N. State, Cosmos and Body in the Last Three Centuries B.C. *Harvard Journal of Asiatic Studies*, 1995B;55(1):5-37.
33- Sommers D. *De Chinese Fascinatie voor de Geest –De Werking van het Innerlijk*. Veghel: Libra & Libris, 2007.
34- Unschuld PU, Tessenow H. Huang Di *Nei jing su wen –An Annotated Translation of Huang Di's Inner Classic –Basic Questions*. Volume I. Berkeley, Los Angeles: University of California Press, 2011.
35- Yang SH. (translator), *The Pulse Classic: A Translation of the Maijing* (by Wang Shuhe). Boulder: Blue Poppy Press, 2002.

## Endnotes

1. The notion of "the Way" is a general idea about a process or a route that was shared by the various groups in early China's population. They used the concept to explain or formalize their specific "way", which could be a manual or recipe to handle with daily affairs, a strategy to cope with difficulties of life or a more formal protocol of a ritual.

2. The texts of Huangdi were first mentioned in the imperial bibliography of the Former Han as the Inner and Outer Classics Yellow Emperor (Huangdi Neijing and Huangdi Waijing). We don't know these books in their original state. The received version has been subject to editing, altering and amending until the 12th century. The invention of printing stopped the continuous changing. We now know the Neijing as divided in three separate books: Basic Questions (Suwen), The Numinous Pivot (Lingshu) and the Grand Basis (Taisu).

3. Huangdi Neijing Lingshu chapter 71. The passage is also found in the Taisu, 5:25-40 and in a parallel passage in Lingshu 12. In: [1:147].

4. The term Confucianism is used here for what in the Chinese language is referred to as Ru [儒], meaning the school or teachings that follow the thoughts of Confucius or the ideals that he represents.

5. Mencius 4A.12, adapted from [19:82].

6. Stone, minerals and jade carry a generative force, an aspect that was used in the mysteries of life and death. The Stone Spirit (Shishen) [石神] was one of the books given to early Han physician Chunyu Yi by his teacher Yang Qing. Stone could be used as powder or mineral medicine (yaoshi) [藥石], as needling stone (more like a probe) or laid on the body or in the room for the special qualities they possessed. Jade, the most refined stone, became the metaphor for physical immortality. See [26:102-103].

7. Xing [型] means "modelling", but also "molding a vessel", as bronze sacrificial vessel that represented the ancestor-descendant relationship [4:14].

8. Shu [數] (literally calculations or numbers) and shu [術] (literally art or technical skill) probably refers to cosmological calculations, since shushu is also the name of the division where books on astrology, the calendar and hemerology, and correlations of yinyang and five phases in the Hanshu bibliographic treatise are found [11:45].

9. The Zuo zhuan chronicle (the year 540 BCE) records the theory of physician He who distinguishes the six types of qi that are produced by Heaven. If excessive activity is generated in one of these Heavenly qi forms in the body, there will be illness. These six types of qi were: yin, yang, wind (feng), rain (yu), darkness (an) and brightness (ming).

10. Although the existence of spirits and demons officially is denied, the next passage shows that a specific presentation of symptoms *resembles* demons and spirits. They don't deny their existence, nor do they specifically say that demons and spirits cannot cause illness. In Lingshu chapter 58 Zei feng [賊風], Huangdi says "What the Master has just stated are all things a sick man himself would know. If, however, he has not encountered an evil qi and further has not experienced horrific shock to his will, and yet suddenly is taken ill, what is the reason for this? Is it nothing other than that the cause lies in the activity of demons and spirits?" Qi Bo said, "In this case there is also old evil that has remained and is not yet released. Because of it, if the will hates something or longs for something, the blood and qi are thrown into disorder inside and the two qi strike one another. The origin of this condition is subtle. Looking one does not see it and listening one does not hear it. Thus it resembles demons and spirits" (translation by Harper [12:99]).

11. The text appears in the Shi ji (Records of the Historian) the universal history written by Sima Qian (145–86 BCE). The biography of Chunyu Yi forms the second part of chapter 105 and is a treasure trove of individual case studies with quite systematic records of each patient's gender, social status and place of residence. The stories further describe Chunyu Yi's prognosis, diagnosis and his therapeutic approach.

12. Both refer to narrow passages or constrictions in the body, as formed between bones and muscles or at the joints [26:119-120].

13. The character [空] (kong) combines [穴] (xue) acupuncture hole, point (empty space) and [工] gong (work).

14. The Neiye or "Inner Workings" is a text compiled about 350 BCE and that showed a new view on humans. While rooted not only in the earth but also in the heavenly realm, the Neiye points out that man has the possibility to develop the characteristics and capacities that belong to the sphere of gods and ghosts. Through inner cultivation and development it is possible to achieve a peaceful and balanced heart, a prerequisite to these divine capacities [33:112].

15. In the Warring States texts the term spirits (shen) refer to gods, divine creatures, ancestors or powers of nature which are present in clouds, mountains, seas and rivers –entities *outside* a human being. The Neiye text explores the conditions of how these divine entities could be persuaded to reside inside man and more specifically in the human heart, and how their divine powers could become part of the human sphere. Later in the Han era shen is already seen as the divine aspect of man, since he is formed out of Heaven and Earth. But still the shen are able to move through diverse gates in the body, circulate through the interior and have their dwelling place in the heart.

CHAPTER FOUR

# THE JINGMAI AND QI

## Acupuncture perspectives

**Stephen Birch**

Human beings have 360 joints, nine body openings and five yin and six yang systems of function. In the flesh, tightness is desireable; in the blood vessels, free flow is desireable; in the sinews and bones, solidity is desireable; in the operations of the heart, mind and will, harmony is desireable; in the essential qi, regular motion is desireable. When this is realised, illness has nowhere to abide, and there is nothing from which pathology can develop. When illness lasts and pathology develops, it is because the essential qi has become static. Analogously, water when stagnant becomes foul; a tree when [the condition of its qi is] stagnant becomes worm eaten; grasses when [the circulation of their qi is] stagnant become withered. Lushi Chunqiu, third century BCE [66:223-224]

Needling regulates (tunes) the qi (tiao qi). Lingshu seventy-five [92:79]

The art of needling is to needle the points of qi and not to needle muscular striations. Lingshu four [130]

In the sky there are yin and yang; human beings have their twelve major mai-channels. The sky has its hot and cold weather, human beings have their depletions (xu) and repletions (shi). He who can model himself on the transformations of sky and earth, yin and yang, will not fail to be attuned to the four seasons. He who can know the pattern underlying the (motions) of the twelve mai-channels will not be surpassed in wisdom even by a sage. Suwen twenty-five [32:8]

Inserting needles and applying moxa, this is an art. Ours is a profession which requires a sense of adventure. Isn't it incredible how all manner of diseases can be cured with nothing more than a needle or a few pieces of moxa? Isn't it grand how needles and moxa can be used to create the effect of all manner of medicine? Acupuncture is of the mind. This should be considered very carefully. One needle can be used to unlock the key to all manner of diseases. It is only natural therefore, that one's technique needs to be perfected. Sorei Yanagiya (1980) [100:237]

Acupuncture is a profession in which we use a thin piece of wire in an attempt to cure conditions which do not respond to medicines. Without a doubt, this is an extremely challenging profession. Denmei Shudo (2003) [100:237]

## Introduction

This chapter will examine how the concepts of qi [氣] and the jingmai [經脈] have influenced and been used in the field of acupuncture. Probably more than in the other medical practices, qi and jingmai have been used extensively in systematic ways in the field of acupuncture. But acupuncture is a diverse field where many ideas and practice models and methods have developed over time, thus the chapter will need to briefly explore the influence of this diversity on the role of qi and the jingmai in acupuncture. It will not be an exhaustive discussion of these topics as that would be too large to include here, but it will present sufficient examples and evidence to capture these themes.

Since acupuncture therapy is usually applied or targeted to the acupoints which primarily lie on the jingmai, and most commonly uses needles to influence the qi of the jingmai, this chapter will briefly explore the relationship of acupoints to qi and jingmai and their combined relationships to the body, and examine discussions in the early literature about how the needling is to be done. The topic of needling is examined further in the next chapter by Chace and Bensky [24]. Some of the issues and themes discussed in the current chapter will be important when we examine problems with how qi and the jingmai are researched by scientists, which is the topic of chapter eight [15].

## What is acupuncture?

A common understanding of acupuncture is that it involves the insertion of needles into acupoints to treat disease and thus help patients recover [62;[1] 72;[2] 83[3]]. However, this understanding of acupuncture does not capture the diversity and range of practice methods and approaches that can be found histori-

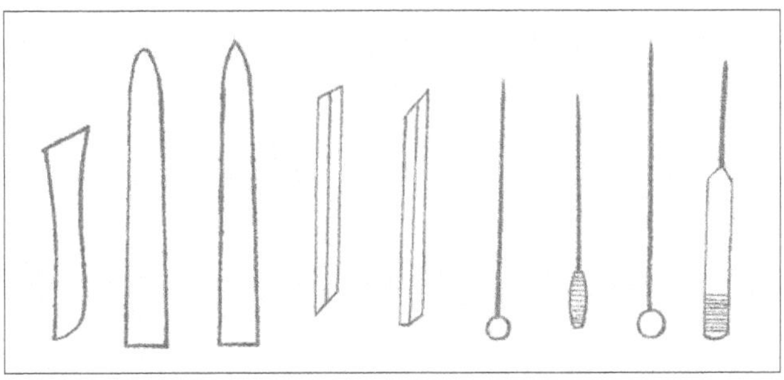

Nine needles from the Lingshu

cally and in the modern period [122[4]]. In order to understand this we will briefly examine historical descriptions and uses that make this kind of simple definition difficult to accept and will briefly outline something of the current diversity of practice styles, methods and techniques that pass under the name acupuncture. The author has written on these subjects before, the reader interested in exploring this further can examine these references [4, 19, 97 and especially 17], see also [73].[5]

Acupuncture is not limited to the insertion of needles into acupoints. The early literature describes nine kinds of needles [九鍼], which not only had different shapes, sizes and functions, but they were not all inserted through the skin –see Figure 1. These nine needles are described in chapters one, seven and seventy-eight of the Lingshu [靈樞] [72:102-103], one of the primary texts that make up the Huangdi Neijing [黃帝內經] corpus. The needle used most by acupuncturists today is the hao zhen [毫鍼], filiform needle, which is a thin needle inserted into the body for treatment. Described in the Lingshu and less commonly used today are the yuan zhen [員鍼] and shi zhen [鍉鍼], round-headed and blunt needles, which are used for rubbing and pressing the skin, they do not penetrate the skin [18:48-54]. The chan zhen [鑱鍼] arrow headed needle was also not inserted into the body, rather pressed in a cutting action to the skin surface [18:46-47]. The feng zhen [鋒鍼] is used for bloodletting[6] and the pi zhen [鈹鍼] for lancing boils etc[7] [18:39-41]. The final three needles, the yuanli zhen [利鍼], round-sharp needle, chang zhen [長鍼], long needle, and the da zhen [大鍼], large needle are inserted to different depths for different purposes [18:54-56].[8] These needles and variations in needling methods have been used in the practice of acupuncture to varying degrees over two millenia [17]. Additionally, the acupuncturist routinely uses jiu [灸] moxibustion. This involves the burning of small cones of moxa (mugwort –artemisia vulgaris) as a form of stimulation therapy. Originally the moxa was burned directly on the skin causing small burns, later alternative methods evolved whereby the moxa is placed on an intermediate substance such as ginger, garlic, salt, or rolled into sticks and the lit end held near the body to apply heat without burning [72:170-172]. Today all these and other forms of moxibustion are regularly used. Moxibustion therapy is found in the Mawangdui and Zhangjiashan texts where it is the principal therapy applied to the mai [47:91]. In these early uses of moxa there is some discussion of applying the technique to influence the qi, the Maishu of the Zhangjiashan discusses how to use moxibustion to help correct qi flow in the body [47, 68]. Cupping therapy is also used in the practice of acupuncture, this was known earlier as "horn therapy" and can be found in the Mawangdui texts [47:98].

Thus the practice of acupuncture has from the earliest times involved the use of inserted and non-inserted needles, bleeding, lancing, moxaing and cupping.[9] Different practitioners at different times selected from and combined these treatment techniques with theories that were developing, that they developed or based simply on observation and experience [17]. On the whole the techniques of moxa, cupping and bloodletting were not directed so much to addressing disturbances of the qi, they have generally been considered to affect the more physical system of the xue or blood.[10] Needling is the principle method in the practice of acupuncture and it is used in the regulation of qi, Lingshu seventy-five tells us: "Needling regulates (tunes) the qi (*tiao qi* [調氣])" [92:79].[11] Rochat de la Vallee considers this as a kind of definition of acupuncture.[12] Needling is principally applied to correct disturbances of the qi[13] and their circulation tracts, the jingmai, Lai and Tong describe how the main purpose of acupuncture is "for regulating qi activities in the human body" [57].[14] This was certainly the main target of treatment in the influential acupuncture text the Nanjing [難經] of circa 106 CE [71:385; 112] and as the quote above shows, probably the Lingshu as well. Thus in this chapter we will focus on needling in the discussions.

While this focus of needling to regulate the qi is clearly articulated in the early texts of the Neijing and Nanjing,[15] the target of treatment by needling was already diverse from the earliest times, as we would expect given the range of opinions and ideas expressed in the Neijing texts.[16] For example we find repeated cautions about how the superior physician[17] is the one that focuses on correcting disturbances of the qi,[18] targeting the jingmai,[19] thereby targeting the circulation tracts of the qi (jingmai) and their access holes (acupoints –xue). An implication from this repeated caution is that there must have been many practitioners using needles in different ways than this. The developing literature, especially since the time of Huang Fumi in his Zhenjiu Jiayijing [鍼灸甲乙經] of 282 CE, started systematically describing symptoms in relation to each acupuncture point, leaving the not unreasonable supposition that there were many that needled the acupoints according to symptoms rather than the regulation of qi.[20] Thus acupuncture needling does not always appear to have been directed towards influencing only the qi in the jingmai, but also as a way of addressing symptoms. This shift of focus to the symptoms is accompanied[21] by an increasing focus on the anatomical body and its structures as target of treatment,[22] a trend that became highly influential with the introduction of Western anatomical concepts of the body into Asian medical thinking.[23] The development of acupuncture after the third century CE is marred by problems, it became known as a dangerous therapy, falling into disrepute up until the Song dynasty[24] where it saw a significant revival [43]. Historically and especially in the modern period many conceptions of the nature and thus target of acupuncture treatment can be found.[25] Another example is seen in the innovations of the Neijing that bring the internal weakness or vacuity, xu [虛] into discussions of how evil qi, xieqi [邪氣] can cause injury, Lingshu sixty-six states: "Therefore, evil alone cannot harm a person. It is invariably only when the two vacuities of vacuity wind and vacuity in the body combine with each other that wind is able to settle in the body" [63:1120]. Given that an internal vacuity or weakness takes on a dominant role, it is thus not surprising that some texts highlighted vacuity as the primary target of treatment. Nanjing sixty-nine is explicit about this: "one must fill first and drain after" [112:583], which has become a core treatment principle for later traditions of practice such as the Keiraku Chiryo or Japanese Meridian Therapy movement that started in the 1930s [17, 41, 99]. While not the focus of this chapter, these different influences, trends, interpretations and foci need to be acknowledged and discussed.

## Summary of historical influences and development of qi and jingmai concepts in acupuncture

As we have seen in previous chapters [16, 20], at the time that the early medical literature developed (circa 200-150 BCE) early models of the body employed the mai [脈] as a kind of primitive physiological model using the tools of bleeding and moxa to treat them.[26] The mai were seen in their relation to xue, blood [血] and qi [氣] [32, 47, 114],[27] but these models of physiology were not well developed, leaving a gap for more detailed explanations. In the push to develop more comprehensive physiological and pathological models that would be of greater use to medical practitioners, the concept of qi was expanded to include multiple subsets.[28] As we saw in chapter one, the concept of qi provides a foundation for understanding the body and mind, the effect of moral conduct on the body and society, relationships between emerging environmental models and the body, emergent cosmological models and the body and a basis for discussing different aspects of the body in more detail. In this latter aspect, it has been noted how in early medical discussions we find reference to a qi that is undifferentiated and whole [29, 92], but that this needed to be differentiated into multiple subsets most likely to allow doctors to start to identify which parts of the whole had become disordered thereby allowing more differentiated treatment approaches [29, 114]. The association of qi with the mai is seen to have strengthened as discussions of the "mai" are replaced by discussions of the "jingmai" [經脈] in the Huangdi Neijing texts, the Suwen [素問] and the Lingshu.

In the pre-Neijing texts (such as the Mawangdui texts) the "mai" are a kind of physiological system that can be stimulated to treat certain symptoms. With the Neijing's introduction of the new term, the "jingmai" and all their extensions through the theory of systematic correspondence, we see not only the ability to apply treatment to target symptoms, but also the ability to target internal organs and through the addition of five-phase correspondences, the ability to import order into the otherwise disordered body and thus "regulate qi". This idea of the extended and usually implicit role of the theory of systematic correspondence as a system that permits the import of the ordering properties of nature (heaven and earth) into the body is introduced in chapters one and two [16, 20]. We will see below that in acupuncture this role appears to reach a kind of pinnacle. It becomes most obvious with the introduction of the acupoints and specific classes of acupoints (see below).

Chapter two described the development of the jingmai [20], Table 1 summarises the twelve jingmai, their principle associations, numbers of acupoints, etc. The two other mai that have acupoints directly associated with them (renmai and dumai) are also listed.

## Qi movements within and associated with the jingmai

We saw in chapter two that the mai contained qi in some of the Mawangdui and Zhangjiashan texts but that there was no circulation of the qi. The trajectories of the mai are centripetal from the periphery to the center, but it is not clear that qi was thought to naturally move in these trajectories. Lingshu chapter seventeen and Nanjing chapter twenty-three contain descriptions of similar centripetal trajectories for the jingmai. These are not part of the circulation of qi described elsewhere in the Lingshu and Nanjing. We suggested in chapter two that perhaps these centripetal trajectories were intended to capture the idea of how the ordering qi of the environment (the qi of heaven and earth) is imported into the body to help produce order within the body and in a sense express the connection of the body to the cosmos of which it is a product. This idea is thus different than that of a (physiologically derived) qi that circulates within the body, running through the jingmai in a continuous circuit where it circulates also inside the body to connect with the major organs, the zang-fu. If this distinction is correct this circulating qi is likely to be described more as a product of things in the body, more a kind of physiological qi and should

**Table 1: The accepted twelve jingmai and their major correspondences**

| arm/ leg | yin/ yang | Five Phase | primary organ | secondary organ | number acupoints |
|---|---|---|---|---|---|
| arm | taiyin | metal | lungs | large intestine | 11 |
| arm | yangming | metal | large intestine | lungs | 20 |
| leg | yangming | earth | stomach | spleen | 45 |
| leg | taiyin | earth | spleen | stomach | 21 |
| arm | shaoyin | fire | heart | small intestine | 9 |
| arm | taiyang | fire | small intestine | heart | 19 |
| leg | taiyang | water | bladder | kidneys | 67 |
| leg | shaoyin | water | kidneys | bladder | 27 |
| arm | jueyin | fire | pericardium | san jiao | 9 |
| arm | shaoyang | fire | san jiao | pericardium | 23 |
| leg | shaoyang | wood | gallbladder | liver | 44 |
| leg | jueyin | wood | liver | galbladder | 14 |
| renmai* yin | yin | - | - | - | 24 |
| dumai* yang | yang | - | - | - | 28[29] |

have description(s) of its production. This is what we find with the descriptions in the Lingshu of how yingqi [營氣] circulates within the jingmai and is produced as a result of organ physiology.

## Ying qi circulation –continuous circulation within the jingmai

Lingshu chapter fifteen and Nanjing chapter one explain how the jingmai circulate the yingqi in a continuous cycle propelled by the breath (see chapter two above for further discussions of this [20]). This circulation of yingqi was linked to astronomical movements and theories such as the twenty eight celestial mansions or constellations, xiu [宿].[30] The yingqi starts at the stomach[31] then passes through the dachang [大肠] (large intestine), from here up to the fei [肺] (lung)[32] to come out at the lung channel [手太陰] flowing from chest to thumb; from here it returns via the large intestine channel [手陽明] rising up to the face, besides the nose, with a branch running from the supraclavicular

* The ren mai was described much later as the "ocean of yin", the dumai as the "ocean of yang" by Li Shizhen in 1578 [77:27&41]. Of the eight qijingbamai, the ren and du are the only two that have their own acupoints, the other six have been described as trajectories that intersect the regular jingmai or ren and dumai at acupoints on them [77].

fossa at ST-12 inside to the fei (lung) and down to the dachang (large intestine); from the face it continues on the stomach channel [足陽明] to descend down the chest, abdomen and leg to the second toe, with a branch entering at ST-12 to pass inside to the wei [胃] (stomach) and pi [脾] (spleen); from the foot it passes to the spleen channel [足太陰] and rises up the leg to pass across the abdomen and chest to end below the axilla, with a branch that runs interiorly from the abdomen to the pi (spleen), wei (stomach) and xin [心] (heart); from the heart it passes to the chest wall to run down the arm to the small finger along the heart channel [手少陰], with a branch inside also running down to the xiaochang [小肠] (small intestine); on the hand it connects to the small intestine channel [手太陽] and runs back up the arm up the neck to end on the face, with a branch running inside from ST-12 to the xin (heart) and xiaochang (small intestine); from the face it connects to the bladder channel [足太陽] and runs down the neck, back and back of the leg to end at the fifth toe, with a branch passing inside at ST-12 to the pangguang [膀胱] (bladder) and shen [肾] (kidney); on the foot it connects to the kidney channel [足少陰] rises up the inside of the leg to run up the abdomen and end just below the clavicle, with a branch that runs inside to the shen (kidney) and pangguang (bladder) and another inside the chest; it continues inside the chest to the xinbaoluo [心包絡] (pericardium) and thence out to the chest wall to follow the pericardium channel [手厥陰] down the center of the forearm to the middle finger, with a further branch running down through the sanjiao [三焦] (triple burner); on the hand it connects to the triple burner channel [手厥陰] and runs up the arm to the side of the head, with a branch running inside from ST-12 to the xinbaoluo (pericardium) and sanjiao (triple burner); from the side of the head it connects to the gallbladder channel [足少陽], runs back across the head down the neck, side of the body to end at the fourth toe, with a branch that runs interiorly from ST-12 to the gan [肝] (liver) and dan [胆] (gallbladder); on the foot it connects to the liver channel [足厥陰] and runs up the inside of the leg to the abdomen and lower chest region, with a branch that runs interiorly to the dan (gallbladder), gan (liver) and thence up to the fei [肺] (lungs)... from where it repeats the cycle.[33]

The yingqi is not the only form of qi that circulates in the body. Another form of qi, the "weiqi" [衛氣] was emphasized alongside the yingqi in several early passages about the yingqi. In the passage we saw above from Lingshu seventy-five that seems to define acupuncture (or at least needling) the passage states: "Needling regulates (tunes) the qi, Qi accumulates in the stomach in order to circulate as nutrition (ying) and defence (wei) each according to its own paths" [92:79]. Lingshu eighteen addresses the question of the origin of the yingqi and weiqi [78:98-99]. Lingshu seventy-six describes how the yingqi's counterpart, the weiqi [衛氣] circulates in the body. Thus for a more complete examination of qi and its circulations in acupuncture theory and practice, we need to briefly examine the weiqi. Its circulation is different from that of the yingqi and yet it is said to meet or reunite with the yingqi once a day and is routinely juxtaposed alongside the yingqi in theoretical discussions.

## The weiqi –qi movements outside the jingmai

The weiqi, defensive or protective qi was described in the Neijing as running over the body surface to help protect the body against external influences.[34] There are a number of different passages about the movements of the weiqi and the origin of the weiqi. While Lingshu eighteen states that the weiqi is formed in the lower jiao, later authors argued that this is a transcription error and that it should have said that it originates in the upper jiao [78:98-99]. It is said to be formed from the more impure elements of food products during digestion [101:152]. Lingshu chapter ten describes how the weiqi "the most impetuous party of the rough ch'i (zhuoqi –turbid qi) is sent forth and circulates first in the extremities, the interstices in the flesh (fen jou), and between the flesh and the skin, never ceasing" [101:154]. Lingshu chapter forty-seven describes the movement as "the weiqi therefore keeps the segments of the flesh warm, gives the skin a full condition, nourishes the tissues between the skin and flesh and controls the opening and closing [of the sweat glands]" [78:150, 129:349]. But the circulation of weiqi is most concretely described in Lingshu chapter seventy-six. Here the circulation is not only linked to astronomical movements, but it describes how during the day the weiqi circulates twenty five times on the body surface and twenty five times at night among the zang organs in the ke or restraining cycle of the five phases [129:554]. The movement of the weiqi is one of bursting out of the eyes upon opening them first thing after waking. It settles simultaneously onto the six yang channels on the head and face and follows their trajectories down to their corresponding fingers and toes. The weiqi that arrives at the fingers passes to the center of the palms and thence to the center of the soles of the feet.[35] The weiqi that arrives at the toes passes to the center of the soles of the feet. From the soles of the feet the weiqi is said to ascend on the yin aspects back to the eyes to make one complete circulation, from where it repeats these movements. The weiqi is described as doing this twenty five times during the day.[36]

The yingqi and weiqi, following astronomical analogies were also said to unite once a day [72:30, 101:152] so as to compose a mutual grand circulation.[37] The movement of weiqi in the body has thus been described with some variation, passages explicitly stating how it flows outside the jingmai and other passages along with the yang jingmai from head to hands and feet. It does seem that the weiqi runs independently of the jingmai. As a form of qi in the body it is highlighted as being very important, in part because of its repeated contrast with yingqi, the nutritive qi that flows within the jingmai. Its movements are also interesting as they appear to flow on the surface of the body as a kind of rhythmic movement associated with being awake or conscious. At the very least its movement is to do with the opening of the eyes. Various speculations can also be found about how needling, for example, might affect either weiqi or yingqi levels or both.[38] The cycle of weiqi movement described in Lingshu seventy-six is notable since it appears to be the first centrifugal type of movement, moving outwards towards the periphery. The mai and jingmai are variously described as having centripetal direction and later an up-down circular flow (see chapter two [20]). In the Nanjing we find discussion of another kind of centrifugal movement of qi, the movement of yuanqi [原氣], source qi, discussed next.

## Yuanqi –source qi, radiating from the center to the jingmai at the periphery

Nanjing sixty-six describes the movement of yuanqi [原氣] source qi[39] from its source at a center in the body, the "shenjian dongqi" [腎間動氣], the "moving qi between the kidneys" via the "sanjiao" [三焦] or triple burner to the organs and jingmai, specifically the yuan or source points. Nanjing chapter eight describes a kind of center or root for the important systems of the body at the "moving qi between the kidneys." This discussion arises in the context of a discussion of how sometimes the pulses feel normal yet the patient dies the next day. The explanation describes how sometimes the roots of a tree are dead yet the leaves still look alive and then goes on to describe this metaphorical root in the body as "All the twelve channels (jingmai) are linked with the origin of the vital qi [生氣]. The 'origin of the vital qi' refers to the root and foundation of the twelve channels –that is to the 'moving qi' between the kidneys. This (qi) is the foundation of the [body's] five depots and six palaces (zang and fu); it is the root of the twelve channels; it is the gate of exhalation and inhalation, and the origin of the triple burner. It is also called the 'spirit guarding against the evil'. Hence the [moving] qi [between the kidneys] constitutes a person's root and foundation" [112:130].[40] This root, the "moving qi between the kidneys" is said to be below the navel in Nanjing sixty-six [112:560] and is the place where yuanqi [原氣], source qi is produced and from where the source qi is transported by the triple burner to the source points of the twelve channels. The triple burner is said to be the "alternate messenger" for the source qi, this transportation from the root of the body (an almost literal center of the body [78:111] to the source points at the wrists and feet represents an unambiguous centrifugal movement of qi in the body. While not directly a movement within the channels or jingmai, this movement is related to them via the connection at the source points, where the source qi is introduced into the channels. Presumably this is intended to enrich that which is already moving in the channels.

## Summary of major qi flows

In the historical literature we find a number of different movements of qi directly or indirectly related to the jingmai. One runs through them from the periphery to the center (Lingshu seventeen, Nanjing twenty-three –see chapter two above [20]), another runs from the root in the center to join the jingmai in the periphery (Nanjing sixty-six) another that runs up and down the jingmai in a continuous circuit (Lingshu ten, fifteen and Nanjing one –see chapter two above [20]) and another that runs from the eyes along the surface of the body roughly around the (yang) jingmai to the fingers and toes and thence back to the eyes [Lingshu seventy-six] see table 2. Clearly early thinking about qi flows and movements in the body were complex evidencing a range of competing ideas in an effort to describe different phenomena. The practice of acupuncture has, following different rules laid out by different authors, attempted to take advantage of these different descriptions.

One of the more practical extensions of the jingmai that we find with the rise of acupuncture in the Neijing is the introduction of the acupoints, the places to which the needling techniques are to be directed.

## The acupoints

We saw above that by the time of the Neijing (circa 150-100 BCE), the jingmai were said to be pathways for the circulation of qi. The xue [穴][41] or acupuncture points developed after the concepts of the mai and jingmai.[42] In the pre-Neijing discussions of the mai there were no acupoints [47:87] see table 3. It is not

**Table 2: qi flow and the jingmai**

| Text | Flow | Purpose? | Treatment implied |
|---|---|---|---|
| Lingshu 17, Nanjing 23 | In the jingmai from the periphery to torso | To import the ordering influences of heaven-earth into the body? | Unclear –but possibly related to the five shu [俞] points –see below |
| Nanjing 66 | From the body central core to periphery to join the jingmai | To distribute yuanqi, source qi to the jingmai and? | Through use of yuan points |
| Lingshu 10, 15, Nanjing 1 | In a continuous up-down, in and out circulation through the jingmai and their corresponding zang-fu organs in a fixed sequence | To circulate yingqi, nutritive qi and help maintain order in the jingmai and the (qi of the) body –linked to cosmological theories and cycles* | Articulated in the Neijing and especially the Nanjing |
| Lingshu 76 | Outside the jingmai on the body surface following the trajectory of the yang jingmai from eyes to fingers and toes back to the eyes | To provide a protective layer through the distribution of weiqi, protective qi –linked to cosmological theories and cycles* | Unclear if treatment ideas are directly associated |

clear how or when precisely the concept of the xue emerged. On the one hand, Harper, agreeing with Yamada, speculates that they probably arose out of the practice of moxa therapy (such as we find in the Mawangdui manuscripts), where we can imagine that practitioners might observe greater effects at certain sites compared to others and started naming those sites [47:92]. This seems quite reasonable, but then on the other hand we find discussion in the

* Tying these cycles to movements in the greater natural environment implies a continuity with or extension of the natural order of things into the body through these cycles.

Lingshu of the xue as being non-anatomically based. Lingshu chapter one, in a brief discussion of the nature of acupoints describes them in their association to the movements of "shenqi" [神氣], "places where the jie (joints) intersect, 'where the qi of the shen (or alternatively qi and shen) travels in and out'" [69:88].[43] The passage further describes the acupoints as being "neither in the skin nor the flesh, neither in the muscles nor the bones" (ie are not anatomically based) [72:14]. Sivin renders this passage as "'At the articulations within the body there are 365 points of communication... 'articulations' refers to where the divine ch'i (sic) travels freely and moves outward and inward, not to skin, flesh, sinews, and bones'.[44] A modern Westerner expects these points of communication, where the physician's needles can affect the circulation, to be places in tissue, but here we find them related instead to processes" [101:51].[45] Lo goes on to explain how this distinction helps us grasp the difference between "crude and skilled practitioners", the latter pay attention to the shen, spirit (rather than the anatomical structures) [69:88-89]. This passage in the Lingshu is among the earliest to define the nature of the acupoints. This passage offers an alternative explanation for how the acupoints may have developed as well as the idea of observing greater efficacy of moxa when applied to specific anatomical sites. In further support of the notion of the acupoints associated with qi rather than as experiential moxa sites, Lo presents evidence for the potential role of the yangsheng literature, especially the metaphoric language of the sexual cultivation literature and its occurrence in the naming of the acupoints [67].[46] We can, from the historical evidence say that from early in their historical descriptions, we see an interlinking of the acupuncture points, the jingmai on which they lie and the movements of qi.

But does this mean that the concept of the xue, acupoint emerged in the Neijing out of its innovations of the qi circulation model, i.e. as an outgrowth of that model, or is this only a kind of temporal coincidence? Is it another temporal coincidence that the Neijing places much greater emphasis on the use of metal needles to stimulate the jingmai and their circulation rather than using moxa to do this [47:92] as is found in the Mawangdui text treatments of the mai? Is the Nei Jing's increased focus on needling related to the concept of the xue, acupoints as sites of qi movement which are strongly influenced by correct needling methods –see the next chapter by Chace and Bensky [24], i.e. do we see the development of the xue in part out of the introduction of needling techniques on the jingmai?[47] We must wait for new evidence to answer these questions. However the concept of the xue arose, they exhibit important historical developments that have encouraged quite different approaches to the practice of acupuncture, partially, we can speculate, out of different interpretations of the early literature on them. Traditions have emerged that focus on the xue as anatomical sites for stimulation with specific anatomical, pathological or symptom treatment targets described, while other traditions have emerged that use the xue as more movable access points into the jingmai and their qi movements. In appendix one I document a number of different styles of acupuncture to illustrate this variety of interpretations and uses.

Table 3 shows the development of named jingmai related acupoints over time. In the Neijing, only 160 acupoints were actually mentioned by name [72:100], but the Neijing described them in more ideological terms related to "shushu" [數術], the "arts and calculations". Suwen chapter nine states how there are three hundred and sixty-five acupoints (obviously based on the number of days in the year), but in the description it discusses numbers related to heaven, earth, the seasons etc [see 125:57]. Even today where we see the largest number of named acupoints associated with the jingmai[48] the number does not reach the numerically ideal number of three hundred and sixty-five. We saw in chapter two that Suwen fifty-eight describes how the three hundred and sixty-five acupoints "serve as passage[ways] of the camp (ying) and protective (wei) [qi]" [114:166]. Lingshu chapter one gives two different descriptions of how qi is supplied to the three hundred and sixty-five acupoints. The first description, as to be expected, is of the "twenty-seven qi" (qi of the twelve jingmai and fifteen luomai) "flow and pour into" the five shu [俞] points (see below) of the twelve channels and thence to the three hundred and sixty-five meetings (acupoints) [125:497]. The other passage relates to the qi related with the yuan [原], source acupoints (see below): "The twelve sources can give qi and taste (nourishment) to the three hundred and sixty-five nodes (acupoints)" [78:99].[49] However one looks at these ideas, the acupoints were associated with qi that which circulates through the jingmai. The "shu" and "yuan" acupoints were seen as being important in this, suggesting that they might have strong effects to influence the acupoints, their related channels and their associated qi movements (see below).

Is the early lack of anatomical definition for the acupoints due to a lack of anatomical knowledge? This is unlikely since we have clear evidence that dissection was performed on political prisoners at the time of the emperor Wang Mang (circa 15 CE) [51, 56:155-156]. Further, chapter twelve of the Lingshu describes how through anatomical study of corpses one can determine the correct depth of needling and numbers of moxa for each jingmai [51, 56:155-159, 78:133-134].[50] Although these can hardly be said to be extensive references to anatomical studies [114:169], it is clear that anatomical studies,

**Table 3: Development of the Acupuncture Points**

| **Text** | **Number named channel acupuncture points** |
|---|---|
| Mawangdui (Zubi shiyi jiujing & Yinyang shiyimai jiujing –circa 168 BCE) | 0 |
| Mianyang lacquer figure (circa 118 BCE) | 0 |
| Huangdi Neijing (circa 150 BCE) | 160 |
| Zhenjiu Jiayijing (282 CE) | 349 |
| Shisi Jingfahui (1341 CE) | 354 |
| Zhenjiu Dacheng (1601 CE) | 359 |
| Now accepted | 361 |

(After [72:100])

albeit different than those in the West [56:159-161], were performed in China and known at the time that the jingmai and their acupoints were being articulated. The early Chinese attention to anatomy was more related to functional systems rather than the details of the anatomical structures themselves.[51] What are we to make of the Suwen fifty-eight passage that clearly implies that the three hundred and sixty-five "xue" [穴] acupoints "meet" [會] with the sunluo [孫絡], grandchild luo [孫絡三百六十五穴會亦以應一歲] "The 365 holes of the meeting points of the tertiary network (sunluo) [vessels], they too correspond to one year" [114:166]. Does this innocuous passage inform us that the acupoints are in the sunluomai? I have not come across anyone else that has picked up on this idea, but it is interesting. The interpretation of the Lingshu one passage above about the nature of the acupoints is that they are process-function related rather than structurally related [101:51]. Does the Suwen fifty-eight passage imply a kind of model for the structural basis of the acupoints? If so it could lend support to the process based nature of the acupoints rather than their structural basis. While the sunluo appear to be localized within the "meetings of the flesh"[52] the sunluo are not given any definite fixed location in the same way that acupoints are beginning with Huang Fumi in the late third century CE. In principle there are a great many sunluo scattered across the body. The passage in Suwen sixty-three about the invasion of "evil qi" into the body (see chapter two above [20]) implies that the sunluomai are more superficial than the luomai which are in turn more superficial than the jingmai [114:271]. The sunluomai thus appear to be numerous and possibly superficial. If the acupoints are at meeting places with them, then the acupoints may well not be limited to fixed anatomical positions, which can be understood from the Lingshu one passage that states they are not of the anatomical structures. The passage mentioned before table three above about the flow of qi into the three hundred and sixty-five acupoints from Lingshu one immediately precedes this statement in Lingshu one about the acupoints being places of qi movement rather than anatomy. The interpretation I have made here is reinforced by both the proximity and sequential ordering of the Lingshu one passages.[53] That the acupoints meet with the sunluo additionally implies that the acupoints themselves may be quite superficial or, like the sunluomai have superficial connections and thus can be accessed at the surface of the body. The fact that they were stated to be "neither in the skin nor the flesh, neither in the muscles nor the bones" [72:14] doesn't give any hint as to their potential location relative to the body surface. Their association with the superficial sunluomai may provide the first evidence of their location relative to the body surface. Is there any other evidence of this? One could argue that the existence of seemingly successful acupuncture styles that employ very shallowly (< 2mm) or even non-inserted needling[54] lend support of this idea [75].[55] The fact that the Lingshu one passage describes the acupoints as places where the qi "travels in and out" [69:88] can also be seen to imply a surface location for the points, they serve as gates between the interior of the body and the external space around the body.[56] While interesting, these arguments and data do not support that this is "the" correct interpretation of the nature of the acupoints, rather it supports a more open-ended approach to understanding the acupoints and provides potential explanations for why certain styles and approaches to the practice of acupuncture can be deemed "traditional" and why they might work. The notion of the acupoints having presence and thus depth within the body is also reinforced by the Nanjing's description of bu [補] and xie [寫] needling techniques which appear to describe a kind of transfer of qi from the surface (yang) to the interior (yin) for bu, supplementation and from the interior to the surface for xie, draining technique [112:639], see below for further discussions. Huang Fumi's systematization of the naming and location of the acupoints in the Zhenjiu Jiayijing [鍼灸甲乙經] of 282 CE appears to start fixing the acupoints in the body, which further reinforces the appearance of the acupoints in the anatomical body. With the advent of the systematization of the acupoints in the Song dynasty bronze statue and its related text, the acupoints can be seen to be increasingly anatomically related. In the modern period with the increasing influences of Western anatomical thinking about the body, the acupoints are now routinely seen to be rooted in that body. There are thus long traditions that have employed acupoints based on ideas that they are deeper in the body, maybe anatomically based and employed deeper needling to stimulate them. All these traditions co-exist, see appendix one for examples of different treatment styles. What do they tell us of the nature of the acupoints? I leave this question here to be addressed at a later time. The number of jingmai acupoints evolved over hundreds of years to the currently accepted total of three hundred and sixty-one. The total number on each of the jingmai and the additional ones on two of the qijingmai (renmai and dumai) are listed in Table 1 along with yinyang, five phase and organ relationships.

## *Acupoint classifications*

The literature has described a number of classifications of the acupoints on each of the jingmai. Every jingmai has one of each of the following types of acupoints: five shu [俞] –transporting points, yuan [原] –source points, luo [絡] –connecting points, xi [郄] –cleft points. Some of the jingmai have points at which trajectories of other channels intersect, such as "sanyinjiao" [三陰交] on the spleen channel where the liver, kidney and spleen channels are said to intersect. Each channel also has associated points on other channels, sometimes on its own channel, such as the mu [募] points on the anterior portions of the torso and the shu [俞] points on the back. The associated points on the back, the shu points are, by name, associated with the zangfu, for example BL-13 is the feishu [肺俞], lung shu.

Of interest to us are the five shu [俞] transporting points which are classified as: jing [井] –well, ying [滎] –spring, shu [俞] –stream, jing [經] –river, he [合] –sea/uniting.[57] Here we see an explicit water flow analogy; the water wells up to become a spring, from where it starts to flow like a stream and then to become a larger flow, like a river and finally to end up in the ocean.[58] The sequence and its naming is interesting for a number of reasons.

First, the sequence of these acupoints on each channel is centripetal from toes to knees and fingers to elbows. Some commentators see them as a different subset of small channels [112:549-550]. Generally though this sequence is seen to overlay and be unrelated to the circulatory flow of the channels described above. We suggested in chapter two that the centripetal flows that were associated with the jingmai were related to the downward moving influences of heaven and the upward moving influences of earth [20]. These two converging flows help bring order into the body, helping align the person with heaven and earth. How was this achieved in the acupuncture literature? The early literature associated these acupoints with the five phases (see Table 4). The correspondence with the five phases allows the practitioner to associate the selection from among these important acupoints with the jingmai and zangfu, each of which was also given five phase associations (see Table 1).

**Table 4: shu –transporting point phase associations**

| [俞] **shu-acupoints** | **yin jingmai** | **yang jingmai** |
|---|---|---|
| [井] jing-well | wood | metal |
| [滎] ying-spring | fire | water |
| [俞] shu-stream | earth | wood |
| [經] jing-river | metal | fire |
| [合] he-sea | water | earth |

Various strategies were described in the Neijing and Nanjing on how to use these correspondences. Nanjing sixty-nine for example describes simple systematic treatment principles that allow the practitioner to select specific acupoints in order to help correct disturbances of qi flow and distribution in the jingmai and thus help restore the natural order.[59] Some of these treatment approaches are based on examining the state of the jingmai and assessing the physiological condition of the patient in order to select treatment acupoints, some utilise these acupoints based on temporal or biorhythmical changes. Biorhythmic influences will be examined in a little more detail below, here I address the question of "why"?

Once the five shu-transport points were associated with the five phases this allowed for a number of more cosmologically influenced associations to be made. For example Nanjing chapters thirty-three and sixty-four explicitly associates the shu-five phase correspondences on the yin and yang channels with the system of the "shi tian gan" [十天干] or ten "celestial stems" [112:361, 554]. The system of ten stems can conveniently be seen numerologically as two systems of five (of the five phases), thus each stem was associated with a phase and yin-yang quality. This set of correspondences is seen in table 5.

Looking at table 5 one can easily see an association. Wood yang will correspond to the wood point on the yang channels (the shu-stream points). Wood yin will correspond to the wood points on the yin channels (jing-well points). Nanjing thirty-three describes the interaction of wood and metal normally seen as the "ke" [剋] or controlling cycle instead in terms of how the tiny qi of metal yang (geng) reaches out to contact the tiny qi of wood yin

**Table 5: Ten stem –five phase/yin-yang associations**

| | |
|---|---|
| Stem 1 [甲] (jia) –wood yang | Stem 2 [乙] (yi) –wood yin |
| Stem 3 [丙] (bing) –fire yang | Stem 4 [丁] (ding) –fire yin |
| Stem 5 [戊] (wu) –earth yang | Stem 6 [己] (ji) –earth yin |
| Stem 7 [庚] (geng) –metal yang | Stem 8 [辛] (xin) –metal yin |
| Stem 9 [壬] (ren) –water yang | Stem 10 [癸] (gui) –water yin |

(yi).[60] This is important for a number of reasons. The incorporation of these cosmological correspondences and their mechanisms of interaction introduce another layer of ordering effects that might be achievable through the use of these points. Over a millenium later the "ziwuliuzhu" "midday-midnight streaming biorhythmic acupuncture systems described a ten-day cyclical system called the "najiafa" [納甲法], which is still used today as a kind of higher order treatment system [75], we return briefly to this below.[61]

## *Effects of the acupuncture points*

We find an evolving and gradually changing use of the acupoints as they have collected reputations through hundreds of years of recorded use by different people in different places. These accumulated experiences and uses would become increasingly selected from in order to use them within the context of the system of practice of particular styles or schools of practice. Thus we find some using points based on their systematic correspondence, others for their location and the pathways they affect, others for their effects on the internal milieu. Examples of the different ways of thinking, organizing information and rationale for selecting points and applying techniques to them can be found in Understanding Acupuncture [17]. Other texts have documented the diversity of practice in historical and modern periods [4, 73, 95, 97], see also appendix one. We can imagine that part of what contributed to this range of different ideas about the practice of acupuncture and the nature of and how to use the acupoints will be the fact that they can manifest different levels of effect, some of which are related to their effects on the qi, their effects on the jingmai they lie on, and some based on what part of the body they lie on. The following is a preliminary list of effects that may have influenced how people think about acupuncture, qi, the jingmai and their treatment foci, the acupoints:

1. Effects that manifest as a result of stimulation of local anatomical structures. These will include both local and more global effects depending on the structures stimulated –for a good summary of some of the local structures see [135]. –all points will have some degree of local effect when treated– effects on surrounding tissues [e.g. needle LI-11 for elbow pain, ST-35 for knee pain] and potentially can manifest more general analgesic effects depending on the structures stimulated, needling depth [135].

2. Effects that manifest as a result of the treatment technique that was applied at that location (shallow versus deep needling, needling versus moxa, etc.) [135].

3. Effects that manifest as a result of the treatment technique that was applied at that location (supplementation versus draining technique)
–in principle each point has some degree of effect on other channels due for example to the yin-yang, 5-phase characteristics of the channel it is located on (supplement the lung channel –counterbalances repletion in the large intestine and liver channels) [18:13-18]. Depending on which technique and how well it was applied, supplementation, for example can both affect the channel treated with regulatory effects on other channels, but more general supplementation of the body's qi can occur (see the discussion of needling techniques below.

4. Effects that manifest due to the channel that the treated acupoint lies on –trajectory effects, yin-yang effects, 5-phase effects, original condition of the channel, etc.
–in principle each point has an effect that manifests through the channel it is located on (e.g. needle ST-44 (on the foot) for dental problems, BL-62 (below the ankle) for neck pain, treating the lung channel for example can help increase the condition of the kidney channel and reduce the condition of the liver channel, large intestine channel) [18:13-18].

5. Effects that manifest as a result of discrete properties of the points such as point classifications (water point, source point or he-sea point) and properties implied by the name of the point (eg CV-6 "ocean of qi"). These effects will tend to be more systemic.

–depending on the discrete property of the point (based on point classification –e.g. mother point, source point) there will be systemic effects both throughout the channel system and throughout the whole body, thus with supplementation of LU-9 (a mother and source point) –the channel system becomes more balanced and observable effects are seen to the "sheng qi" (vital qi) throughout the body [9]. Needling a "he-sea" point such as SP-9 can, according to Nanjing sixty-eight [112:577], help reduce counter-flow qi symptoms or loss of body fluids.

6. Effects specific to that acupoint, such as the clinical targets or effects attributed to the non-channel "extra" points.
   –extra points can be local or distant to the region they affect and have specific symptom targets such as asthma (ding chuan) or hemmorhoids (er bai).

However, understanding the nature of the acupoints is complicated by a number of historical facts [17]:

i) their locations vary by text and tradition. Some differences are small, some quite large;[62]
ii) the manner of their use varies by text and tradition compare use of the acupoints in modern Chinese and Japanese traditions;[63]
iii) their clinical indications/uses vary by text and tradition;[64]
iv) their contraindications vary by text and tradition.[65]

These facts about the acupoints make it difficult to make clear the relationships of them to qi and the jingmai. There is a large body of literature available for study, but what lies behind the contradictions and trends found in that literature has been all but ignored by practitioners and scholars. We will see in chapter eight [15] that these facts have been pretty much ignored by researchers rendering much research difficult to accept or digest.

## Rhythms in the qi and jingmai

Qi movements in the body were seen from earliest times related not only to processes and events occurring in the body, but also to external processes and changes. It is natural given the evolution of the concepts of qi in the pre-medical and early medical traditions that influences from outside the body would impact the body via their effects on the qi. Lingshu fifty-five says "the ebb and flow of the qi correspond with the yin yang of heaven and earth, with its four seasons and five elements. The increase in power and the decline of the mai are for the observation of emptiness and fullness, excess and insufficiency, in the blood and qi" [59:83]. We have seen above and in chapter one how certain cosmological models influenced conceptions of the body, in chapter two we suggested that the Neijing's fusion term "jingmai" may have been attempting to capture and express the influences of heaven and earth on the body. Working with models of the body where the qi and its ordering trajectories in the body, the jingmai, are key features of physiology and pathology it becomes difficult not to have a body of literature regarding how heavenly and earthly influences create changes. It is also natural given the rhythmic cycles of change that can be observed in heaven and earth, that some of these influences might be related to rhythmic changes and cycles within the qi and jingmai systems. This is what we find. In the primary chapters that discuss the circulation of qi in the jingmai, Lingshu fifteen and Nanjing one, we find detailed discussions of the movement of qi in the jingmai relative to celestial movements with precisely timed qi movements according to celestial divisions, breath and channel lengths. A good summary of this can be found in Huang Fumi's Zhenjiu Jiayijing [131:29-31], which appears to explain Lingshu fifteen.[66] The twenty-eight xiu [二十八宿] "celestial mansions" or "constellations"[67] are related to twenty-eight channels,[68] the movements of the qi in them which is propelled by the breath, they are numerically matched to the counting of time via the dripping of the clepsydra,[69] timed to the passing of the celestial constellations. In the first description of the circulation of qi in the jingmai system we find explicit correspondences to external cycles in the environment, Lingshu fifteen states: "When the conditions of the fifty cycles circulation of the channel energy is illustrated, it is the comprehensive condition of heaven and earth" [125:594].

The early methods of counting time in China utilised various theories including the "ten heavenly stems" [十天干] and the "twelve earthly branches" [十二地支]. These terms have been found on Shang oracle bones (as early as 1500 BCE) and thus long predate the medical literature [80:396].[70] Many early societies observed nature, classified cycles observable in nature and structured their behaviours and activities around those cycles (such as the timing of when to plant and harvest crops, etc). The early Chinese used numerological systems of ten and twelve to perform these counting of times [80], with, for example the ten stems counting a ten day "week", the twelve branches twelve "hours" of the day, etc.[71] Often the same time unit was counted in both stem and branch units, thus giving a combination of values to each time unit and offering an additional sixty unit cycle (the shortest time period for cyclical systems of ten and twelve to start and return to the beginning), this is seen for example in the sixty year cycle.

Consequently we can find many different discussions in the early and later medical literatures about the influences of the seasons, the weather, the cyclical passage of time. Many of the early discussions in the Neijing relate to precautions and contraindications for treatment according to these such as the phase of the moon (eg Suwen chapter twenty-six), the time of year (eg Lingshu chapter seventy-eight), the time of day in a ten-day cycle (eg Lingshu chapter sixty-one ). The Neijing (Suwen chapters eighteen and nineteen) and the Nanjing (chapter fifteen) articulate models of how the qi of the body changes and manifests in the mai –pulses according to the season [112:200-218].[72] In Wang Bing's eighth century edition of the Neijing Suwen (the oldest extant version), a whole section (chapters sixty-seven to seventy-five) was introduced regarding cyclical changes in a large cosmological model, the "wuyun liuqi" [五運六氣], five transformations and six qi system, involving for example sixty year cycles, seasonal changes, weather changes, constitutional patterns and pathological influences [72:139-149, 114:387-493].[73] The various cycles mentioned here describe how complex changes occur in the qi and how they may manifest in the body. Later cyclical descriptions extend this to include the concept of acupoints "opening" [开] and "closing" according to various temporal cycles [72:137-138]. This level of detailed change led by the twelfth century to tabulation of acupoints that could be treated according to what time of which day it was in a particular cycle. There are, for example, the ten day cycle of five phase and yuan-source acupoints, the najiafa [納甲法] (first described in the Ziwu Liuzhu Zhenjing [子午流注鍼經] circa 1200 CE), the sixty day cycle of the qijingmai eight acupoints, the lingguibafa [靈龜八法] (first articulated in the Zhenjiu Daquan [鍼灸大全][74] of 1437).[75] I mention these cycles and their associated methods here not only to expose diversity in the practice of acupuncture, but also to reveal something about the movements and cycles of qi in relation to the jingmai and their acupoints. I return to this topic briefly at the end of this chapter where I try to show what these systems were probably trying to achieve.

## Variations in the language of needling techniques

When we examine descriptions of needling techniques in the Huangdi Neijing [黃帝內經] and the Nanjing [難經] we find interesting variations in how the core techniques of "bu" [補] and "xie" [寫], supplementation and draining techniques were conceived and to be applied. The principles of bu and xie are clearly articulated in the Neijing in Lingshu chapter ten [盛則寫之虛則補之] "If abundant then drain it, if vacuous then supplement it."[76] Many chapters in the Suwen, Lingshu and Nanjing describe different techniques for how one is to accomplish these important goals. Not only were different techniques described for bu and xie, but how the very nature of what is involved in accomplishing bu and xie also varies, this is most obvious in a contrast of the needling model of the Nanjing with that of the Neijing.[77]

In the Neijing the dominant model appears to be one of the body filled with healthy qi (many terms for this are used[78]) which circulates within. Lingshu sixty-six tells us that if this becomes weak, it allows "xieqi" [邪氣] evil qi to penetrate into the body and cause symptoms [63:119]. Bufa is applied to strengthen the body's healthy qi and xiefa is applied in such a way as to allow the xieqi to leak out of or be drained out of the body. For the draining technique we find in Suwen twenty-seven "... When the exhalation is completed, [the needle] is removed. Large [quantities of] qi leave" [114:278] and in Suwen sixty-two

> Do not close the outside gate, so that the qi is made to leave. Widen its way by moving [the needle] here and there, as if its road were made passable [This is called "massive drainage."] It is essential to squeeze [the arm] and make [the qi] leave. [As a result], large [quantities of] qi will yield [114:280].

For the draining needle technique the image is clearly one of causing the qi to leak or escape from the body. For the supplementation technique Suwen twenty-seven tells us "Wait for an inhalation and pull the needle. The qi must not leave. At each place [where a needle was inserted], push [the hole] and close the door, and thereby let the spirit qi be preserved. Large [quantities of] qi stay where they are. Hence this is called 'supplementation'" [114:283]. With the draining needle technique care is taken to not leak the body's healthy qi and to let out only the xieqi, evil qi. With supplementation the needling technique causes "qi far away will arrive", the "essence qi is preserved", which can make "the evil qi will disperse"[79] [all from Suwen sixty-two, see 114:281].

The Nanjing model describes bu and xie in quite different terms [10].[80] Unschuld describes the core idea of needling in the Nanjing as "the concept of filling (bu) and draining (xie) through internal exchange" [112:639]. The "internal exchange" is achieved via both the needling techniques and the choice of acupoints. The technique itself is described in Nanjing seventy-six and especially seventy-eight,[81] and also in Nanjing seventy-one in a discussion of the importance of protecting the ying and wei in the techniques of bu and xie.[82] The act of bu involves needling shallowly at the level of the weiqi [衛氣], getting qi to arrive, then pushing the needle deeper to the level of the yingqi [營氣] which flows in the jingmai, while the act of xie involves needling a little deeper to start with to the level of the yingqi in the jingmai, get the qi to arrive then pull the needle up to the more superficial level of the weiqi. This is fundamentally about trying to restore yin-yang balance as represented by the balancing of qi distribution between the yang (wei) and yin (ying) levels.[83] The Nanjing also introduces the notion of using the shu [腧] points based on five phase theory to supplement or drain "in the case of depletion, fill the respective [conduit's] mother. In the case of repletion, drain the respective [conduit's] child" [112:583]. In the case of vacuity one can supplement the mother point of the channel that is weak; for example in vacuity of the lung, LU-9 is the mother point of the lung channel since it is the earth point and earth is the mother of metal, thus supplementing LU-9 will strengthen the lung channel. Additionally, one can also supplement the mother channel (in this case the spleen channel, at an acupoint such as SP-3. The choice of acupoint and channel combined with supplementation technique directs the effects to the channel that is vacuous.[84] In both the bu and xie techniques it appears that one is not only increasing and balancing qi in the body, rather one is taking advantage of the natural regulatory influences associated with the five phase cycles which deal with the regulatory interactions between the channels-organs and the yin-yang regulatory influences that work between the surface (weiqi) and deeper (yingqi) levels. It seems as though the Nanjing model is more one of balancing and allowing the natural healing power of the body to carry out its job, consistent with its innovative emphasis on the theory of systematic correspondence.[85] This description of needling techniques also implies a model of the yingqi and weiqi as basically the same thing: qi [氣] –in yin and yang manifestations. The techniques of bu and xie are not about changing one form of qi into the other by moving the two qi between their two levels, rather it seems to be one of manipulating qi in terms of its depth and location so that it can act differently according to where it is and also create (yin-yang) balance. Unschuld drew attention to this [112:639] but I have found no other author that has focused on this [10].

What kind of description of this natural healing power does the Nanjing give? It is likely that the Nanjing's model is based on the idea of the shengqi [生氣], the vital qi described in Nanjing eight (see above). The shengqi is rooted in the "moving qi between the kidneys" and is the foundation for all the major systems (qi, zang-fu, jingmai, sanjiao) in the body. Presumably when the shengqi is in a healthier condition the body's systems are better able to take care of what needs to be done. It seems in the Nanjing's model that the job of an acupuncturist is to move qi from one place to the other so that something (probably the shengqi) can do this –seen with the idea of moving qi between the level inside the jingmai and above the jingmai and the regulatory agency of five phase interactions. The Neijing on the other hand has a less well developed idea of the body taking care of itself and relies more on the imagery and language of adding influences (qi) into the body as needed and if not enough to also remove disturbing influences (qi) from the body rather than waiting for the body to try to resolve them. Evidence for these differences lies in the practical descriptions of how the bu and xie are to be carried out and the more general background imagery and models employed in the different texts. Another possible rationale can be proposed for how these natural healing is enhanced with needling.[86] We saw in chapter one a passage from the Mawangdui sexual cultivation treatise the "Heyinyang" [和陰陽] which describes the arrival of qi thus: "The qi arrives, blood and qi flow freely, the ears and eyes are keen and bright, the skin gleams, the voice is clear, and the back, thighs and buttocks are sturdy, so that one 'attains divine illumination'" [71:381]. We will see below that for all needling to be effective, the qi must arrive. Perhaps there was a common understanding based on passages like this from the Heyinyang, that the arrival of qi itself promotes vitality (qi and blood flow, the senses are keener, the skin lustre improves, the physical body stronger), while the actions of bu and xie, which are applied after the qi arrives, help restore balance and order. I will return to this theme later.

In later periods different practitioners read and then cite these different passages as they attempted to (re)construct the techniques of bu and xie in their own practical way according to their own understanding, observations, preferences and judgments. This is discussed further in appendix two with a specific example of how bu was constructed through the interplay of traditional text, practical and theoretical interpretation, observation and experience. What has usually been important to practitioners is to find practical methods that work. The fact that the texts they have cited may or may not have been conceptually congruent and even at times may have been seemingly contradictory would be of little concern to most practitioners. Some may have chosen to follow their understanding and model of one approach or another, others would pick practical ideas, try them out until they had woven methods that worked for them [11]. Attempts to reproduce traditional descriptions naturally create the diversity of treatment approaches evidenced in the field today and in historical times.

## Needling and the qi

I hinted above at the idea that the relationship between qi, the acupoints and jingmai was strengthened by the introduction of metal needles for applying treatment. The tip of the needle becomes a clear focal point or pivot for creating change. The idea of the needle being the pivot may indeed have been the inspiration for the renaming of the "Zhenjing" [鍼經] "Needle Classic" to the "Lingshu" [靈樞] "Spiritual Pivot" in the Tang dynasty (see the next chapter [24]). There are many discussions in the Neijing to support this, remember the passage from Lingshu seventy-five "needling regulates (tunes) the qi", this is the purpose of needling. The next chapter by Chace and Bensky examines a highly significant passage from Lingshu chapter one about the core aspects of needling. Below I touch on a few other issues to highlight two main types of discussion: first, discussions of the importance of the practitioner's inner state and the focus of treatment on the qi and shen of the patient, this sets the stage for the needling descriptions. Second, the inner states of the practitioner needed to successfully needle and the role that the needle plays in treating the qi. Following this I present a model of how to think about these different aspects in relation to the stages of development of the practitioner and the natural variety of practice styles and experiences that flow from this. Today the practitioner who attempts to reproduce "traditional" acupuncture techniques in clinical practice typically cites passages from the classical texts such as the Suwen, Lingshu and Nanjing and says that they are reproducing those ideas. Naturally there are different interpretations given to the same passages and thus naturally many different needling "styles" can be found citing the same passages or utilizing competing, or alternate passages about needling. Appendix two describes the needling techniques of "bu" (supplementing) used in the Toyohari [東洋はり] (East Asian Needle) traditional Japanese "Keiraku Chiryo" [経絡治療] or Meridian Therapy system and then disassembles the technique according to the source texts that were likely to have influenced those reproduced techniques. I have included this because Meridian Therapy practitioners have, since the 1920s, explicitly tried to reproduce the needling methods found in the classics so that they can be used in the modern period. This process has involved a kind of systematic critical re-evaluation and practical reproduction. In Toyohari, this has been reinforced with efforts to seek a consensus description of the techniques so that they can be systematically reproduced and at the same time demonstrate clinical effectiveness. Thus appendix two gives an example of how different ideas described in the classical literature have been given attention to construct the traditional needling techniques used in a modern "traditional" system of acupuncture. This compilation can in principle be made for all other "traditional" types of acupuncture found in use today.

### *The focus of needling and the inner state of the practitioner*

Larre and Rochat de la Vallee cite a passage from Suwen chapter fifty-four about the inner posture of the practitioner as he approaches the patient:

> Whether it is near or far it is all one: it is in the observation of the qi through the depth or the surface. Be as if looking into the abyss: take care not to fall. Make your hand like one that would seize a tiger: do not lack strength. Do not allow your spirits to be disconcerted by anything: with a quiet will consider your patient without shifting your gaze to the left or right. Do not allow your movement to deviate, since your own uprightness will allow for rectification. First of all, rectify your spirits, since your regard to the patient will call for the regulation of his spirits. Hence the qi circulates with ease [58:52-3].[87]

Chace discusses the same imagery and state of mind outlined in Lingshu chapter nine [23]. In the Lingshu passage we find

> [The practitioner must] deeply reside in a place of stillness and divine the comings and goings of the spirit with one's [sensory] doors and windows shut. [The practitioner's] ethereal and corporeal souls must not be scattered, his mind must be focused, and his essence qi undivided, and undistracted by human sounds. By concentrating his essence, he must unify his mind and direct his will entirely toward needling. [In this way, the practitioner may skillfully practice] shallow insertion while retaining the needle, or gentle, superficial insertion so as to successfully transform the patient's spirit and as the qi arrives then one stops [23].

Shudo summarizes this Lingshu passage with the following "When inserting the needle, do not look, do not listen, do not speak, and do not move. Simply pay close attention to focus on the tip of the needle to feel for the coming and going of qi" [100:239].[88] Chace reasons that the kind of mental focus that comes through residing in a place of stillness with exclusion of sensory input of the external environment is a reference to a Daoist cultivation practice that is clearly articulated in the Neiye of the fourth century BCE [23]. This idea of stillness also seems to appear in an early pre-Neijing medical text in the Zhangjiashan [張家山] Yinyangmai Sihou [陰陽脈死候] which says "When the mai are full empty them; when empty fill them. **Be quiescent in**

**order to treat them** [淨則侍之][89]" (emphasis added) [32:96]. The author(s) of this text appear to have adopted a similar idea about the inner state of quiescence that is needed in order to carry out the therapeutic action correctly. Is this an intermediary step between the earlier Neiye and the later Neijing descriptions? The meditative practice described in the Neiye allows the person practicing to cultivate and refine their qi to become like jing qi (essence qi) and thus like shen (spirit) [88:113-6]; it allows the person to have knowledge of, connect to and influence other things or beings in the cosmos [88:115], and creates change without expending energy [94:62].[90] The Lingshu's reference to the essence qi probably follows the Neiye's use of the term (as a more refined and concentrated form of qi). Likewise the reference to the mental quieting practices during needling in order to contact or trigger and feel the arrival of qi strongly parallels the Neiye which describes: "therefore this vital energy cannot be halted by force, yet can be secured by inner power (de). Cannot be summoned by speech, yet can be welcomed by the awareness (yi)." [94:48].[91] The qi arrives not by physical action but is welcomed by one's "yi" [意] (translated here as "awareness"), a quiet inner state of the practitioner, inseparable from the state of the body of the practitioner.[92]

This focus on the "yi" is paralleled by Guoyu of the Han dynasty who described:

> Medicine is attention (yi) [意]. The regions of the skin are very finely divided. Following the flow of qi requires consummate skill. When inserting needles, an error of a hair's breadth will mean failure. A kind of spirit connects the physician's heart with his hand, and that is something I can know but cannot explain" [95:176-177].[93]

The relative importance of focusing the mind while needling is described in many other acupuncture texts early and late [9, 41:156-157, 78:38, 100:237, 130].

Citing Lingshu chapter seventy-three Yang tells us "It is essential when using the needle to not forget the spirit" as you "subtly rotate and slowly push" the needle [130]. Yang also cites Lingshu chapter four "The art of needling is to needle the points of qi and not to needle muscular striations. When the needle enters a point, it is like a ship entering a harbor, needling a muscular striation just causes pain on the skin" [130]. This passage not only describes what the focus of treatment is with needling treatment, but it further stresses the issue raised above that the acupoints were originally conceived as places of qi movement and not anatomically based structures.

In these descriptions it appears to be important while needling to be able to remain aware of the total state and change of the patient while focusing on the tip of the needle. Ames and Hall pointed to the dependency and interconnectedness of "focal" and "field" awareness in the effects of our actions on the world, especially if we are to achieve the goals of our actions [2].[94] The needle gives a focal point for the qi while acting on the patient. Thus the needle can be seen to represent a focus that requires "focal awareness", applying which requires a sense and awareness of the whole of the patient "field awareness". This aspect becomes clearer in the next section.

### *The inner state and arrival of qi*

The Lingshu describes what can only be understood to be some of the most subtle aspects of treatment. Two key ideas can be found about effective needling. Treatment only becomes effective after "qi zhi" [氣至], the qi has arrived (at the needle). Yang translates the key passage from Lingshu chapter one thus: "the important thing in needling is that the qi arrives, then there will be an effect - and the sign of the effect will be like the wind blowing away the clouds, as clear as the blue sky that appears" [130].[95]

This reference to the "blue sky" and "blowing away the clouds" can be found in other Neijing passages. Suwen chapter twenty-six makes the following statement: "Although it is appropriately obscure, it is clear to me alone, like the wind blowing the clouds. For this reason it is called the spirit" [24]. Here the analogy of the clouds being blown away is one of making something clear, like the "spirit", shen [神]. Suwen chapter three makes another statement in this regard that additionally associates the blue sky with higher mental states (will and attention –yi [意] and zhi [志]) and physiological conditions: "When the qi of the azure sky is clear and calm, then the will and attention are ordered. Normalize it, and then the yang qi is secure. Although a thieving pathogen may be present, one cannot be injured" [C. Chace May 2009, Amsterdam]. It seems reasonable to link the reference to "blue sky" to similar references that are found in other traditions, especially contemplative traditions where, like these Suwen passages, the reference is to increased clarity of perception and mind. The use of this analogy is found in other parts of the world, especially in meditation traditions (see for example the discussion in [39:164]). Let us also recall the passage from the Heyinyang above about the arrival of qi:[96] "The qi arrives, blood and qi flow freely, the ears and eyes are keen and bright, the skin gleams, the voice is clear, and the back, thighs and buttocks are sturdy, so that one "attains divine illumination" (tong shenming [通神明])" [71:381].[97] The concept of shenming, here translated as "divine illumination" is important for a number of reasons. While the term shenming has had various meanings[98], it is a term associated with the heightened state of consciousness that the sage has attained, and with various practices to achieve that state. The purpose of the sexual cultivation techniques of the Heyinyang and related texts[99] were about trying to attain this heightened state, similar to what is commonly called "tantric yoga". Thus it is possible to see the discussion of the arrival of qi with reference to shenming in the Mawangdui text and the discussion of the arrival of qi with the clear blue sky analogy of the Lingshu as being related.

The relevance of this becomes clear when we examine the role of the practitioner when needling. In order to accomplish the tasks of needling correctly the practitioner must be able to feel the arrival of the qi. This requires sensitivity, training and mental focus[100] [5, 99, 100]. There is also a four character phrase in Lingshu one related to the core aspects of needling therapy describing how mental/spiritual aspects are essential and stresses the importance of focusing on the needle tip. The passage "shen zai qiu hao" [神在秋毫] is translated by Yang as "the spirit must be focused on the tip of the needle" [130].[101] This is usually seen to mean that the practitioner focus their mind on the tip of the needle. In chapter one above, "Qi, mind and body –explorations of the links between qi, the mind, mental and emotional states and the body" [16] relationships between the mind and qi were explored, where it was documented how qi relates to the experience of the world and then suggested that it is a concept related to the mutual interaction of the "observer" and the "observed". The proper focus of the mind on the tip of the needle is (at least part of) how qi focuses or gathers at the tip of the needle, it is a natural consequence of that focus. Another supporting example can be found in the Maishu: "As for vapor (qi)... it follows warmth and departs from coolness." [47:81], qi is made to descend from above in a vessel with excess qi in it by applying moxa to the waist [47:91]. What is important is that the application of heat causes qi to move towards where the sensations of heat are felt which naturally draws one's mental focus.[102] While the heat of moxibustion can have this effect, the Neijing descriptions suggest that the tip of the needle seems especially useful in this regard.

## *The perception of the arrival of qi*

While there is a dominant view in the modern Chinese acupuncture literature that the patient is the one who should experience the qi (deqi)[103] during needling [3, 28, 57, 130], this appears to be a departure from earlier ideas about who experiences the arrival of qi [130]. There is a distinction drawn by some authors between "deqi" [得氣] as something experienced by the patient and "qizhi" [氣至] as something experienced by the practitioner [99:181, 117:533]. Yang argues that the current trend in modern China to focus on what the patients feels is not in accord with the classics, he argues that qizhi is felt by the practitioner not the patient [130]. But even this does not tell the whole story. There are clear examples in the historical literature of seeing both "qizhi" and "deqi" as referring to experiences that the practitioner experiences, not the patient. Nanjing seventy-eight is quite explicit about this [99:181, 112:635, 117:523]. It is instructive to examine the Nanjing passages.

In a discussion of the difference between those "who know how to apply the needle" and those who "do not know how to apply the needle" Nanjing seventy-eight states: "those who know how to apply the needle rely on their left [hand]; those who do not know how to apply the needle rely on their right [hand]" [112:635]. The needle is to be held at the acupoint by the left hand, while the right hand grasps the handle of the needle to advance and manipulate it. In an explanation of this the Nanjing describes how once the qi is felt to arrive then the needle is inserted and the needling technique begins: "as soon as the arrival of the influences [felt below one's left hand] resembles the [pulsation of the influences at the usual location] where the movement [in the] vessels [can be felt below the skin] insert the needle" [112:635].[104] Nanjing eighty states it thus: "as soon as one notices with one's left hand that the influences (qi) appear, one inserts the needle" [112:646].[105] Clearly for the author of the Nanjing, the "arrival of qi" is something that the practitioner feels at the acupoint to be treated (with their left hand) *before* the needle is inserted and the techniques of needling begun. This makes more sense when one recalls the descriptions of Lingshu chapter one above about the nature of the acupoints as being "where the qi of the shen (or alternatively qi and shen) travels in and out" [69:88], and not being anatomically based structures. In other words the acupoints (the target of needling) are places where the qi comes in and out of the body and are thus directly palpable by the practitioner. The skilled practitioner can feel this movement of the qi and encourage the qi to start to arrive through the touch of the left hand and additional techniques to prepare the acupoint[106], following which the needle is introduced and the needling technique begun. These are quite subtle phenomena, the feelings associated with the arrival of qi are very delicate and subtle [5, 14, 57, 99, 100, 126, 130, 134].

In order to explore this issue further I think it is helpful to examine how one interprets the term "de" [得]. There is mounting evidence that the Neiye was very influential in laying the groundwork for the development of the physiological systems laid out in the Huangdi Neijing [47, 91, 104]. There is also strong evidence that the Neiye influenced Huangdi Neijing discussions about how to use a needle to influence the qi of the patient [23, 24]. Thus, when interpreting ideas such as "de" [得] of "deqi" [得氣] which is important in the discussions of needling and influencing qi, it could be helpful to examine whether and how the term was used in the Neiye. What we find is a consistent use among scholars of the Neiye to render the term "de" as a cognitive term. This is quite different from modern translations of the term "de" in the acupuncture literature as to "obtain". Of course one can obtain an understanding of something, but more commonly the term "obtain" is used in contexts such as "obtaining a license", "obtaining a painting". Experts on the Neiye have rendered the term "de" with a variety of English words such as "grasp", "achieve", "realize" [94], "sense" [60:91] and more explicitly as "comprehend", "understand" [91]. This distinction is important as it may help us understand the language of the Huangdi Neijing better. The principle issue is that it is due to changes inside the practitioner that "qizhi" [氣至], qi arrives. The practitioner must understand or grasp "de" [得] that fact in order to respond appropriately and with correct timing.[107] The issue of timing is found to be strongly stressed in the early discussions of needling. For example Lingshu one and Nanjing seventy-eight tell us that needling techniques begin only after the qi has arrived[108] and that "the subtleties of needling lie in its speed" [24]. Suwen sixty-two states "To move the qi, wait for the [proper] time" [114:281] while Suwen twenty-seven tells us: "When the qi has arrived, this is exactly the moment for which one has to be on the alert" [114:283]. From these and the two passages from the Nanjing above we can see that first one must get the qi to arrive and one must be cognizant or aware of that, then the techniques of needling begin. This awareness of the arrival of qi, which itself is a very subtle phenomenon [57, 99, 130] cannot be something the patient is to experience, it must be something that the practitioner experiences, otherwise how could one possibly respond in a timely manner "the subtleties of needling lie in its speed"? This understanding on the part of the practitioner is "deqi" [得氣], one "de's" (understands, grasps) the arrival of qi.[109] To understand more about this it is helpful to focus again on the "yi" [意].

We saw above and especially in chapter one [16] understanding about the "yi" is very important in relation to how one is able to engage and the extent to which one influences the qi. This is obvious once one accepts the important influence of the Neiye on the Lingshu and passages about needling contained there "therefore this vital energy cannot be halted by force, yet can be secured by inner power (de). Cannot be summoned by speech, yet can be welcomed by the awareness (yi)." [94:48]; in other words the qi arrives at the needle because it has been welcomed by one's "yi".[110]

In chapter one, we drew a distinction between three stages of development of "yi", as a parallel to Zhuangzi's ideas about three stages of perception and knowing. Zhuangzi wrote:

> Make your will one! Don't listen with your ears, listen with your mind. No, don't listen with your mind, but listen with your vital energy (qi). Listening stops with the ears, the mind stops with recognition, but vital energy is empty and waits on all things. The Dao gathers in emptiness alone. Emptiness is the fasting of the mind. [128:93].

In this discussion perception arises at three levels. In the lowest level one merely listens with one's ears (physical action). In the second one listens with one's mind, which Yang characterises as using a kind of underlying deeper form of perception and knowing through the "common sense" [128]. In the third one simply embodies the act of perceiving and knowing through the qi, which is integral to the nature of both mind and body, here the actions are simply natural. We extended this idea in order to understand "yi" [意] on three progressive levels:

–"yi" at the beginner level as *intention*[111] –one is not yet entirely sure or confident how to engage and act directly, thus one starts by intending it to happen, which is a guide to the actions that one wishes to make, but is still one that requires effort. Actions on and through the qi are less;[112]

–"yi" at the intermediate level as *attention* –after a lot of experience (and often further training), the actions one wishes to take become more natural and require less effort, they are achievable by becoming more focused on what one wishes to act on and the action one wishes to make, and holding those foci. While more actively engaging and using the qi than the previous "intention" to carry out the actions and achieve the desired end, it is still less than in the third state;

–"yi" at the more advanced level as *awareness* –after much more experience, the actions are fully embodied and effortless ("wuwei" [無爲]). Drawing awareness to patient and action, the process naturally unfolds, here engagement and actions on and through the qi are to a much higher degree as they are mediated precisely through the qi.[113]

It can be seen as a process of integration of going from the duality or multiplicity to one-ness. Qi would in this context be understood as both the means to and symbolic of one-ness.

The "yi" of which the Neiye speaks "therefore this vital energy cannot be halted by force, yet can be secured by inner power (de). Cannot be summoned by speech, yet can be welcomed by the awareness (yi)." [94:48] is likewise the higher of the three levels of yi. The importance of this in relation to acupuncture cannot be stressed enough: the papers by Chace [23] and Chace and Bensky [24][114] clearly illustrate that the early descriptions of needling in the Lingshu are influenced by the Neiye. Thus the descriptions of how an individual can "welcome the qi with their yi" and the steps and actions he must take in order to do this are essential. Attention to good posture, closing the sensory doors so as not to be distracted, mental acuity and calmness, lack of effort and tension are integral factors. These thus need to be cultivated in order to carry out the actions of needling correctly. The better carried out, the more the needling acts at the level of the qi and can influence the qi in the desired direction.[115] This does not deny the existence of the actions of needling on the biological or bio-psycho-social systems of the patient. The act of inserting a needle of course affects the body, acting upon and thus through a cascade of different anatomical-physiological systems[116] according to what is done, how it is done and where it is done. By this means, beginners are able to help their patients, but the extent to which traditional models of qi and the jingmai play a role in these effects is debatable. It is possible that the relative contribution of them varies due to practitioner skill levels. This is clearly an important issue for research [15] and needs more discussion.

These three stages characterize the differences between the student and relative beginner, the more experienced practitioner and the very experienced practitioner, the "master". At all levels "yi" is important (Guoyu said "Medicine is attention (yi). The regions of the skin are very finely divided. Following the flow of qi requires consummate skill. When inserting needles, an error of a hair"s breadth will mean failure. A kind of spirit connects the physician's heart with his hand, and that is something I can know but cannot explain" [95:176-177]. The consummate skill spoken of here is not something which the student or beginner has developed, nor even the experienced practitioner mastered. This is not something unique to acupuncture, it permeates all activities. Through studying the piano one can start to place fingers on the keys at the right time so that what is played starts to sound what it is supposed to sound like (student and beginner). Continuous practice and studying with a skilled teacher allows these skills to continue to develop over time so that the student can start to play the piece better and better. But it is only through extensive experience, practice and training combined with developed and incipient talents that allow the master pianist to play the piece at the level of a concert pianist. Even the intermediate level good pianist after many years of practice still cannot do this. These stages of development are normal and take time, they cannot be by-passed. There is no "matrix-like" program that can be plugged into the back of the head and downloaded. Incipient talent and diligent effort can accelerate such things, but otherwise they take time to mature naturally. Denmei Shudo, considered by many to be a highly developed expert acupuncturist wrote that it took him thirty years of practice before he could understand the arrival of qi properly, but suggested others might start to grasp it after five to ten years or even sooner with diligence and proper training [100:236].[117]

This does not mean that one should make no effort as a beginner to cultivate and eventually master these skills, treatment will still be effective, but likely for other reasons than just the effects one has on affecting and regulating the qi.[118] This has a number of important implications:

First, in order to cultivate and develop these skills diligent study and practice is necessary. But alone it can take time, even with talented practitioners, thus a number of exercises and practices can be helpful to try to accelerate this process. The final chapters of this book describe a number of such exercises that will be helpful for cultivating, developing and accelerating this process of learning [22].

Second, if we are to investigate qi in the practice of acupuncture, there will be a number of key issues to which attention must be paid. Among these are how to ensure that we are confident that we are investigating the effects of qi or a person that can clearly influence changes in the qi of the patient. What kind of qi influences are being accessed or stimulated with treatment? Here there will likely be an advantage to focus efforts on investigating what is happening when a really experienced practitioner or "master" is working, where it is more likely that they use their "yi" as "awareness", that is they naturally and without effort influence the qi. This will be discussed further in chapter eight [15]. In order to help put the discussions above into context, I next present a simple model into which much of what has been described can fit. This model may also assist further investigations.

## A preliminary model

Given the descriptions of needling, how the needle might affect the qi, and the role of the consciousness of the person needling, it is useful to propose a preliminary model in order to make these things clearer.

A key to understanding the following model is the definition of acupuncture offered by the Lingshu in chapter seventy-five: "Needling regulates (tunes) the qi (tiao qi [調氣])" [92:79]. We apply needles in order to regulate the qi.

We have seen that qi is said to flow along the jingmai, one of the primary functions of which is to help bring order to or help regulate the body's qi. If one can regulate the jingmai with needling one can regulate the qi of the body better, hence diagnosis and treatment focuses on identifying and correcting conditions of xu-vacuity and shi-repletion of the jingmai. Regulation of the qi and jingmai helps bring about greater ordering and efficiency of the functional systems in the body such as the zang-fu. Greater efficiency of the functional systems helps improve overall qi production, distribution and usage. The jingmai appear to play an intermediary role between the functional systems and the person's qi (the one or unitary qi discussed above). The consciousness of the practitioner is of fundamental importance for this to happen –the Neiye informs us how the "yi" welcomes the qi. In a recently published paper I proposed a three level model for starting to understand these descriptions [9]. In this model a series of concentric circles are used to represent the functional systems (inner circle), the jingmai (middle circle) and the body's unitary qi/vitality (outer circle) –see figure 2 [9].[119] To this I add here another level, that of the mind. For the sake of simplicity, we will say that this four level model is embedded into the environment (level five), both ecological and cosmological, such that the individual (represented by the four levels) continuously interacts with these background environments –see figure 3.[120] In this simple five-level model[121] the fourth level, the mind is now the outer circle, the environments (level five) are the background surrounding the outer circle. This allows us to capture what Sivin describes as "life is maintained not merely by the internal circulation of qi, but by a continuous dynamic interchange between body and cosmos. Shared vital rhythms make the body correspond to heaven and earth, and keep them in accord" [102:16].[122] In this model a few basic rules apply, the logic and reasoning of which are presented elsewhere [12], see also various discussions in chapter one above, [16]:

a- higher levels help control or regulate the levels below
b- lower levels help provide the support for the levels above

The more that level four (the mental level) is engaged appropriately during treatment, the greater the ability to bring about regulatory influences on level three (vitality), level two (jingmai) and thus level one (functional systems). Thus, "tiao qi" [調氣] "regulating qi" is most effectively realized when the men-

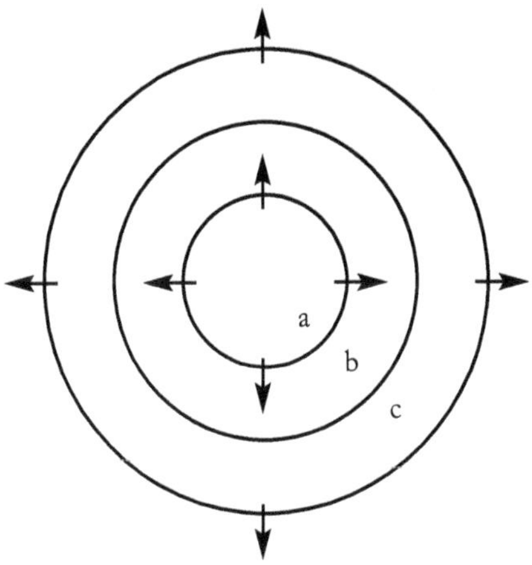


**Figure 2: Three level model**
A = Functional systems (Zang Fu, etc.)
B = Channel systems
C = Vitality: Global Qi of the body

tal level (eg the "yi") is operating at more advanced stages ("awareness" rather than "attention" or "attention" rather than "intention"). Cultivation of the mind (this includes the "shen" [神]) requires many things and can occur along many pathways over time. Quieting of the mind, calming the emotions, remaining undistracted by sensory input, quietly focusing and allowing awareness to arise, maintaining an aligned good posture, remaining relaxed etc, are all involved. The practical chapters of this book describe a series of exercises and procedures that can help in this cultivation [22]. Figure 3 gives a simple model for grasping the relationships between the four levels of the mental, vital, jingmai and functional systems and the ecological and cosmological environments in which they are embedded. This can be used to model what is happening within any individual including both the person needling and the person being needled.[123] Because, as the historical literature discussed above clearly implies, the inner state of the practitioner is necessary to optimally engage qi during needling, thus it is helpful to acknowledge the necessary inter-relationship between qi and the mind discussed in chapter one. An important concept made explicit here following historical texts and confirmed by experience is that the *mental or internal state of the practitioner influences the qi of the patient.* This idea is at odds with how many have conceived of acupuncture in the modern period, where the practitioner having made a decision of what to do, applies the needles to achieve those things, he is more the mechanic applying his tools (the needles) and less an integral part of the process. As we have seen above, in the historical descriptions of needling to influence the qi, the inner state of the practitioner is a necessary feature. The five-level model is constructed in order to start mo-

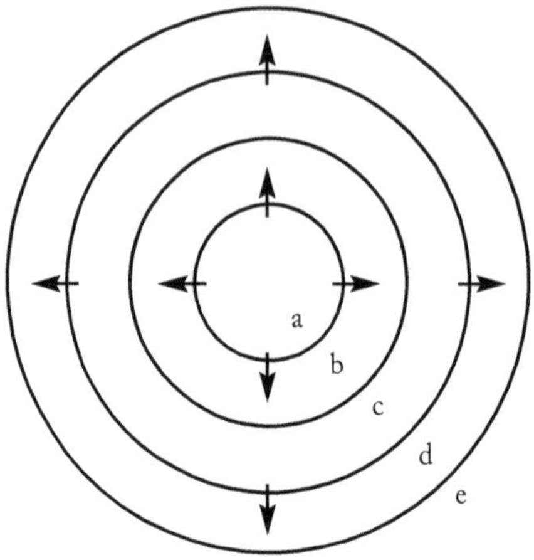


**Figure 3: Five level model**
A = Functional systems (E.g. Zang-Fu)
B = Channel systems
C = Vitality: Global Qi of the body (E.g. Zheng Qi, Sheng Qi, Yuan Qi)
D = Mind -Heart/Mind (E.g. Yi: intention/attention/awareness;)
E = Environmental systems (E.g. ecological/social systems –including "earth"; cosmological systems –including "heaven".)

deling how the mental state of the practitioner can do this. For the sake of simplicity here, I assume that levels one and two do not interact much between individual people, while levels three and four have less well defined boundaries and can mutually interact between people. In addition to any physical movement or manipulation of the needle, the vitality and mental levels of the practitioner can act directly on all four levels within the patient. In a sense, this is to be expected once we acknowledge the nature of qi in relation to the experiences of the mind. This understanding of qi was discussed in chapter one. Since there is an intimate relationship between the very nature of the mind and qi, it is thus natural that it is this aspect that would be influential in how the practitioner engages qi with the needle. How this may occur is discussed in the next section as we examine the engagement of qi during treatment.

## *Qi engagement*

On the basis of the above considerations we can also begin to speculate about what kind of qi might be involved in the needling of different level practitioners. I propose that there are at least three **qi-levels** that can be engaged depending on the stage of development of the practitioner. In the first, only the qi of the patient or "physiological qi", from levels one and two in figure three is engaged. In the second, there is more interaction between the practitioner and patient so the qi that is engaged is not limited to that of the patient, I call it "interactional non-physiological qi", from levels three and four in figure three. In the third, the practitioner is able to engage qi that has its origin in the background environment, which I call "matrical non-physiological qi"–from level five in figure three.

Clearly the insertion of a needle into the body delivers some form of physical stimulation that will create change. Simply inserting a needle will effect a stimulation of the normal physiological qi of the patient. Manipulating that needle to achieve the action of "bufa", supplementation implies that we try to increase in some way the qi (at that point, in that channel). At the very least a successful needling will maybe stimulate a flow of physiological qi towards the place where the needling occurs, which will serve through a kind of physiological redistribution to increase (bufa) that point or channel. According to theory, the change of one channel will trigger re-balancing through yin-yang and five phase mechanisms [18:13-18]. We can also imagine that as a channel experiences an increased qi content this might in turn influence the degree of functioning of associated functional systems (zang-fu), which in turn could trigger a slowly acting increase of qi through the improved/increased functioning. In this simple model of needling with the supplementation method, the needle acts on the physiological qi of the patient to create change. The practitioner does not contribute directly to these qi flow and content changes. Any beginner can insert a needle to influence the physiological qi of the patient and with minimal training can create this slowly building physiological change. But the descriptions of needling in the Neijing and Nanjing and the role of the practitioner's inner state necessary to realize the effects described with this needling necessarily involves something other than the physiological qi of the patient. I present here proposals for a more comprehensive model of what may be happening.[124]

### *Thoughts about how the three stages described by Zhuangzi might manifest and act in treatment*

Treatment can work at all three **qi-levels** with observable changes created in the patient depending on the stage of development of the practitioner.

The practitioner at the first developmental **stage** helps create change in the diagnostically named targets of treatment (intended [意] actions and targets), the tissues/region needled and the channel system. Actions are limited to using techniques to stimulate and manipulate the physiological qi of the patient, that is **qi-level** one. A certain degree of "balancing" can be achieved due to the auto-regulatory effects among the channels on which treatment is applied explained by five phase and yin-yang correspondences and theory.[125] The effects of needling one point on one channel can thus trigger some degree of change on other channels. The primary theories of acupuncture that are used to formulate diagnoses and treatments relate mostly to these effects.[126]

The practitioner at the second **stage** of development brings into play more of the resonating (ying/ganying) [應/感應] effects of the practitioner. Thus "interactional non-physiological qi" (interactions at the level of the "vitality"–shengqi [生氣][127]/zhengqi [正氣]) is introduced (i.e. **qi-level two**) which helps create additional and higher-level regulatory effects in the patient. With practice and greater skill the intention becomes more naturally focussed as attention [意] and manipulation helps bring about additional regulation of the channel system and physical/functional systems. The specific theories of acupuncture used to diagnose and select treatment (yin-yang, five phase, zang-fu functions, etc) do not explicitly describe actions and qi influences from this level. These qi influences become apparent through practice and analysis of the details of needling techniques. They are thus implicit in treatment, developed through practice rather than in only in imitation of textbooks.

The practitioner at the third **stage** of development brings into play the dynamical effects of acting naturally through stillness, non-action (wuwei) [無爲]. This accesses qi from the third **qi-level** "matrical non-physiological qi". One mechanism likely involved in this is resonance (ying [應], especially "total ying" [感應]) which allows the person more at the third stage to access influences from heaven.[128] Cosmological qi, tianqi [天氣][129] or yuanqi [元氣][130] is the matrix in which is embedded all systems with their locally appearing movements and actions. Through tuning to this with the correct dynamic (ji) [機] and more reflexive/integrated and passive focus, or awareness [意], the natural (ziran) [自然] state of these systems as being embedded within this (cosmic) qi matrix emerges or becomes apparent, allowing a higher level ordering and regulating effect, and the infusion of (background) "matrical non-physiological qi" (tianqi/yuanqi) into the patient. Like the second **qi-level**, these qi influences and sources are not explicitly described in the traditional theories of acupuncture that are used to guide and select treatment, Instead, these qi influences and actions are implicit. They become apparent through the practice of developed practitioners, they are hinted at in the background theories of acupuncture and become clearer through detailed analysis of the requirements for "proper" needling techniques, the needling techniques of the superior physician. Table 6 summarises this. The three practitioner development **stages** in table 6 describe how the mind through different states of cultivation is able to access different levels of qi, each of which has different actions and functions. Table 6 primarily relates to the stage of cultivation of the practitioner, but, as we will see can be used to understand similar influences of the patient during treatment.

In a single treatment at least the first and up to all three **qi-levels** can be activated or engaged in differing degrees. The absolute beginner (practitioner **stage** one) will activate **qi-level** one only so that qi from that level will be the primary mediator of treatment effects. Only when that person starts to relax and get into a rhythm of treatment will **qi-level** two effects begin to activate or engage so that the qi from that level starts to play more of an influence mediating the gradually increasing treatment effects of the practitioner. Then with more training and repeated experiences over many years of practice effects from **qi-level** three naturally can start to play more of a role as the individual merely needs to draw awareness to the process. Qi from this level now plays more and more of an influence to mediate the treatment effects of the practitioner.

Some individuals may, because of their background and prior experiences, be able to use qi from **qi-levels** one and two from the start and access qi from **qi-level** three sometimes quite early on in their career. There will be an enormous variety of manifestations of these **stages** in treatment depending largely on the stage of development of the practitioner. How well qi from each of the three **qi-levels** participates in or is brought into the treatment will depend on many factors. An advanced practitioner with a lot of experience (**stage** three) will more likely be able to bring qi from all three qi-levels into play routinely. The intermediate experienced practitioner (**stage** two) will more likely be able to bring qi from the first two **qi-levels** into play routinely during treatment, and occasionally (and probably with increasing frequency) from the third qi-level. The beginning practitioner (**stage** one) will be able to marshal qi from the first **qi-level** from the beginning in treatment, occasionally (and with gradually increasing frequency) bringing qi from **qi-level** two into play. Very rarely will the beginner be able to bring qi from **qi-level** three into play.

The factors that influence this for each and every practitioner during each and every treatment are likely to be many and complex. Among these will be the state of the patient. It is likely that part of the learning and development process that each practitioner goes through will involve encounters with different patients, some of whom are likely to influence the process. At first the practitioner may not understand these influences, but gradually over time an understanding through experience will develop. It is also possible that practitioners can lose control of this, or "have a bad day". A very skilled practitioner operating at level 2 or 3 might have difficulty due to personal or health issues that make it difficult to reproduce their normal treatments effects.

Many patients come for treatment in poor condition so that their manifestations are limited more to the levels at **qi-level** one; with such patients the beginning practitioner is unlikely to be able to draw on qi influences from **qi-**

**Table 6: three stages of yi, needling and qi[131]**

| Practitioner Stage | Qi-level influences | Possible actions and mechanisms |
|---|---|---|
| 1st stage (yi [意] as *intention*)<br><br>listening with the ears [耳] | Physiological qi of the patient is stimulated<br><br>qi-level one<br><br>*[physiological qi]* | Needling directly affects/stimulates physical systems and their physiological components + acts on the channel system to increase (bu) or decrease (xie) qi flow, triggering yin-yang and 5-phase balancing/counterbalancing actions all of which help to regulate and thus improve functioning of the internal systems (zang/fu etc) –supplementation occurs as a movement and increased physiological functioning |
| 2nd stage (yi [意] as *attention*)<br><br>listening with the heart/mind [心] | Interaction between practitioner and patient, triggers a mix of physiological and non-physiological qi (vitality) interactions and influences<br><br>qi-level two<br><br>*[interactional non-physiological qi]* | The role of touch; the role of the acupoint as the gate for flow of qi (vitality) in and out; role of shengqi (生)/ zhengqi (正氣)/yuanqi (原氣) interactions; role of shen/spirit (神) and heart/mind (心) interactions/influences; probable role of simple (gan) ying/resonance (感應)[132]<br>–supplementation occurs as a result of even greater regulation of and increased physiological functioning |
| 3rd stage (yi [意] as *awareness*)<br><br>listening with the qi [氣] | Opening up to environmental/cosmological qi cycles, influences, movements (the matrix-like basis for everything) produces non-physiological qi interactions and influences, which enhance and regulate physiological qi[133]<br><br>qi-level three<br><br>*[matrical non-physiological qi]* | Naturally tuning to the natural movements and rhythms spontaneously –ziran (自然), without intention –wuxin (無心), through nonaction –wuwei (無為);<br>probable role of total/cosmic (gan) ying (感應) and ji/dynamic (機)<br>–supplementation occurs both due to higher level regulation of and increased physiological functioning and a realigning or tuning into the matrix of background qi, thus allowing qi to suffuse into the body[134] |

**levels** two and three. Some patients are very "sensitive" and thus show manifestations acting at **qi-level** two; with such patients the beginning practitioner may experience qi influences from **qi-level** two (but not be able to reproduce this easily on other patients). Occasionally a patient comes who is in a higher state themselves so that they show manifestations from **qi-level** three; with such patients, beginning and intermediate practitioners may be able to experience qi influences from **qi-level** three (but not be able to reproduce this easily on other patients). The interaction between patient and practitioner will probably enhance or damp down these higher **qi-level** effects. On some patients the practitioner will be able to access qi from higher **qi-level** sources "accidentally"/"unintentionally" because of the inner state of that patient, and not be able to access the same on other patients. Only the more developed practitioner will be able to overcome these damping effects so as to access higher **qi-level** effects routinely, regardless of the patient they are treating. Less developed practitioners are likely to take time to develop an understanding of what is happening with those patients and how to reproduce that on other patients. The rate at which these patient encounters and their ensuing experiences can be assimilated, reproduced and acted upon by the individual practitioner will vary tremendously.

While the state of the patient is not modelled here,[135] we can thus see how this may also play a role in how and from which level qi effects manifest during treatment, depending on how their physical and inner development stages manifest. The role of qi and the jingmai during acupuncture treatment and their impact on the patient can thus be modelled using the four-level model of each individual (patient and practitioner) combined with the **stages** of development of the practitioner and the levels of qi access through the three "**qi-levels**".

## Tying the threads together

Now that we have examined how the concepts of qi and the jingmai have been used in the early and later acupuncture literatures, I would like to offer a final model for understanding why the jingmai were developed with their extended correspondences at the same time as the acupoints and the act of needling. The following model is, like some other ideas above, speculative, but it fits with many established facts.

We saw in chapter one that as the concept of qi evolved, the various systems of thought that employed this concept held a model of nature that places humans in the centre in relation to "tian" [天] and "di" [地] heaven and earth. We saw that various authors (Confucius, Xunzi, Mencius, Zhuangzi, etc) envisioned different ways that "heaven" imposes order on humanity, or can be accessed through correct rituals and actions, especially the actions of the enlightened sage or ruler (the son of heaven with tianming [天命], heaven's mandate) to help bring order, restore order, impose order on themselves, those around them, the empire and the environment.

With the early literature that describes acupuncture, the Neijing corpus, we see models of the body in a diseased state as being that of a body that has basically lost the way, is no longer enmeshed within the stream of nature imposed by heaven and earth. The human being through his own actions has created states whereby he is no longer tuned in with, properly influenced by, properly aligned with the natural flow of the cosmos and has allowed himself to become disordered.[136]

The role of the doctor thus is to help restore this natural alignment, to help restore order, to "zhi" [治] (re-)order the patient, as Lingshu chapter seventy-five puts it to "tiao qi" [調氣], "regulate the qi". The very purpose of acupuncture is to regulate the qi in order to help the person return to a more naturally aligned and regulated state.

We have also seen that early instructions on needling techniques to influence the qi are to very subtle and not easy methods, these are the methods of the "superior" doctor (see discussions in the previous [105] and next chapter [24]). We have seen that needling techniques to influence the qi have probably been influenced by earlier traditions whereby the individual attempts to cultivate their qi, as is found in the Neiye.[137] Thus, although the needling techniques have become the focus of treatment as a needle doctor (acupuncturist), the ability to "tiao qi", regulate the qi is difficult for the beginner. I speculated above how the very experienced practitioner is able to tap into or access the non-physiological qi of the environment "qi-level three" (influences of heaven) and thus, through themselves, help import order into the patient to aid their recovery. But for the practitioner who is only able to access qi-levels one and two, how can this be achieved or at least approximated? Influencing the qi with a needle is easy and necessarily will occur, but "regulating qi", this is another thing altogether.

It is here that we see the role of the jingmai and some of their acupoints corresponded to yin-yang (Mawangdui), then five phase (Neijing) and then later ten-stem (Nanjing) correspondence systems. While the principles at work do not appear to have been explicitly described (and here is where my speculation begins), these correspondences are not only about giving the practitioner ways of organizing data into diagnoses and making treatment choices,[138] but as (if not more) importantly about having systematic ways of importing and imposing order within the body. This was already hinted at in chapter two with the model of understanding the centripetal flows of the mai and jingmai as being about this. I speculated that these represent the flow of non-physiological qi into the body downwards from heaven and upwards from earth.[139] The Neijing and later Nanjing describe extended uses of yin-yang and five-phase correspondences that also allow for the systematic importing and imposition of order in the body.

In the pre-Neijing texts the mai were already seen to be linking human ailments to cosmological patterns.[140] The six-fold categorization of jing that we see with the taiyang-taiyin etc labelling of the twelve channels refers to a cosmological model of classifying for example the course of the year in terms of yin-yang stages. In other words the very act of using needles to regulate the jingmai (bu [補] what is xu [虛] and xie [瀉] what is shi [實]) already starts to trigger a reordering of the body according to the norms of heaven.[141]

The Neijing correlations of the twelve jingmai to the five phases (see table one above) and the five shu [腧] acupoints to the five-phases (see table four above) then allows for additional ordering to be imported through these extended correlations in nature.[142] The subject of how to do this in the Neijing is not so systematically addressed, rather there is a focus on difficult to reproduce needling techniques in order to try to achieve this or maximise this. The Nanjing seems to have tried to address this issue in two ways. First it extended correlations of the five shu acupoints further by correlating them also to the "shi gan" [十干] ten-stems of heaven (see table five above). This extended correlation implies an even greater import of order into the body from heaven through treatment of these acupoints. The Nanjing also adapted the needling techniques of bu and xie by describing how one moves qi from one level to another as an additional kind of yin-yang regulation and thus ordering. Finally the Nanjing described a treatment principle in difficulty sixty-nine: "for vacuity supplement the mother, for repletion drain the child". In appendix two we have seen how the treatment principles described in Nanjing seventy-nine are extended interpretations of important needling techniques described in Lingshu chapter one[143] (see the next chapter [24] for extended discussion of the Lingshu passage in which this is embedded). The Nanjing adapts needling techniques from the Lingshu further and replaces them with a systematic rule and thus treatment principle that uses an extended version of five-phase theory to both choose what channels to treat and also which five shu acupoints to treat. This gives a systematic approach for figuring out what to treat and applying treatment in order to both counterbalance disturbances in the body and import order into the body through the principle of the extended correlations.

Later authors extended these treatment principles further as they tied qi flow and the jingmai through their extended yin-yang and five phase correlations to broader cosmological concepts and the cyclical changes of qi movements and flows that were already in use outside the medical field. With Wang Bing in the seventh century we see the development of the extensive "wuyun liuqi" model of practice, with He Ruoyu of the twelfth century we see the application of these theories in the "ziwuliuzhu" systems, the "najiafa", the "nazhifa" and then later with Xu Feng in the fifteenth century the "lingguibafa" system. These are introduced above. The application of these cyclical systems allows for a systematic importation of cosmological order into the body to help return the patient to a healthier state.

In the last paragraphs I have tried to explain why the early theories of acupuncture employed the theories of systematic correspondence in order to help achieve the goal of needling, the restoration of a more ordered state of qi inside the patient. I have tried to describe how, as Sivin put it: "life is maintained not merely by the internal circulation of qi, but by a continuous dynamic interchange between body and cosmos. Shared vital rhythms make the body correspond to heaven and earth, and keep them in accord" [102:16]. While I have speculated here on the reasons why the jingmai and their acupoints were classified and used the way they were and thus the role of needling, perhaps other researchers can investigate this further.

## Conclusions

In this chapter I have explored some of the ways that the early literature described the role of qi and the jingmai in the practice of acupuncture. This has been fundamentally an effort to expose the variety of practice styles that have emerged and can be found today in the field of acupuncture. Rather than try to describe every variation that has developed or even exists in the modern period, itself a huge task, I have tried to expose descriptions in the historical literature and show by example how that has led through different interpretations and models to different utilisations of the qi and jingmai concepts in different styles of practice. I have also tried to show how the use of the needle to accomplish the goals of treatment draws attention to the role of the practitioner, thereby exposing different models of practice according to the stages of development and skill of the practitioner. Themes that emerged in chapter one re-emerged in this chapter regarding the role of "yi" and effects of the practitioner in engaging qi. I have also tried to tie these different aspects together to show how the application of the theory of systematic correspondence may well have been incorporated and used in the early acupuncture literature to help achieve the qi regulating effects that define the nature of acupuncture during its emergence in the Neijing corpus.

For many this chapter will be surprising since it does not make the usual descriptions or assumptions about acupuncture that are commonly found in modern books. I have tried to be more scholarly than acupuncture textbook authors tend to be so as to develop credible evidence about these different descriptions of acupuncture and its historical context. I have also tried to set the stage for two practical explorations of the issues discussed in this chapter. First, how to do what is being described, and here the reader is referred to the practical exercises in chapters nine and ten which give a range of ideas about how to accelerate one's development as a practitioner of "qi" related therapies [22]. Second, I have tried to lay a foundation for establishing valid research approaches to acupuncture that attempt to investigate acupuncture more on the basis of the early descriptions of it and their modern practical applications, the reader is referred to chapter eight for these discussions [15].

## Appendix one: Diversity of theoretical, diagnostic and therapeutic methods

Several texts document the variety of styles of acupuncture that can be found in the modern period [4, 17, 73]. Below is a table that illustrates this variety.

**Table 7: examples of different schools of acupuncture from China, Japan, US, UK and France: their theories and needling foci**

| Acupuncture "style" | Theoretical foci | Needling foci | Acupoint location concepts |
|---|---|---|---|
| TCM acupuncture (1) | zang-fu;<br>qi-blood;<br>8-principles –yin-yang theory;<br>etc.<br>Acupoints have "functions" | Patient feels "qi" reaction "deqi" | Anatomically defined and located in the anatomical structures –located by measurement and palpation |

| | | | |
|---|---|---|---|
| Japanese Meridian (2) Therapy | 12 channels; yin-yang theory; 5phase theory; acupoints as access points to qi circulation | Practitioner feels "qi" reaction "qi zhi"/"deqi" | Anatomical structures guide finding the "live point", points move –located by soft touch |
| Yin-yang channel balancing (3) | 12 channels; 8 extraordinary vessels; yin-yang theory Acupoints as access points to qi circulation | Nothing specified about feeling "qi" reaction | Anatomical structures guide finding the "live point", points move –located by pressure (pain) |
| Chinese Acupuncture (4) | 12 channels; various channel systems; Acupoints as access points to qi circulation | patient feels "qi" reaction "deqi" | Anatomical structures guide finding the "live point", points move –located by pressure |
| Biorhythmic acupuncture "ziwuliuzhu" (5)* | Daily, ten day and sixty day cycles of rhythmic "opening" of specific acupoints, which gives access to the internal systems | Needling reactions vary by country of practice | Point location concepts vary by country |
| "Traditional acupuncture" (6)** | twelve officials; 5 phase theory; Acupoints as sites of stimulation | Patients feels "qi" reaction | Anatomical structures guide finding the points –located by measurement and palpation |
| Ryodoraku (7)*** | 12 channels; ANS**** balance; Acupoints as sites of stimulation | Nothing specified about feeling "qi" reaction | Points can be found by electrical measurement or palpation |

| | | | |
|---|---|---|---|
| Akabane balancing (8)*** | 12 channels balancing Acupoints as sites of stimulation | Nothing specified about feeling "qi" reaction | Anatomical structures guide finding the point, points located by pressure |
| Terrain acupuncture (9)***** | Character "terrains"; 12 channels; Acupoints have "functions" | Patient feels "qi" reaction "deqi" | Anatomically defined and located in the anatomical structures –located by measurement |
| Okyu –Japanese moxibustion (10) | Treat acupoints to relieve symptoms | Patients feel heat of burning moxa, no discussion of "qi" reaction | Anatomical structures guide finding the "live point", points move –located by pressure pain |

* this style is not physiologically based nor based on pathophysiological processes, rather on cyclical fluctuations in the body due to the rhythmically changing environment;
** this style is not so much physiologically or channel based, rather it take advantage of the close relationships between qi and mind in emphasizing the psychological and emotional characteristics of the patients;
*** these styles used non-traditional methods (electro-dermal skin measurements, acupoint heat sensitivity) to make diagnosis and choose treatment;
****ANS = autonomic nervous system;
***** this system combines psychological and physiological character types

(1) for example: [3, 28, 33, 89]
(2) for example: [41, 49, 85, 99]
(3) for example: [74, 75]
(4) for example: [106, 117]
(5) for example: [64, 75]
(6) for example: [30, 123]
(7) for example: [79, 84]
(8) for example: [1]
(9) for example: [90]
(10) for example: [40, 98]

# Appendix two: modern construction of "traditional" needling methods, an example from Japan –the supplementation technique of the Toyohari school of Keiraku Chiryo

I have chosen this needling technique because I am very familiar with it in my acupuncture practice and because I teach this method. As such I can elaborate details more clearly and naturally than the techniques of another school or style. This needle technique is described from the perspective of the practitioner using the language that describes for him what is happening. Other untrained observers watching the needle technique will probably want to describe the technique in different terms. I feel it more suitable to use the more natural language rather than the language of another interpretive model. After describing the needle technique I then cite relevant passages from the historical literature, especially the Suwen, Lingshu and Nanjing upon which the details of the needling technique are based. Others familiar with the same historical passages may have different interpretations or practical applications of the same passages,[i] but that is one of the purposes of this appendix –to illus-

i. Take the example of "needling with the flow of the channel" as an important historical idea about how to apply the "bufa" or supplementation method that is cited by many [33:13, 41:151, 76:164, 99:184, 136:163]. Of this and a number of other historical ideas about needling Ellis, Wiseman and Boss state "The above methods are not a subject of unanimous agreement. Through the ages different opinions have been proffered. We present them here as an introduction to the subject, realizing that each practitioner must develop his or her own preferences on the matter" [33:14]. One of the original passages that is interpreted as discussing the idea of needling with the flow is found in Lingshu chapter one which says [追而濟之惡得無實]. The term "zhui" [追] is similar in meaning to "sui" [隨], to "follow" and is usually interpreted in this passage as needling along with the flow of (qi in) the channel, but many alternate interpretations can be found that appear to depend on the style of needling and which historical literature the translator is familiar with: "To tonify means to follow, to assist, to agitate" [124:2]; "In invigorating, the pricking can be carried out at any time" [125:495] –though the same phrase in Lingshu nine is rendered by the same translators Wu and Wu as "when one twists the needle along with the running direction of the needle, it is the invigorating therapy" [125:546], and a similar phrase in Lingshu three as "'assisting along with it' means to prick in the direction similar to the channel's circulation" [125:511]; "Supplementation may be defined as tracking. Tracking implies (insertion of the needle) in a seemingly casual way" [131:291 –this passage is a translation of text from the Zhenjiu Jiayijing that is clearly based on the original Lingshu text]. Different styles of practice interpret historical passages within the context of that practice style. The three cited translations are from modern practitioners influenced by the modern TCM style of acupuncture where the needling is done more deeply to get "deqi". In the TCM literature, the angle of insertion is less important in relation to bufa [3:306, 28:329, 83:409, 89:192] since the needling tends to be deeper in comparison to historical descriptions [17:53-54 + 81] and changes of needle angle from perpendicular needling are to do with constitution, age, condition of the disease and location of the acupoints [89:192] not the application of the technique for trate how over time and through clinical practice different needling techniques that are based on practical interpretations of the classical texts have and can develop. The following is published in more elaborate form as a paper [11].

## *The needling technique*

In this needling method, the needle does not penetrate into the body, the needle tip is held at the skin surface or perhaps touches the skin, it does not penetrate the skin.[ii] The methods described here cannot be learnt from textbooks but only through highly structured supervised training with regular feedback. In the Toyohari Association, one of the founders, Mr Kozato found that it is possible to monitor the radial pulses throughout the needling techniques and that based on the changes that are felt in the pulses, one can give continuous feedback to the technique. This is the "Kozato hoshiki" or Kozato method [5, 41]. Given that the "mai" were said to reflect the state of qi in the body, that Lingshu ten describes how one must palpate the mai in order to understand the xu-shi of the jingmai [See 125:570 + 574, and 76:153] and that the theory of pulse diagnosis in the Nanjing informs that one can read the radial pulses to understand the condition of qi in the body and in the jingmai, channels, it is natural that one would feel the radial artery pulses to ascertain how well the needling has affected the condition of the qi. In the Kozato method, one can give feedback to every stage of the needling as different changes occur at each

bufa. On the understanding of the term "sui" in relation to needling, differences of opinion can be found in the historical texts as well. Nanjing seventy-two discusses the principle of "sui" when needling, Zhang Shixien (1510 CE) and Xu Dachun (1727 CE) interpret this passage as meaning to needle with the flow of the channel [112:602-603], while other commentators of the same passage see other interpretations [112:599-603]. Meanwhile Nanjing seventy-nine offers a completely different explanation of the idea of "sui" in relation to its theory of systematic correspondence and thus explaining the treatment principle from Nanjing sixty-nine "In the case of depletion fill the respective mother" [112:583]: it is seen in relation to five phase engendering cycle and acupoint selection rather than the angle of the needle [112:641]. I have published a paper discussing this among other themes [10]. As Chace and Bensky illustrate in the next chapter [24], passages from historical texts often have different layers of meaning that can be picked up on by different practitioners, this has been in part responsible for generating the historical variety we find in the field of acupuncture.

ii. Non inserted needling methods are not uncommon in Keiraku Chiryo, Japanese Meridian Therapy, several authors describe their routine use with specialized terminology for variant techniques such as "sesshokushin" (touch or contact needling) and "sanshin" (rapid contact needling over an area) [41, 53, 76:170 + 176, 86, 99, 100]. It is helpful to recall discussions above of how two of the nine needles from the Lingshu (shizhen, yuanzhen) were also not inserted in order to influence the qi. While non-inserted needling methods are not how "acu-*puncture*" is normally thought about today (given the assumption about "puncturing"), they are a routine part of the larger field of acupuncture practice in both historical and modern contexts.

stage. For the technique described below I assume that it was applied well and that the desired changes in the radial pulses were each step by step achieved and confirmed by other qualified practitioners.[iii]

## *Bufa (Japanese hoho) [補法] –the supplementation technique*

A silver needle (40mm long, 0.18mm gauge) is used for this technique.

After selecting the appropriate acupoint to be treated, the practitioner stands in the correct position relative to that acupoint.

Holding the needle in the right hand (sashide), the practitioner places their left hand on the patient in order to find the acupoint.

Touching very lightly the left index finger is softly and slowly stroked along the (flow of) channel (jingmai) to be treated looking for the acupoint to be needled, paying attention to find signs of vacuity to identify the exact location. The vacuous point has certain physical characteristics (is soft, loose, etc) but more subtle feelings are also detected, the (experienced) practitioner becomes aware of something –touching or contacting the qi of the patient (at the "live point").

After finding the exact ("live") location to be needled, and still touching very softly, the practitioner places the thumb of the left hand next to the index finger, pressing the pads of finger and thumb gently together directly over the acupoint to be supplemented. This forms the "oshide".

In order to stabilise the oshide, the other fingers of the left hand are placed lightly so as to secure the "oshide". These movements are done all the while retaining the awareness of the qi at the point to be treated.

The practitioner relaxes and adjusts their posture so as to relieve any unnecessary tension and then introduces the needle into the space between the index finger and thumb over the acupoint, angled along with the flow of the channel and directed towards the acupoint.

Very carefully and slowly and the practitioner advances the needle tip towards the acupoint with their right hand (sashide) paying special attention to feeling when the needle tip contacts or engages something (contacts the qi). This can occur with the needle tip a small distance above the actual surface of the skin or at the skin surface. The practitioner feels this contact in their left hand (though other sensations elsewhere in their body may also be detected).

iii. This stipulation is intended as a counter-argument to the claims that pulse diagnosis is incorrect or unproven and therefore of doubtful value [110]. If there is at least agreement to the observations then those observations can be considered to be reliable, the first step towards validating the method scientifically [81, 82]. Hence for the sake of argument I assume that two or more observers have agreed upon all observations. This theme is touched upon again in chapter eight [15].

Once the practitioner has ascertained that the needle is at the correct "depth" (here the language of depth is within the flow of qi, not within the body), the right hand stops advancing the needle and holds the needle handle very softly while the left hand finger and thumb are pressed slightly more together (this is "left-right pressure" to seal the space around the needle tip to prevent qi leakage).

Throughout these actions the practitioner remains calm and quietly focused noticing and relieving any tension that develops in their body.

With the needle no longer advancing the practitioner seeks a change in the feeling (of qi) at the tip of the needle. If this change does not come automatically the practitioner may apply additional subtle manipulations with the right hand very gently until this change of feeling starts. As the change starts and the feeling (of qi –usually felt in the left hand) increases, the practitioner monitors it, then at the last moment increases the pressure of the left finger and thumb and as the patient inhales he rapidly removes the needle from the acupoint while simultaneously rolling the index finger or thumb over the acupoint (to close the "hole" or space where the needle had been). The timing of this increased "left-right pressure", needle removal and closure of the "hole" is very precise and takes time to learn.

The pressure is maintained on the acupoint for about one breath, then the digit is removed and the technique finished.

## Historical origins

The following are a list of fourteen classical concepts or descriptions that have been employed in one practical form or another in the above needling technique. For each I cite relevant chapters from the Suwen, Lingshu or Nanjing, translations of the same passages can be found in the footnote.[iv]

### *Mechanical factors*

**1a.** Insert the needle at an angle in the direction of flow of the channel treated [e.g. Lingshu 1, 9][v].

iv. For each factor one can see relevant translations: 1a (24, 76:164; 125:546); 1b (112:583+641); 2 (115;2:126); 3 (115;2:126); 4 (24, 125:494); 5 (115;2:133); 6 (115;2:126); 7 (125:495); 8 (112:635+ 646); 9 (112:635+ 646); 10 (112:635); 11 (115;2:126); 12 (115;1:431+452 & 115;2:126, 72:91, 24); 13 (115;1:430+ 432+451-2 & 115;2:19-20+126, 72:91, 23, 24, 95:176-177); 14 (23, 112:589+ 595, 115;2:106, 125:496).

v. Given the recurrent use of hydrological flows that are found in the theories of the jingmai and qi flow (see chapter two), it is difficult to resist the further application of those to explain the role of angling the needle with the flow of the jingmai for bufa and against the flow of the jingmai for xiefa. Inserting an object like a piece of wood into a flowing stream can be used to encourage that

**1b.** Needle the mother point of the vacuous channel [e.g. Nanjing 69, see Nanjing 79].
**2.** Insert the needle on the exhalation and remove on the inhalation. [e.g. Suwen 27, 62].
**3.** Place one's finger over the point immediately upon removal of the needle from the point. [e.g. Suwen 27, 62, Lingshu 1].
**4.** Advance the needle slowly, withdraw the needle quickly [Lingshu 1]
**5.** Apply the needling to one side of the body [Suwen 63][vi].
**6.** Obstruct the "needle hole" on four sides (so that the essence qi cannot leak) [Suwen 62][vii].

*Skill based factors*

**7.** Insert the needle so that it is completely painless, (literally like a mosquito {bite}) [Lingshu 1][viii].
**8.** Feel the arrival of qi before inserting the needle [Nanjing 78, 80][ix].
**9.** Feel the qi arrival with the left hand [Nanjing 78, 80].
**10.** Begin the supplementation needling technique after the arrival of qi (has started) [Nanjing 78][x].
**11.** At the exact moment when the (feeling of) qi is at its maximum (feels replete) remove the needle [Suwen 62].

*Internal factors of the practitioner*

**12.** Focus on the timing of needle removal as the qi "arrives" [Suwen 25, 27, 62, Lingshu 1] also described as the mechanism/dynamic ("ji") associated with the movements of qi, [Lingshu 1].

flow when placed along with the flow (bufa), while it can sluice out of the flow when placed against the current of that flow (xiefa).
vi. See Wilms translation of Suwen sixty-three [119:104].
vii. In the Toyohari system, following initial investigations by Mr Kozato and then confirmation by his colleagues, an important part of the supplementation technique is "left-right pressure", where the index finger and thumb pads are pressed together so as to close the space around the needle. This concept clearly copies this Suwen passage and the role of the left hand described in Nanjing 78, 80 (see "skill based factor" 8).
viii. Although the needle is not per se inserted, it can touch the skin, the important feature being that the needling is painless.
ix. The finding of the "live point" is experienced as contacting and touching the qi with one's fingers, this is necessary before the needle is placed and advanced to the acupoint.
x. See endnote 81 below.

**13.** The inner state of the practitioner must be quiet, focused, undistracted by sensory input or emotions [Suwen 54, Lingshu 9], the intentions must be stable [Suwen 62], the focus and attention correct [Lingshu 1] since what is observed is very subtle [Suwen 25] and one has to remain very alert and focused [Suwen 27].

### *Needling style*

**14.** Needle shallowly [Suwen 62, Lingshu 9, Nanjing 70, 71] or with non-insertion [Lingshu 1, 7, 78]

## Conclusion

What is important here is that in this technique, the approach has attempted to establish a practical interpretation and clinical application of the historical sources. Others may look at the same historical sources and make a different interpretation of the various texts, that is alright, but it in no way demonstrates that what is done above is somehow wrong. Following historical trends in East Asia, knowledge is practice-based (see discussions in chapter one), *interpretations of the same passages are correct if they lead to a practical application that can be reasonably related to the original text*, not only a scholarly translation of the text. This is of fundamental import as this is one of the major reasons why the field of acupuncture has manifest both historically [43:6] and in the modern period [4, 17] with such variety. In this example, the interweaving of techniques from the Neijing and Nanjing is accomplished despite the fact that the needling techniques of the Neijing and Nanjing are conceptually quite different.

## Bibliography

1- Akabane K. *Chinetsukando Niyoru Shinkyu Chiryoho - Acupuncture and Moxibustion* by Heat Sensitivity Method, Yokosuka, Ido no Nippon Sha 1985.
2- Ames RT, Hall DL. *A Philosophical Translation: Dao De Jing –making this life significant*, New York, Ballantine Books, 2003.
3- Anon. *Essentials of Chinese Acupuncture*. Beijing, Foreign Languages Press, 1980.
4- Birch S. Diversity and acupuncture: Acupuncture is not a coherent or his-

torically stable tradition. in AJ. Vickers (ed.) *Examining Complementary Medicine: The Sceptical Holist*. Cheltenham: Stanley Thomas, 1998, pp. 45-63.
5- Birch S. Grasping the sleeping tiger's tail. *NAJOM*, 2004:11, 32:20-23.
6- Birch S. Improving vitality –a case history. *Thieme Almanac 2007: Acupuncture and Chinese Medicine*. Stuttgart, George Thieme Verlag, 2007:80-87.
7- Birch S. Channels and points? A brief review of jing mai and kong xue theories, historical and modern ideas about their nature and evidence for their existence. Lecture given at University of Victoria, Melbourne, April 10, 2007.
8- Birch S. The problem of acupoint contraindications in pregnancy, published online, 2007, see http://www.paradigm pubs.com/Birch Contra
9- Birch S. Filling the whole in acupuncture. Part 1:1 What are we doing in the supplementation needle technique? *European J Oriental Medicine*, 2009:6(2):25-35. Part 1:2, 2009:6(3):18-27.
10- Birch S. Perspectives on ho-sha and kyo-jitsu: historical and modern clinical reflections. *NAJOM*, 2012;19(56):3-6.
11- Birch S. Traditional needling techniques as practical constructions from reading historical descriptions. *Eur J Oriental Med.* 2013;7(3)26-33.
12- Birch S. (In preparation). Filling the whole in acupuncture. Part 2: The "treatment space" –modeling the treatment process in acupuncture.
13- Birch S. (In preparation). Filling the whole in acupuncture –Part 3: researching acupuncture and traditional East Asian medicine (TEAM).
14- Birch S, Azzopardi J, A pilot study investigating practitioner based deqi experiences, (in preparation).
15- Birch S, Bovey M. Chapter eight - Qi, Jingmai: Scientific investigation of concepts based in traditional East Asian medicine: challenges to cross-paradigm research. In this volume.
16- Birch S, Cabrer Mir MA, Rodriguez M. Chapter one: Qi and the mind –explorations of the links between qi, the mind, mental and emotional states. In this volume.
17- Birch S, Felt R. *Understanding Acupuncture*, Edinburgh, Churchill Livingstone, 1999.
18- Birch S, Ida J. *Japanese Acupuncture: A Clinical Guide*, Brookline, Paradigm Publications, 1998.
19- Birch S, Lewith G. Acupuncture research, the story so far. In MacPherson H, Hammerschlag.R, Lewith G, Schnyer R (eds). *Acupuncture Research: Strategies for Building an Evidence Base*. London, Elsevier, 2007:15-35.
20- Birch S, Rodriguez M, Cabrer Mir MA. Chapter two: The jingmai –a summary of their development and nature. In this volume.

21- Cabrer Mir MA. Chapter seven: Qi and stillness –Taijiquan, qigong and acupuncture. In this volume.
22- Cabrer Mir MA, Rodriguez M, Birch S. Chapter ten: Practical Exercises. In this volume.
23- Chace C. On greeting a friend, an approach to needle technique.*Lantern*. 2006:3(3):4-7.
24- Chace C, Bensky D. Chapter five: An axis of efficacy. The range of meaning in chapter one of the Lingshu. In this volume.
25- Chace C, Shima M. *Exposition on the Eight Extraordinary Vessels*, Seattle, Eastland Press, 2009.
26- Chae Y, Chang DS, Lee SH, Jung WM, Lee IS, Jackson S, Kong J, Lee H, Park HJ, Lee H, Wallraven C. Inserting needles into the body: a meta-analysis of brain activity associated with acupuncture needle stimulation. *J Pain*. 2013 Mar;14(3):215-22. doi: 10.1016/j.jpain.2012.11.011. Epub 2013 Feb 5.
27- Chen WC, et al. The determination of the depth of puncture for the development of needling sensation. *National Symposia of Acupuncture and Moxibustion and Acupuncture Anesthesia*. Beijing, June 1-5, 1979, pages 113-114.
28- Cheng XN. *Chinese Acupuncture and Moxibustion*. Beijing, Foreign Languages Press, 1987.
29- Chiu ML. *Mind, body, and illness in a Chinese medical tradition*. Ph.D. thesis, Harvard University, 1986.
30- Connelly D. *Traditional Acupuncture: The Law of the Five Elements*. Columbia Maryland, The Centre for Traditional Acupuncture, 1979.
31- Csikszentmihalyi M. *Material Virtue: ethics and the body in early China*. Brill, Leiden, 2004.
32- Daly NP. *Hybridizing the human body: The hydrological development of acupuncture in early Imperial China*. Masters thesis, Department of East Asian Studies, McGill University, 1999.
33- Ellis A, Wiseman N, Boss K. *Fundamentals of Chinese Acupuncture*; Brookline, Paradigm Publications, 1988.
34- Epler DC. Bloodletting in early Chinese medicine and its relation to the origin of acupuncture. *Bull Hist Med*; 1980; 54:337-367.
35- Field SL (translator). The Zangshu, or Book of Burial by Guo Pu (276 324). July 26, 2009, http://www.fengshuigate.com/zangshu.html
36- Field SL. In Search of Dragons: Fengshui and Early Geophysical Notions of Qi. May 9, 2003, http://www.trinity.edu/sfield/Fengshui/Dragons.html
37- Filshie J, White A. eds. *Medical Acupuncture*. Edinburgh, Churchill Livingstone, 1998.

38- Firebrace P, Hill S. *New ways to health; a guide to acupuncture*, London, Hamlyn publishing group limited, 1988.
39- Forman RKC. *Mysticism, Mind, Consciousness*, Albany, SUNY Press, 1999.
40- Fukaya I. *Kadenkyu Monogatari -Family Recipes in Moxa Therapy*, Tokyo, Sankei Publishing Company, 1982.
41- Fukushima K. *Meridian Therapy*, Tokyo, Toyo Hari Medical Association, 1991.
42- Golding R. *The Complete Stems and Branches*, Edinburgh, Churchill Livingstone, 2008.
43- Goldschmidt A. *The Evolution of Chinese Medicine: Song dynasty, 960-1200*, London, Routledge, 2009.
44- Hall DL, Ames RT. *Thinking from the Han*, Albany, State University of New York Press, 1998.
45- Hammerschlag R, Langevin HE, Lao LX, Lewith G. Physiological dynamics of acupuncture: correlations and mechanisms. In MacPherson H, Hammerschlag.R, Lewith G, Schnyer R (eds). *Acupuncture Research: Strategies for Building an Evidence Base*. London, Elsevier, 2007:181-197.
46- Harper D. *The "Wu Shi Erh Ping Fang": Translation and Prolegomena*. Doctoral Thesis, University of California, Berkeley, 1982.
47- Harper D. *Early Chinese Medical Literature: the Mawangdui Medical Manuscripts*. London, Kegan Paul, 1998.
48- Holloway KW. *Guodian – the newly discovered seeds of Chinese religious and political philosophy*, Oxford, Oxford University Press 2009.
49- Honma S. *Keiraku Chiryo Kouwa –Lectures on Meridian Therapy*. Yokosuka, Ido no Nippon Sha, 1949.
50- Hsu E. Pulse diagnostics in the Western Han: how mai and qi determine bing. In Hsu E, (ed). *Innovation in Chinese Medicine*, Cambridge, Cambridge University Press, 2001:51-91.
51- Hsu E. Tactility and the body in early Chinese medicine. *Science in Context*, 2005:18(1):7-34.
52- Irie T. *Rinsho Toyo Igaku Genron*, Osaka, published privately by the author, 1990.
53- Kobayashi S. *Acupuncture Core Therapy –Shakujyu Chiryo*, Taos, Paradigm Publications, 2008.
54- Kosodo T, Hamada Y. *Ishaku Kotei Daikei Reisu –Explanation of the Huang Di Nei Jing Ling Shu*; Tokyo, Tsukijishokan K.K, 1972.
55- Kuriyama S. Between mind and eye; Japanese anatomy in the eighteenth century. In Leslie C, Young A. (eds); *Paths to Asian Medical Knowledge*, Berkeley, University of California Press; 1992, pages 21-43.

56- Kuriyama S. T*he Expressiveness of the Body and the Divergence of Greek and Chinese Medicine*, New York, Zone Books 1999.
57- Lai XS, Tong Z. A study on the classification and the "catching" of the "arrived qi" in acupuncture. *J Trad Chinese Med*, 2010;30(1):3-8.
58- Larre C, Rochat de la Vallee. *The Seven Emotions*. London, Monkey Press, 1996.
59- Larre C, Rochat de la Vallee E. *Essence, Spirit, Blood and Qi*, London, Monkey Press, 1999.
60- Le Blanc C. *Huai-Nan Tzu –Philosophical Synthesis in Early Han Thought*. Hong Kong, Hong Kong University Press 1985.
61- Lewis ME. *The Construction of Space in Early China*. Albany, SUNY Press, 2006.
62- Lewith GT, Machin D.On the evaluation of the clinical effects of acupuncture. *Pain*. 1983; 16:111 127.
63- Li Jianmin. They shall expel demons: etiology, the medical canon and the transformation of medical techniques before the Tang. In J Langerwey, M Kalinowski (eds). *Early Chinese Religion*, Leiden, Brill, 2009, pages 1103-1150.
64- Liu BQ. *Optimum Time for Acupuncture*; Jinan, Shandong Science and Technology Press, 1988.
65- Lloyd G. The techniques of persuasion and the rhetoric of disorder in late Zhanguo and Western Han texts. In Nylan M, Loewe M (eds). *China's Early Empires –A Re-appraisal*, Cambridge, Cambridge University Press, 2010, pages 451-460.
66- Lloyd G, Sivin N. *The Way and the Word*, New Haven, Yale University Press, 2002.
67- Lo V. The influence of nurturing life culture on the development of Western Han acumoxa therapy. In Hsu E, (ed). *Innovation in Chinese Medicine*, Cambridge, Cambridge University Press, 2001:19-50.
68- Lo V. Spirit of Stone: Technical Considerations in the Treatment of the Jade Body. *Bulletin of the School of Oriental and African Studies*, University of London, 2002; 65:1:99 128.
69- Lo V. Huangdi Hama jing "The Yellow Emperor's Toad Manual" in a special edition of Asia Major, 2001;14(2):61-99, edited by Nathan Sivin: Essays Contributed in Honour of Michael Loewe [published in Spring, 2004]. See also http://www.ihp.sinica.edu.tw/~medicine/ashm/lectures/Lo.pdf.
70- Lo V. The territory between life and death. *Medical History,* 2003, 47: 250-258.
71- Lo V, Li Jianmin. Manuscripts, received texts and the healing arts. In Nylan M, Loewe M (eds). *China's Early Empires –A Re-appraisal*, Cambridge, Cambridge University Press, 2010, pages 367-397.

72- Lu GD, Needham J. *Celestial Lancets*; Cambridge, Cambridge University Press, 1980.
73- Macpherson H, Kaptchuk TJ. *Acupuncture in Practice*. New York, Churchill Livingstone, 1997.
74- Manaka Y. *Ika no Tameno Shinjutsu Nyumon Kuoza*; Introductory Lectures on Acupuncture for Medical Doctors; Yokosuka, Ido no Nippon Sha, 1980.
75- Manaka Y, Itaya K, Birch S. *Chasing the Dragon's Tail*, Brookline, Paradigm Publications, 1995.
76- Matsumoto K, Birch S. *Five Elements and Ten Stems*, Brookline, Paradigm Publications 1983.
77- Matsumoto K, Birch S. *Extraordinary Vessels*, Brookline, Paradigm Publications, 1986.
78- Matsumoto K, Birch S. *Hara Diagnosis Reflections on the Sea*; Brookline, Paradigm Publications, 1988.
79- Nakatani Y, Yamashita K. *Ryodoraku Acupuncture*; Tokyo, Ryodoraku Research Institute, 1977.
80- Needham J. Ling W. *Science and Civilisation in China –Volume III*, Cambridge, Cambridge University Press, 1959.
81- O'Brien KA, Birch S. A review of the reliability of traditional East Asian medical diagnoses. *J Alt Complem Med*, 2009:15(4):353-366.
82- O'Brien KA, Abbas E, Movsessian P, Hook M, Komesaroff PA, Birch S. Investigating the reliability of Japanese Toyohari Meridian Therapy Diagnosis. *J Alt Compl Med*; 2009:15(10):1099-1105.
83- O'Connor J, Bensky D. *Acupuncture a Comprehensive Text*; Seattle, Eastland Press, 1981.
84- Oda H. *Ryodoraku Textbook Osaka*, Naniwasha Publishing Company, 1989.
85- Okabe S. *Shinkyu Keiraku Chiryo*. Tokyo, Kobunsha, 1974.
86- Ono B. *Keiraku Chiryo Shinkyu Rinsho Nyumon*. Yokosuka, Ido no Nippon Sha, 1988.
87- Pomeranz B, Berman B. Scientific basis of acupuncture. In: G Stux, B Berman, B Pomeranz. *Basics of Acupuncture*. Berlin, Springer-Verlag, fifth edition, 2003, pp 1-86.
88- Puett MJ. *To Become a God: cosmology, sacrifice, and self-divination in early China*. Cambridge, Harvard University Asia Center, 2002.
89- Qiu ML. *Chinese Acupuncture and Moxibustion*. Edinburgh: Churchill Livingstone, 1993.
90- Requena Y. *Terrains and Pathology in Acupuncture*; Brookline, Paradigm Publications, 1986.
91- Rickett A. Nei Ye.Inner workings and introduction to the four "xin shu"

chapters. In *Guanzi, Volume Two*. Princeton, Pinceton University Press, 1998:15-55.
92- Rochat de la Vallée E. *A Study of Qi in Classical Texts*, London, Monkey Press, 2006.
93- Rodriguez M. Chapter six: Qi, jingmai, yaoyi –a study of their relationships. In this volume.
94- Roth HD. *Original Tao –Inward Training (Nei Yeh)*. New York, Columbia University Press, 1999.
95- Scheid V. *Chinese Medicine in Contemporary China*, Durham, Duke University press, 2002.
96- Scheid V, Bensky D. Medicine as signification. *European J Orien Med*, 1999:2, 6:32-40.
97- Schnyer R, Birch S, MacPherson H. Acupuncture practice as the foundation for clinical evaluation. In MacPherson H, Hammerschlag.R, Lewith G, Schnyer R (eds). *Acupuncture Research: Strategies for Building an Evidence Base*. London, Elsevier, 2007:153-179.
98- Shiroda BS. *Shinkyu Chiryo Kiso Gaku*; Yokosuka, Ido No Nippon Sha, 1986.
99- Shudo D. *Introduction to Meridian Therapy*, Seattle, Eastland Press, 1990.
100- Shudo D. *Finding Effective Acupoints*, Seattle, Eastland Press, 2003.
101- Sivin N. *Traditional Medicine in Contemporary China*, Ann Arbor, Centre for Chinese Studies, University of Michigan, 1987.
102- Sivin N. State, cosmos and body in the last three centuries BC. *Harvard J. Asiatic Studies*. 1995:55(1):5-37.
103- Slingerland E. *Effortless Action*, Oxford, Oxford University Press, 2003.
104- Sommers D. *De Chinese Fascinatie voor de Geest*, Veghel, Uitgeverij Libra and Libris, 2007.
105- Sommers S. Chapter three: How to become a shang yi or "superior physician," An exploration on the influence of the practitioner in early China. In this volume.
106- Soulie de Morant G. *Chinese Acupuncture*. Brookline, Paradigm Publications, 1994 (translation of *L'Acupuncture Chinoise*, 1956.)
107- Sterckx R. *The Animal and the Daemon in Early China*, Albany, State University of New York, 2002.
108- Sunu K, Lee Y. *The Canon of Acupuncture: Huang Ti Nei Ching Ling Shu*, Seoul, Korea Acupuncture Society, 1985.
109- Tessenow H, Unschuld PU. *A Dictionary of the Huangdi Neijing Suwen*, Berkeley, University of California Press, 2008.
110- Ulett GA. *Principles and Practoce of Physiologic Acupuncture*, St Louis, Warren H Green Inc, 1982.

111- Unschuld PU. *Medicine in China: A History of Ideas*, Berkeley, University of California Press, 1985.
112- Unschuld PU. *Nan Ching: The Classic of Difficult Issues*, Berkeley, University of California Press, 1986.
113- Unschuld PU. Epistemological issues and changing legitimation: Traditional Chinese medicine in the twentieth century. In Leslie C, Young A, (eds) *Paths to Asian Medical Knowledge*; Berkeley, University of California Press, 1992, pp. 44-61.
114- Unschuld PU. *Huang Di Nei Jing Su Wen –nature, knowledge, imagery in an ancient Chinese medical text*. Berkeley, University of California Press, 2003.
115- Unschuld PU, Tessenow H, Jinsheng Z. *Huand Di nei jing su wen: An annotated translation of Huang Di's Inner Classic –Basic Questions; volume 1 and volume 2*. Berkeley, University of California Press, 2011.
116- Vincent CA, Richardson PH, Black JJ, Pither CE. The significance of needle placement site in acupuncture. *J Psychosom Res*. 1989:33, 4:489-496.
117- Wang JY. *Applied Channel Theory in Chinese Medicine*. Seattle, Eastland Press, 2008.
118- Wilber K. *Integral Psychology*, Boston, Shambhala Publications, 2000.
119- Wilms S. *The Great Compendiunm of Acupuncture and Moxibustion*, volume 1, Portland, Chinese Medicine Database, 2010.
120- Wiseman N, Feng Y. *A Practical Dictionary of Chinese Medicine*, Brookline, Paradigm Publications, 1997.
121- Wolpe PR. The maintenance of professional authority: Acupuncture and the American physician. *Social Problems*, 1985:32(5):409 424.
122- World Health Organization. *Acupuncture: Review and analysis of reports on controlled clinical trials*. Geneva, WHO division of traditional medicine, 2003.
123- Worsley J.R. *Is Acupuncture For You*. Leamington Spa, England, College of Traditional Chinese Acupuncture, 1973.
124- Wu JN. *The Spiritual Pivot*, Honolulu, University of Hawaii Press, 1993.
125- Wu NL, Wu AQ. *Yellow Emperor's Canon Internal Medicine*, Beijing, China Science and Technology Press, 1997.
126- Xu RD, Zhang JW. The original meaning of "arrival of qi" in the Huangdi Neijing (in Chinese). *Zhongguo Zhen Jiu*. 2005;25(6):445.
127- Yanagiya S. *Shinkyu Ijutsu no Mon; An Introduction to the Medical Arts of Acupuncture and Moxibustion*; Yokosuka, Ido no Nippon sha, 1948.
128- Yang RB. From "merging the body with the mind" to "wandering in unitary qi": a discussion of Zhuangzi's realm of the true man and its corporeal basis. In Cook S (ed). *Hiding the World in the World*. Albany, State University of New York, 2003:88-127.

129- Yang WJ. *Huangdi Neijing Lingshu Yijie*, Taipei, Chinese Republic Publishing company 1978.
130- Yang ZY. On presence of mind and subtle sensations. *The Lantern*, 2007;IV(2):28-30.
131- Yang SZ, Chace C. *The Systematic Classic of Acupuncture and Moxibustion*, Boulder, Blue Poppy Press, 1994.
132- Zhang K, Lu SK. *Ziwu Liuzhu Method and Its Application*, Shanghai, Shanghai Scientific and Technological Publishing House, 1992.
133- Zhang YH, Rose K. *A Brief History of Qi*, Brookline, Paradigm Publications, 2001.
134- Zhang F, Wang HD. Discussion on needling sensation, arrival of qi and needling response (Deqi) (In Chinese). *Zhongguo Zhen Jiu*. 2012;32(12):1132-4.
135- Zhang ZJ, Wang XM, McAlonan GM. Neural Acupuncture Unit: A New Concept for Interpreting Effects and Mechanisms of Acupuncture. *Evidence-Based Complementary and Alternative Medicine* Volume 2012, Article ID 429412, 23 pages doi:10.1155/2012/429412.
136- Zmiewski P, Feit R. *Acumoxa Therapy,* Brookline, Paradigm Publications 1989.

## Endnotes

1. "Real acupuncture involves the use of acupuncture needles inserted into acupuncture points supposedly therapeutically effective, for the condition being treated, and can be considered to be properly performed acupuncture." [62].

2. "Acupuncture and moxibustion are two of the most ancient and characteristic therapeutic techniques of Chinese medicine. The one may be defined broadly as the implantation of needles to different depths at a great variety of points on the surface of the human body, points gathered in connected arrays according to a highly systematised pattern with a complex and sophisticated, if still essentially medieval, physiological theory behind it... The other technique consists in the burning of Artemisia tinder, either in the form of incense like cones (whether or not directly on the skin), or as cigar shaped sticks held just above it, the points chosen for application being in general identical with those of the acupuncture system." [72:1].

3. "Acupuncture and moxibustion are methods of treating disease by stimulating certain points or loci on the body... Acupuncture involves the use of needles, ordinarily inserted beneath the superficial layers of skin, to provide mechanical stimulation of the underlying points. Moxibustion on the other hand, utilizes the dried powdered leaves of the moxa plant... which are burned on or above the surface of the skin to provide thermal stimulation." [83:397].

4. "Acupuncture literally means to puncture with a needle. However, the application of needles is often used in combination with moxibustion –the burning on or over the skin of selected herbs– and may also involve the application of other kinds of stimulation to certain points. In this publication the term "acupuncture" is used in its broad sense to include traditional body needling, moxibustion, electric acupuncture (electro-acupuncture), laser acupuncture (photo-acupuncture), microsystem acupuncture such as ear (auricular), face, hand and scalp acupuncture, and acupressure (the application of pressure at selected sites)" [122:3].

5. We should be mindful of the comments of other authors who are critical of the rather limited way that the literature on acupuncture has been portrayed. Their comments while now slightly dated are still rather pertinent: "In approaching acupuncture through the works of representatives of the present day practitioners in the Western world some reserve should be exercised, for the following reasons: (a) very few of them have had reliable linguistic access to the voluminous Chinese sources of many different periods, (b) it is often not quite clear how far their training has given them direct continuity with the living Chinese clinical traditions, (c) the history in their works is liable to be minimal or unscholarly, (d) their accounts of theory are generally very inadequate, (e) they tend to adopt a too simplistic assimilation of classical Chinese disease entities to those of modern Western medicine, (f) the cardinal importance of sphygmology in Chinese differential diagnosis is almost ignored, and (g) their works are naturally so much influenced by modern Western concepts of disease aetiology and semeiography that they seem not to practice the classical Chinese methods of holistic classification and diagnosis." [72:11 12]. Also, "because serious research in Chinese studies has been devoted to an exploration of the contents and foundations of traditional Chinese medicine, only for a rather short time now, our knowledge in this regard should still be considered as preliminary and open to frequent reassessment," [113]. But these reservations are not limited to Western authors and representations they also include modern Asian authors: "As a graduate from the mathematics department of my university, it was always necessary to provide the proof of one's answers. I can't help thinking that current Chinese medicine (TCM) tries to give answers without providing proof, (because of this,) perhaps the medical doctors of ancient China are crying (in their graves)" [52:35].

6. References to the use of bloodletting were quite numerous in the Neijing [34, 114].

7. Harper discusses the incorporation of lancing with stones described in the Mawangdui text the "Maifa" [經法] to lancing with special needles in Lingshu chapter seven as evidence for how the older tradition was incorporated into the newer [47:93], and next discusses [47:94] how the use of the lancet for bleeding appears to be a novel therapy that perhaps arose out of the newer trend of inserting needles, in contradiction to arguments from Epler [34].

8. Lo discusses how only the "haozhen" "chanzhen" and "yuanlizhen" are explicitly described for use to influence conditions of qi pathology [68].

9. After examining a range of different opinions and definitions by a number of Japanese practitioners and authors, and partly from his own perspectives, Manaka had the following

to say about a definition of acupuncture: "Based upon the above considerations, we can draw the following conclusions: 1 acupuncture is an ancient Oriental medical therapy based on empirical observations and transmitted from then to now continuously; 2 as tools, needle like things called 'zhen' are used; 3 the focus of treatment is on the 'acupoints' which have particular significance and meaning." [74:4-7]. He specifically recognised that the needles are not necessarily inserted.

10. Although in the some of the Mawangdui texts such as the Maifa [47:91 + 429] we find descriptions of how moxa influences the qi, in the later Neijing medical literature [114], the use of needles takes on the more dominant role as qi influencing therapy so that moxibustion, in contradistinction is seen to act in different ways.

11.The term tiao [調] is variously translated. Rochat de la Valle as "regulate", "tune" [92:79], Tessenow and Unschuld as "be in agreement", "to harmonize", "to adjust", "to regulate" [109:424]. There is general agreement among translators on how to understand the passage, Wu and Wu render it thus "In the law of pricking; it is mainly the adjusting of the energy" [125:795].

12. "So the definition of acupuncture here is tiao qi [調氣]. You do something with the qi which is like tuning a piano, and you try to make it more harmonious" [92:79-80].

13. It is useful to recall the premedical literature about self-cultivation and life enhancement techniques (yangsheng). The Lushi Chunqiu makes a clear statement about how when there is a free flow in the interstices of the flesh and the jingqi renews daily, pathogenic qi is expelled and healthy life is maintained [101:49]. In other words if proper circulation and movement of qi can be restored and maintained, one remains healthy and can resist negative influences, the stated goal of treatment at the start of the medical tradition in Suwen chapter one [114:198-199]. Such ideas help us understand why one would want to "tiao qi" or "regulate the qi".

14. Writing about the influence of the yangsheng culture on the early development of acupuncture, Lo states "I differentiate 'acupuncture' from bloodletting and other minor surgery by the target of medical intervention. Acupuncture, as I define it, is the act of piercing the body with the intention of moving qi in the channels" (jingmai) [67:29].

15. Lo presents evidence for the influence of the yangsheng literature "in the construction of the acumoxa body" which she defines as "a body delineated by channels through which qi moves and on which are points where qi can be influenced" [67:33]. The thesis is that the earliest developments of acumoxa therapy in the Neijing evidences a new model of the body, where the jingmai with qi flowing in them and on which the acupoints are first described forms a novel understanding of the body, deriving some of its language from earlier yangsheng literature. These themes were extensively discussed in chapters one and two [16, 20].

16. Of the Suwen, Epler said: "The Plain Questions (Su Wen) does not embody a single coherent, logical system of medicine that served as a contemporary standard of orthodoxy.

There was no such system prior to and during the Western Han, early Chinese medicine consists of assorted, sometimes contradictory, theories and practices that were in a considerable state of flux for many centuries. The extent of conceptual change is revealed as early as the third century A.D. by medical writers who were stating that what they called the 'ancient texts' were obscure and difficult to understand; for instance Huang Fumi, author of a text on acupuncture, says of the Plain Questions that its import is 'profound and mysterious, not easily perceptible.' This means that all later texts and commentaries are of very limited value for a historical interpretation of the Plain Questions. Their authors, writing for a medical audience, were able to select specific passages for inclusion in their own works or for comment; when these same passages are considered in their historical contexts, their meaning may be quite different." [34:338].

17. The "superior physician" is discussed by Dianne Sommers in the previous chapter [105].

18. See for example Lingshu chapter one where a repeated contrast of the superior physician and the crude or inferior physician is made with regards the art and subtleties of needling. "The crude attend to the form, the superior to the spirit... the crude attend to the junctures, the superior to the dynamic" [24]. A full translation with extended commentaries of the passage can be found in the next chapter by Chace and Bensky [24].

19. Lingshu chapter eleven discusses this, here is Lu and Needham's marvelous translation: "Whether a man goes on living in health, or whether a disease arises; whether it is in human power to control it, and whether the patient can be cured; whether one is only at the beginning of study of acupuncture (and moxibustion), or whether one has come to the fullness of it –all depends on (an understanding of the functions of) the twelve-tract network system of yang and yin channels (jingmai). To the slap-dash practitioner or the tyro it all seems very easy; only the great physician knows how difficult it really is" [72:28]. This contrast of the superior and inferior physician continues in the medical literature. Citing the Neijing (Lingshu fifty-five, see Unschuld [112:631-633]) Nanjing seventy-seven tells us: "The superior practitioner treats what is not yet ill; the mediocre practitioner treats what is already ill" [112:630].

20. Was this a parallel to the earlier Mawangdui descriptions of the use of moxa on the mai based solely on the presence of specific symptoms?

21. Whether there is a causal link or it is coincidental is a question for others to resolve.

22. Authors as early as Huang Fumi in the third century CE sought to systematise and standardise the acupoints which had not been so clearly described in the Han canonical texts of the Neijing and Nanjing. Naturally the anatomical body would become a target for describing their location. The revival of acupuncture triggered during the Song dynasty also occurred after efforts to standardise the variable locations of the acupoints up till that time, the Tongren Yuxue Zhenjiu Tujing [銅人腧穴鍼灸圖經] and the accompanying Bronze statue of Wang Weiyi [43:26-33] focused the description of the acupoints to anatomical structures to fix and standardise their locations. These changes were important for the history and development of acupuncture. In the Song dynasty they were instru-

mental in the revival of Classical medicine and its theories of the twelve channels and their circulation of qi as an important target for treatment [43:30-37].

23. Influence of the Western anatomical body penetrated into Japan by the 1700s with Sugita Gempaku's translation of the Dutch anatomical text "Anatomische Tebellen" in his highly celebrated Kaitai Shinso (1774) [55], while the anatomical body found fertile soil in China after Wang Qingren reported on the dissection of corpses in his text Yilin Gaicuo of 1830 [51, 111:79]. It could be argued that much of the modern literature on acupuncture in these countries has been influenced by these developments. This theme is briefly discussed by Birch and Felt [17:39-40, 50 and following].

24. In the middle of the eighth century CE Wangtao stated "acupuncture can kill healthy people... If one desires to adopt this technique, I am afraid he will harm life" [43:29]. It seems that the loss of traditional texts after the Han led to disparate systems of sporadic practice, some of which was poorly performed, giving acupuncture the reputation of being something dangerous [43: 29-30, 72:127-135]. The classical doctrines upon which early acupuncture had been founded were largely lost "none of the canonical works was in wide circulation, and practitioners largely shunned needling" [43:30]. During these centuries we see a rise in interest, recommendations and the use of moxibustion, presumably because it was not seen to be so harmful [43:29, 72:128] and could easily be directed to the acupoints.

25. As examples I cite three very different models from the modern literature. In the first acupuncture is purely preventative: "Acupuncture is foremost a philosophy of preventive medicine, of intervention to correct the body's energy balance before pathology becomes manifest. To restore correct energy flow, the Chinese employ a variety of needles of varying widths, lengths, and metals, and base the correct depth, rotation, and duration of needle use on the diagnosis" [121]. The second promotes another kind of ideological approach where the therapist is principally involved in persuading the patient's body to fix itself by regulating the qi: "Acupuncture sees the body as a self rectifying dynamic whole, a network of interrelating and interacting energies. Their even distribution and flow maintains health, but any interruption, depletion or stagnation leads to disease. Acupuncture is a system of medicine which seeks to aid these natural processes, helping the body to correct itself by realignment or redirection of energy, which the Chinese call Qi.' [38:9], "Acupuncture is a technique whereby the movement of the ch'i influences through the body's transportation channels is regulated" [111:92]. The third lacks any of these ideological perspectives and targets instead the disease rather than the patient and his natural abilities: "Acupuncture is essentially a treatment based upon actions of the nervous system" especially for treating pain [110:v]. Interestingly from the earliest times acupuncture practice based on classical theories of the channels and qi flow can be found, as can acupuncture based on treating points to relieve symptoms, with little attention to channel theory or qi regulation [43:7-8]. Acupuncture has always been a heterogeneous medical system [17, 43:6], "Medicine was clearly not a monolithic edifice of scholarship but there must have been two thousand years ago just as now, a multiplicity of points of view" [50:62].

26. This is seen in the Mawangdui [馬王堆](168 BCE) and Zhangjiashan [張家山] (186 BCE) texts [32, 47, 68].

27. The first mention of blood vessels appears to be in the Zuozhuan description of a distraught horse (mid fourth century BCE) [47:82, 107:74], the first mention of the idea that "qi flows along with blood through the vessels inside the body" occurs in first half third century BCE [107: 74]. Then we find discussions of the compound term xueqi [血氣] (blood-qi or blood and qi) in relation to living animals [107:74]. Sivin cites the first usage of the term "xueqi" to be in the Analects of Confucius [101:46] where he translates the term as "physical vitality" or "physical powers". While there might be an inclination to see "xueqi" as referring to the blood and qi, many argue against this: Kuriyama argues, they are "essentially the same. Doctors did, to be sure, occasionally spotlight distinctions. Blood had form, for instance, while qi was formless... blood and qi were complementary facets of a unique vitality, its yin and yang manifestation" [56:229; see also 101:51-52]. Sterckx traces this inseparability of the two into the later Han: "According to Wang Chong, human beings live by the agency of refined qi (jingqi) which is made possible by the blood vessels. He further defines blood as the 'jingqi during one's life period' and describes 'blood and qi'(xueqi) as the seat of one's jingshen, hereby again associating the development of spiritual energy with the presence of a physiological substrate of blood vapor" [107:75]. This association helps us understand why Lingshu chapter eighteen states "the blood (xue) is the shenqi" [78:98]. The blood and qi together are vital to living things which are animated by "shen" [神], hence their close association. Kuriyama points to this natural type of association in other traditional systems, such as that of the Greeks with blood and pneuma, but there a polarization of the two gradually increased [56:229].

28. Harper comments that while both qi and bood were seen as essential components of life, qi came to be seen as being "more necessary to human existence than blood: it was the air that man breathed, it was the nourishment extracted from food; it was what suffused the body and made man alive; it was what connected the human organism to the larger operations of nature" [47:77].

29. Even as late as 1980 Lu and Needham list twenty-seven rather than twenty-eight acupoints on the dumai [72:56].

30. See below. The following description is a summary of the pathways of the yingqi following the up and down trajectories and interior pathways of the jingmai.

31. Lingshu chapter eighteen [78:97-99].

32. Internal trajectories of the jingmai are summarised by Matsumoto, Birch [78:49-65].

33. The details are more complex, but this summary captures the basics of the yingqi circulation through the jingmai and their corresponding zang-fu.

34. Lu and Needham called it an "Extravascular protective yang component" since it is explicitly described as moving/circulating outside the jingmai while the yingqi [營氣] circulates within the jingmai [72:28-30].

35. How it passes from the hands to the feet is not described.

36. The passage states: "The yang qi (weiqi) comes out from the eyes when one's eyes open, passes up to the head, the neck and leg taiyang (bladder channel). Coming to the back it passes down to the external corners of the little toes. One of the scattered parts separates from the external corners of the eyes and passes down to arm taiyang (small intestine channel), passing to the external corners of the little fingers. Another scattered part separates from the external corners of the eyes and passes down to leg shaoyang (gallbladder channel), to down in between the fourth and fifth toes. As above (the next) passes around arm shaoyang (triple burner channel) and passes to in between the fourth and fifth fingers. A separated (part), as above, reaches to in front of the ear, unites with the vessel on the chin and passes to leg yangming (stomach channel), passing down to the upper part of the foot and in between the five toes. A dispersing (part) passes from below the ears to arm yangming (large intestine channel), coming to between the thumbs and index fingers. (Those that pass to the hand) pass to the center of the palm, this (then) passes to the feet and the center of the soles. They (probably all six parts) come out to the internal malleolus, passing to the yin parts and returning to the eyes. Therefore this is one cycle" [translated from 129:554], see also translation of the same passage by Yang, Chace [131:32-3] and Wu [124:249-250]

37. Following Lingshu chapter eighteen, Nanjing thirty is explicit about this "the clear [portion] turns into constructive [influences]; the turbid portion turns into protective [influences]. The constructive [influences] proceed inside the vessels, the protective [influences] proceed outside of the vessels. They circulate [through the organism] without a break; [after] every fifty [passages they have] another great meeting" [112:341], see also Lu, Needham [72:30].

38. The Nanjing discusses the depth of needling in relation to applying bufa [補法], supplementation technique and xiefa [寫法], draining technique [78:25, 112:626-629] where the more superficial needling aspects are often said to involve the weiqi and the deeper the yingqi.

39. Unschuld calls this "original influences", I have followed Wiseman and replaced "original influences" by "source qi" in the translation [120:548].

40. Where Unschuld uses "influences" I have rendered "qi", where "conduit-vessels" I have rendered "channels".

41. The acupoints were given various names such as kongxue [孔穴], qixue [氣穴], shu [俞], qifu [氣府], xuedao [穴道] and commonly xuewei [穴位] [72:13-14, 120:6]. The term xue [穴] can be found as referring to the most auspicious burial sites for the dead in pre-Neijing geomancy traditions [35, 36], perhaps implying a similarity of meaning.

42. "So we can only conclude that there is no evidence to show that stimulating the channel network via a mature acupoint system with metal needles was a feature of therapy before the first to second centuries BC." [68].

43. Le Blanc describes three uses of the term "shenqi" during the Han dynasty, the first as "spiritual emanations, having a supernatural character" the second as "the most subtle essence or substance, understood as a naturalistic concept –as used by the theory of yin-yang", the third as "vitality, spirit and breath, morale" [60:118]. The term here most likely is used in the third sense as "vitality", though the second sense could be implied, the third is much more likely. Sivin also sees the term shenqi to refer to the "normal vitality of the body" [102:14].

44. While Lo translates shenqi [神氣] as "qi of the shen" or "qi and shen", Sivin translated it as "divine qi", we remind the reader that compound terms like "shenqi" are often points of disagreement among translators, and that the meaning will probably have varied at different times in different textual sources in China. Probably Sivin's idea of the "normal vitality of the body" is correct, since we find terms like "shenqi" and even "jingqi" used instead of "qi" in some contexts, all of which are probably variations of expression of the same term... something to do with qi.

45. The initial descriptions of the xue, acupoints in the Neijing were often unclear. The post Han author, Huang Fumi (282 CE) in his Zhenjiu Jiayijing began a systematic description of the location, indication, depths of needling and numbers of moxa to be burned for each acupoint. We have already suggested that this new emphasis may have triggered a trend away from interpreting and approaching the xue as non-anatomically based sites for qi to enter and exit that we see in the Lingshu towards more anatomically based interpretations and approaches. It is a natural consequence that the act of codifying information might transform that information and its messages, especially if that information was not entirely clear to begin with. For sure we see by the time of the Bronze statue which emerged in the eleventh century, that the acupoints had become fixed in the body. The sites of each point were located as holes on the surface of the bronze statue. The statute was then covered in wax and filled with fluid. Correct needling of the point would draw fluid from it [43:34-36, 72:133]. Anatomically fixed points serve the function of helping train beginners in addition to providing readily identifiable sites to which one can target treatment. The issue raised here is that we can expect that there would be different interpretations and styles of acupuncture on the basis of how the Lingshu passage is read. This is precisely what we find in different modern styles of practice. As we will see below, there are some styles that take the xue as anatomically fixed (even here there are variations in how different schools of acupuncture locate some of the acupoints), with teaching and practice methods evolving alongside this. Then there are other styles that take Lingshu one quite literally and take the xue as more fluid, even movable, with teaching and practice methods evolving alongside this. See further discussion of this last point below.

46. Writing about a massage text found in the sexual cultivation literature, Lo concludes: "this massage text produces a representation of the body which pre-dates and therefore in its methods of describing the body in metaphorical terms, anticipates the acupoints" [67:39].

47. The point here is that with the early literature on needling techniques we find a strong focus on the role of getting qizhi [氣至] the "arrival of qi", without which the needling

was said (Lingshu chapter one) to be ineffective [9, 24, 130], and where better to get the qizhi to happen than those places where the qi flows in and out of the body (Lingshu chapter one), the acupoints?

48. And of course the renmai and dumai –see table 1.

49. This translation ties together with the theory of Nanjing sixty-six which describes how yuanqi [原氣], source qi is distributed to the source points from the "moving qi between the kidneys" by the sanjiao [三焦], triple burner [112:560].

50. The dissection described in the Hou Hanshu dating from around 16 CE describes how the blood vessels were measured, their connections noted, organ capacities were measured, etc. The dissection of corpses described in Lingshu twelve talks about looking at and measuring the qi of the jingmai, assessing the relative amount of qi and blood, the volume capacity of different organs, etc [51, 56:155-159, 78:133-134, 114:169]. Hsu argues that the Lingshu passage is most likely to date from the period 475-221 BCE, that is it is a quite old passage dating from a time before Confucianism became so widely accepted and was incorporated into the later Lingshu text [51:10]. The point Hsu is making that under strong Confucian thinking, dissection was generally not encouraged.

51. But the Lingshu passage remains puzzling, it explicitly discusses observing and measuring the qi in the channels: "the transparency of his blood, the quantity of his qi (air, breath, vapor), and among the twelve channels, the abundance of blood and the paucity of qi, and the paucity of blood and the abundance of qi, as well as the abundance of blood and qi, and the paucity of blood and qi, all have their "norm"" [51:9]. What it was that was being inspected and called qi remains unclear.

52. In the passage immediately after the statement that the 365 acupoints meet the sunluo the Suwen continues "Good now please tell me [what I asked about in the first place] about the streams and river valleys of the sunluo. Qi Bo said that large meetings in the flesh are the river valleys and the small meetings in the flesh are the rivulets/streams. The spaces between the partings of the flesh are the meetings of the streams and river valleys" [translation from Chip Chace, March 2011]. If the acupoints are related to the sunluo this implies that they lie in the "meetings in the flesh" or "partings of the flesh".

53. There are traditions of acupuncture that explicitly caution the need to palpate for the precise point to be treated once one is in the correct proximity of its "anatomical" location [41, 75, 100, 117].

54. See for example the treatment descriptions from Fukushima [41], Shudo [99, 100].

55. Manaka's argument on this point is interesting: he argues that since descriptions of the qi systems appear to refer to quite subtle, non-visible things, then, were they to have a biological basis, their examination and demonstration may best be performed with extremely light "stimulation" methods –in his text he described numerous such experiments that demonstrate activities related to these qi systems [75]. Based on his results and clinical

utilizations, he then proposed that perhaps the qi systems traditionally described as e.g. the "jingmai" were part of a low-level energy biological system involved in earlier stages of organism development (both embryological and evolutionary) with the principle role of bio-regulation, but that became less functional once higher order structures had developed to perform more efficient bio-regulation [75].

56. Lingshu chapter twelve describes the following needling depths for the twelve jingmai (in numbers of cun [寸]): All arm jingmai -0.2; stomach -0.6; bladder -0.5; gallbladder -0.4; spleen -0.3; kidney -0.2; liver -0.1 [129:154-155, see 125:580-581]. Chen et al. have estimated that the "cun" is a measurement of approximately 2.23 cm [27], while Harper estimated it to be 2.31cm [46]. Needling depths following these would therefore range from 2.3mm to 13.8mm for the twelve jingmai. Huang Fumi started the tradition of stating the depth of needling for each acupoint. Birch and Felt summarized the differences of needling depths found in five historical and five modern Chinese texts [17:53-54] showing that needling today in China generally tends to be deeper than in historical periods. For sure needling was applied more shallowly in historical texts than is generally found in modern China. Does this imply that what was to be needled (the jingmai, the xue) were viewed as being more superficial? In classical Chinese thinking "asking 'what' was inseparable from asking 'how'" [56:96]. This passage about needling depths while describing how to treat the jingmai correctly tells something about what they are, or specifically at what relative depth the channels are located. Taken together the passages from Suwen fifty-eight and Lingshu twelve indicate that the acupoints are superficial lying above the slightly deeper jingmai with which they are connected. This has important implications for how we conceive of the nature of acupuncture, accept its inherent diversity of approaches and how we try to investigate these things scientifically –see [15].

57. The term "he" refers to the place where the river unites with the sea, the "mouth" of the river.

58. This is explicitly discussed in Lingshu chapter one [125:497] and Nanjing sixty-eight [112:577].

59. Nanjing sixty-nine states "for xu (vacuity) bu (supplement/tonify) the mother" and "for shi (repletion) xie (drain) the child" [112:583-588]. These two simple rules have given raise to systematic treatment approaches [17:232-233]. For example Gaowu in 1529 described the mother (supplementation/tonification) and child (draining) points on the basis of this [76:159]. Sa'Am of Korea in the late 1500s described set treatment point combinations that strictly follow these rules [136:139-140]. The first rule "for vacuity supplement the mother" proved to be very fruitful in the twentieth century when Japanese practitioners in the 1920s and 1930s interested in reconstructing traditional methods of acupuncture practice were trying out different historical ideas [17:56]. This latter process helped give rise to the Japanese system called "Keiraku Chiryo" [経絡治療] or literally jing-luo regulation therapy.

60. Nanjing thirty-three poses the following question: "When the liver is brought into water it will sink; when wood is brought into water it will float. When the lung is brought into water it will float; when metal is brought into water it will sink. What are the res-

pective sentiments [of liver and lung]?" [112:361]. Nanjing thirty-three explains this thus: "It is like this. The liver is not pure wood; the I {second stem}, [which is associated with the musical note chiao] is the soft partner of keng {seventh stem}. In macro-terms [I and keng] represent yin and yang; in micro-terms they constitute husband and wife. [The liver] releases its feeble yang [influences] and absorbs feeble yin [influences]. Its sentiment is joy of metal. Furthermore, it proceeds mostly through yin paths. Hence when liver is brought into water, it will sink. The lung is not pure metal. The hsin {eight stem}, [which is associated with the musical note] shang, is the soft [partner] of ping {third stem}. In macro-terms, [hsin and ping] represent yin and yang; in micro-terms, they constitute husband and wife. The lung releases its feeble yin [influences]; through marriage it approaches the fire. Its sentiment is joy of fire. Furthermore, it proceeds mostly through yang paths. Hence when the lung is brought into water it will float" [112:361, see also 76:59-61]. This text specifically associates certain of the shu-transporting acupoints with the extended models of the five phases, the ten stems.

61. Various texts describe the use of this system in the modern period. Some have adapted it to help select times when the acupoints that are suitable for a given patient might be more active [64], others on the basis of the broad general regulatory effects that they have [75:167-175].

62. Shudo [100] has one of the most explicit acknowledgments of this as he describes many examples of variations of the location for the same acupoint. Matsumoto and Birch [77:121] and Manaka et al. [75:50-52] give examples of point location differences in different traditions. Reasons for these variations are rarely discussed [7].

63. Compare for example what is said of treatment techniques between the Chinese need to get "deqi" a sensation experienced by the patient [3, 28] and Japanese approaches that either avoid getting sensations at all or prefer that the practitioner feels the qi [18, 75, 100]. This issue is discussed further below under needling techniques.

64. This can readily be seen in a comparison of the descriptions found in texts from the moxa traditions of Japan [e.g. 40], needling traditions from Japan [100] and China [33].

65. Yanagiya [127] and Manaka et al. [75:355-361] have catalogued the quite remarkable variation in the contraindications of the acupoints. Birch examined this in relation to contraindications in pregnancy and found considerable inconsistency and variability [8].

66. For Lingshu fifteen see Wu, Wu [125:595-6] and for Nanjing one see Unschuld [112:65-80].

67. For a discussion of these see Needham, Ling [80:239].

68. This is usually understood to be the twelve jingmai on the left and right, plus the renmai, dumai, yinqiaomai and yangqiaomai [108:203, 131:30, 124:84].

69. A Clepsydra is a special water clock and used to count the passage of the day.

70. The stem and branch cyclical terms are commonly found on the "oracle bones" of the Shang dynasty [80:396].

71. These temporal units were more than just demarkations of the passage of time, the stems and branches also had elaborate correspondences to the five phases and yin yang, thus layering meanings and implications to each time unit. Hence the system was an extension of the theory of systematic correspondence and extended to give many uses, including general and medical astrological value. Li Jianmin has collected significant evidence that these numerological extensions, which manifest through the system of "shushu" [數術] or "art of numbers" played a significant role not only in these elaborate extensions of the theory of systematic correspondence but also played an important role in the developing models of the body in the early medical literature, and how the concepts of the mai and jingmai evolved (see [70] for a review and brief summary of his work).

72. A good physician is one who understands these normal changes and can identify when what is observed is normal or pathological for a particular patient at a particular time.

73. The wuyun liuqi system is a complex system of medical practice that can still be found in use today [42] and which has had its proponents throughout history [72:139-149, 114:393-493].

74. The first description of the lingguibafa in the Zhenjiu Daquan is also the first articulation of the now commonly accepted four pairs of eight treatment points associated with the qijingbamai [77].

75. Various modern texts can be found that tabulate these and related cyclical systems with explanations of how to use them clinically [64, 75:167-175, 132].

76. See 112: 585 and 125:566. This likely has precedent in the Mawangdui text, the Yinyangmai Sihou [陰陽脈死候] text that says "When the mai are full, empty them; when empty fill them" [32:96] and another Mawangdui text, the Maifa [經法] "The mai are held as precious by the sages... Those who cure illnesses take surplus and segment deficiency" [32:6].

77. Unschuld briefly examines this difference, see [112:639-640] and also [10].

78. See endnote 67 in chapter two for a list of candidates as to what this healthy qi might be called [20].

79. This mirrors the Lushi Chunqiu when it discusses health preserving techniques that enhance one's qi, "using the fresh and casting out the old, so there is a free flow within the interstices of the flesh. The vitalities (jingqi [精氣]) are renewed daily, heteropathic qi (xieqi) [邪氣] is completely expelled, and a full span of life is attained'" [101:49]. The expansion of the qi of the body accomplished by bu, supplementation needling similarly expels the xieqi.

80. "As is typical of the Nanjing, it does not state openly that it reinterprets the old terms, rather, it presents them in a new conceptual context, which claims to be that of the "scripture" (i.e. that of the Neijing)" [112:604].

81. Nanjing seventy-six: "when one fills one removes influences from the protective [influences]; when one has to drain, one releases influences from the constructive [influences]" [112:626] and Nanjing seventy-eight: after the palpating the point to get the qi to arrive and after it has arrived "one inserts the needle. When the influences have accumulated [around the needle], one pushes them towards the interior. That is called 'to fill'. To move [the needle] and withdraw it [from the section of the constructive influences into the section of the protective influences] is called 'to drain'" [112:635]. Note also that the arrival of qi comes in two stages, first following certain palpation methods of the acupoint to be treated, then again after the insertion of the needle, following which it is either pushed in deeper for supplementation or pulled back more superficially for draining.

82. "It is like this when needling the yang [influences], one performs the pricking with a lying needle (i.e very superficial needling), when pricking the yin [influences], one first presses with one's left hand, the location of the transportation [hole] where the constructive [influences] are to be needled. As soon as the [protective] influences are dispersed one inserts the needle" [112:595].

83. It is quite likely that this innovative idea is based on an interpretation of the earlier Neijing. We have seen above how in Lingshu seventy-five needling is said to be for the purpose of "regulating qi," tiaoqi [調氣], seen by Rochat de la Vallee as a kind of definition of acupuncture [92:79-80]. But the full text of the Lingshu passage says: "Needling regulates the qi. Qi accumulates in the stomach in order to circulate as ying and wei, each according to its own pathways" [92]. Here the concept of "regulating qi" is closely associated with the ying and wei. If this idea of regulating qi was seen to define acupuncture, perhaps the needling methods of bu and xie in the Nanjing are a practical interpretation of how to regulate between the (layers of) ying and wei (qi) and that was how the Nanjing author(s) interpreted the Lingshu passage.

84. For further discussion see endnote 59 above.

85. Nanjing seventy-eight gives a kind of definition of the purposes of bufa and xiefa, Unschuld translates the passage as: "The flow of the constructive and protective [influences through the organism] is the major [goal] of the [therapeutic interventions of filling and draining (bu and xie)" [112:626]. This can be seen as a kind of extension of the principle from Lingshu seventy-five "Needling regulates (tunes) the qi" [92:79].

86. While Lai and Tong do not mention needling techniques from the Nanjing, focusing only on the Neijing, they do discuss qizhi and deqi and the techniques of bu and xie making the following statement: "Obviously the 'arrival of qi' (qizhi) and 'obtaining of qi' (deqi) both indicate that the reinforcing (bu) and reducing (xie) needling manipulation can regulate vital-qi of the human body and make it in a favorable state" [57]. They later discuss the "'obtaining of qi' in the real sense" referring to the balance of yingqi and weiqi.

These authors seem to see the needling techniques in relation to creating a greater regulation of "vital-qi" in the body.

87. Yang translates the same passage as follows "as if standing close to the edge of a high cliff, the hold on the needle as if grasping a tiger's tail –you want the grip to be firm. Your mind notes nothing in the surroundings, but calmly and quietly focuses on the patient, without looking left or right. The needle is not inserted at a random angle, but stands straight. Our spirit too should be upright, so that as you look into the patient's eyes their spirit feels the effect [becoming calm, quiet and unified]. In this way the qi moves easily" [130]. While there are some interpretive differences both translations transmit the same basic message.

88. In chapter two we discussed analogies for how we can imagine qi flow in the jingmai, as part of this discussion we cited and discussed many instances where the qi is described as "coming and going". It is the observation of this very subtle phenomenon that the texts discussed here in the current context focus on, as they describe the necessary inner state of the practitioner in order to observe and then engage these qi "movements."

89. Daly following Gao reads 靜 (stillness) for 淨 and 待 (treat) for 侍 [32:96, ref 82].

90. As Puett states it: "Thus since all things consist of qi, that which possesses the most refined qi (as do the spirits) possesses both knowledge about and power over that which possesses less refined qi. By accumulating essence within himself, man becomes like a spirit; able to understand the changes of forms, avoid being harmed by them, and even gain control over them" [88:115].

91. Rickett translates the same passage as: "Thus, this vital force –Never to be restrained by physical strength, it may be brought to rest by spiritual power (de) Never to be summoned by one's call, it may be made welcome by one's power of awareness (yi)." [91:39-40].

92. I remind the reader that in the Neiye, there are extensive discussions about posture, breathing, physical actions and proper alignment to create a state of the body that can engage the qi through the properly cultivated "yi". These are not inseparable from each other.

93. Rodriguez explores how yi might manifest and be employed in the practice of herbal medicine in chapter six [93].

94. "Focal awareness" is the action of the "xin" [心] or "heart-and-mind" while focusing on something. "Field awareness" is the action of the "xin" or "heart-and-mind" while taking in something in the context of the total field of experience or background against which all focal events occur. See discussions in Ames and Hall [2:33-36, 44:23-77 (especially 39-43)].

95. Virtually all translators render this passage the same way [54:5, 108:36, 124:3, 125:497].

96. Which Lo has demonstrated was influential in the language of needling and qi arrival in the Lingshu [67].

97. Harper's translation of the Heyinyang passage is somewhat different, but gives essentially the same meaning [47:417-418].

98. Lo and Li comment it can mean "the gods of heaven and earth" [71:369]. Lewis describes shenming as referring "both to powerful spirits and to the highest state of mental powers which matches those of the spirits" [61:331-332]. Harper describes the concept as having arisen in religion referring to magical spirits with great powers [47:120] mirrored by Csikszentmihalyi who describes shenming as referring to "inspectors from the spirit world who enforce the punishment and reward scheme of tian (heaven)" [31:41-42, also 237]. Later the term came to refer to higher mental states achieved through the import or cultivation of shen, spirit into the body in the cultivation traditions of the Neiye and early Han Mawangdui, Zhangjiashan texts, shenming "is a kind of mana which those who practice cultivation can concentrate in their body" [47:121].

99. For example the Tianxia Zhidaotan of the Mawangdui [47:427], the Shiwen also of the Mawangdui [Harper 1998:391] which both describe similar ideas of sexual cultivation practice. The Neiye and later Huainanzi have a similar description of the condition of the body in the more cultivated state [94:76-77].

100. Although the term "mental focus" is used here, it can be misleading. Often people create tension when they try to focus this is the opposite action for the best results. This topic is discussed in detail in the practical sections of the book [22] and comes up in various other chapters in relation to the quiet still state needed for "welcoming [迎] the qi". In a small pilot study Azzopardi and Birch have attempted to capture the sensations and experiences of the practitioner when needling, these often require a more relaxed state and involve often quite subtle phenomena [14].

101. While many translators render this passage in a similar way [124:2], or that the mind must be focused at the needle tip [108:33, 125:495], others give varied translations [54:5] or give completely different translations "the spirit resides in an autumn hair" but this more literal translation is given a similar interpretation [24]. Another reading can allude to a concept found in the Lushi Chunqiu where it is a "common metaphor for the subtle first stirrings of change that only a sage detects" [65:453, 66:204] and similarly in the Huainanzi [65:456], implying that what is happening is incredibly subtle.

102. As described in chapter eight [15], this is the opposite of energy movements according to the second law of thermodynamics suggesting that qi cannot be understood as energy.

103. Various descriptions of the sensations associated with deqi have been given, these include "soreness, aching, distension, heaviness, numbness or tingling" [33:12] or "sharp, pulling, electric, tingling, heavy, pulsing, spreading, pricking, aching or hot" [116].

104. Is this idea of feeling the "arrival of qi" with the hand that is placed on the body before needling commences presaged by Chunyu Yi's notion of palpating the vessels and "de... qi" [得 X 氣] getting the qi of X? [50]. Hsu describes how Chunyu Yi palpates a vessel and "gets" the qi of for example the liver "the sensation of qi that Yi gets when he rubs the mai informs him about the condition of the five depositories inside the body" [50:76]. Is the Nanjing's description of arrival of qi a merging of ideas from Chunyu Yi and the Neijing?

105. Shudo quotes both of these passages as well [99:181].

106. Nanjing seventy-eight describes these thus: "When one is about to prick, one first presses with one's left hand the transportation [hole] (acupoint) where one [intends to] needle... The pressure to be exerted with full vigor through one's finger nail" [112:635]. Suwen chapter twenty-seven [114:282-283] and Nanjing chapter seventy-one [112:595] likewise describe the methods of palpation for preparation of the acupoints before insertion of the needle.

107. This issue is touched on in the next chapter by Chace and Bensky [24]. We are reminded of the following passage from the Guodian (circa 300 BCE): "Sages know the way of heaven. Knowing something and putting it into practice is righteousness. Practicing something with the appropriate timing is virtue (de [德])" [48:59].

108. For the Nanjing see [112:635] and as an example of the Lingshu see Zhang Jiebin, author of the Leijing who comments on Lingshu one: "One should tonify and one should drain according to the opportune moment in the instant when one meets the qi" [24].

109. This notion appears to be reinforced by Chunyu Yi's use of the term "de" when he "gets" the qi of for example the liver [50]. His usage refers to both a feeling or sensation of something (qi) but that has a quality that informs him about the condition of something inside the body, by which he "grasps" or "understands" the condition of the patient. Although used in a different context than the "deqi" of needling, it seems that Chunyu Yi's usage is both one of sensation and cognition.

110. This is not a discussion about the "power" of one's "yi", like the power of mental concentration, it is about the idea of creating an empty space where the qi can be welcomed and therefore manifest around the tip of the needle. For further discussions of this theme see chapter one "Qi, mind and body –explorations of the links between qi, the mind, mental and emotional states and the body" [16] and especially chapter seven "Qi and Stillness" [21].

111. There is a habit in the modern period to see "intention" as some all-powerful thing, like some kind of mental power, as though the act of having the "intention" to fly to the moon could transport one to the moon. Clearly having an intention alone is not enough. To be realistic, intention is necessary for any action to be carried out successfully and according to one's wishes, but that does not attribute or imply a kind of mental power for doing that action, rather it is at first no more than the guide to what one wants to achieve.

The distinction drawn here of "yi" as "intention", developing to "yi" as "attention" and then further to "awareness" is in part a device to help put aside mistaken ideas of "yi" as some special mental power.

112. The fact of "intending" to contact, influence or affect the qi of the patient in no way guarantees that one will do so. This is obvious to anyone with experience training students of acupuncture, and especially in systems of acupuncture where feedback mechanisms (such as pulse changes) are used as concrete guide to those actions. For many the "intention" creates an act of trying too hard, which is usually counterproductive. Not to belabor the point, but the same is true for the pianist, the artist, the carpenter, etc. This theme is revisited in the final chapters of this book [22] where we lay out a series of exercises that utilise the radial pulses as a feedback tool for monitoring the effects each has on the qi of the person being touched, needled, etc. The better contact and influence on the qi invariably comes through a quieting of the mind, a calm, non-striving focus. The more one can act effortlessly ("wuwei") and naturally (which comes in part through repetitive practice) the more one's "yi" can influence the qi. This is not the intention of the beginner it is the seasoned actions of experience, and especially the actions-as-second-nature, or natural (automatic) actions of the very experienced and "aware".

113. In his summary of the core meaning and message of chapter six of the Huainanzi, Le Blanc makes the following statement: "The most perfect form of government is that of non-action (wu-wei), for it operates through the natural (zi-ran) resonance (ganying) of all things. The perfect ruler is the true man who, being one with the dao is in a state of mutual resonance with all things" [60:192]. Substituting "the highest form of practice" for the "most perfect form of government" and the "highest level practitioner" for the "perfect ruler", Le Blanc's description matches exactly what we think is happening at level three when the practitioner operates with "yi" as "awareness".

114. I recognise that we have used an opposite sequencing of intention-attention-awareness than Chace and Bensky have, but we are making a different point than they do [24].

115. Of course it is possible that relative beginners can perform actions that engage the qi at this level. Often this is non-reproducible and cannot be deliberately repeated, much like the "peak experiences" that Maslow and Wilber discusses [118:134]. A "peak experience" is an altered state of consciousness, a temporary higher state of consciousness. It can be achieved at great effort or accidentally, but is not readily reproducible. In the practitioner whose "yi" operates simply by becoming "aware", the actions on the qi and via the qi are virtually automatic and are entirely natural and unforced, thus reproducible and highly controlled. The practitioner whose "yi" operates by developing "attention" can regularly act on the qi with the needle but must still make an effort to retain this focused attention for these effects to be consistent, but the "peak" effects occur more frequently than in the next. The practitioner whose "yi" has not yet had chance to develop beyond "intention" may or may not act on or much upon the qi when needling, these are more like "peak" or chance effects.

116. The issue of the physiological effects of needling are not the focus of this book, they are discussed in several other places quite thoroughly [17:147-183, 26, 37:69-150, 45, 87,

135]. Chapter eight [15] touches on this issue with regards how one can investigate qi and claims to have measured qi in physiological terms. Manaka addressed this issue to some extent, stressing the importance of separating the physical actions of needling from the more subtle influences one can have via the qi and jingmai system [75:17-37 and later chapters]. The fact that physical objects (needles) are inserted into the body triggering physiological events and changes cannot be denied, but understanding how those events and changes relate to qi is a different matter entirely.

117. Shudo comments the following when acupuncturists complain that they do not the patience or time to wait five to ten or more years to start to feel the arrival of qi: "'Perhaps you should give up acupuncture and try another profession.' Becoming a skilled acupuncturist requires that much dedication" [100:236].

118. Such as the physical stimulation physiological effects of inserting a needle mentioned above.

119. In a passage about life and death Nanjing eight discusses a concept "shenjian dongqi" [腎間動氣], the "moving qi between the kidneys", which is seen as "the 'source of vital qi'", it is "fundamental to the five viscera and six bowel organs, is the root of the twelve channels, the gate of breathing, the source of the triple burner. Another name for it is the shen that protects against evil," [9, 78:110, 112:130]. The idea of the various systems of the body being centered around something can be understood in this passage, which describes how they either are rooted there or have their origin there. See Matsumoto, Birch [78] for extensive discussion of this concept. Additionally the arrival of qi with needling is, by its very nature, health promoting according to the quote cited earlier from the Mawangdui Heyinyang text "blood and qi flow freely, the ears and eyes are keen and bright, the skin gleams, the voice is clear, and the back, thighs and buttocks are sturdy" [71:381]. Thus not only is there an idea of a common underlying form of (undifferentiated) qi, seen in Nanjing chapter eight, but if one can access it, it naturally helps produce or promote greater health, greater order. In 2007 Birch published a case history illustrating the effects of "improving vitality" [6].

120. The traditional model from China was of heaven-earth-person as a triadic system of influences, usually with the "person" in the middle as a product of the interactions of heaven and earth. The circular model of four levels pertains only to the "person". Naturally the person is embedded in their ecological (earth) and cosmological (heaven) environments, these are represented here as "level five".

121. This five-level model is a simplified version of a seven-level model that is being developed to help structure theories of TEAM, model treatment and model the role of the practitioner through practitioner-patient interactions [12], so that more precise and testable models can be developed to assist pursuing more valid scientific investigations of TEAM [13]. In the seven-level model, levels six and seven represent the physical, social and cultural environments.

122. This description captures also the idea that the proper accord or maintenance of resonance between heaven-earth (level five) and the body (levels one to four) helps

maintain proper order. The outer level helps regulate the inner levels –a theme developed in chapter two above in an examination of variant descriptions of the mai and jing-mai trajectories.

123. Elsewhere I describe these in more depth and how interactions between individuals might occur [12, 13].

124. Many of the ideas discussed above from the historical literature support the model presented here. For example, the idea in Lingshu chapter one that the acupoint is the place where qi is accessible, where it flows in and out as the principle nature of the acupoints, the definition from Lingshu seventy-five of acupuncture as "tiaoqi" –"the regulation of qi" and the statements in Nanjing seventy-eight and eighty, that the qi must arrive before the needle is inserted and the intended techniques carried out, all support the qi based descriptions here. It seems clear that Lingshu one and Nanjing seventy-eight associate the action of touching the acupoint as connecting with the qi, that this qi is not a normal "physiological qi" as the needle has not yet been inserted to stimulate that, rather it is to do with the act of touching, an interactionally based action. It seems clear that not everyone can do this as the text of the Lingshu and Nanjing state this is what the advanced practitioner can do, thus there must be degrees of skill and therefore different types of effect on the patient. Further the ideal type of influence to be created by treatment is one of regulation, a concept explicitly associated with influences that arise outside of the body and that can be imported into the body (through a well ordered mind, through "resonating" with environmental influences (qi) that provide the matrix for everything that is). The model presented here not only accounts for fundamental concepts described in the historical literature related to the (correct) practice of acupuncture, but it integrates ideas about the fundamental actions of how qi operates (ganying –resonance) and the ac-tions of the accomplished practitioner (ji –dynamic) in order to accomplish this (such as is described in Lingshu one –see the next chapter by Chace and Bensky [24]).

125. There will likely be auto-regulatory actions at a "tissue" level as well, governed by more general yin-yang, etc rules. The influence of these is not as explicit (or clear) as how these rules operate on the channels as auto-regulatory mechanisms, so I leave them out of the description here.

126. It is important to recognise the nature of thinking and thus the role of theory in TEAM. In chapter one [16] and again in chapter eight we touch on this issue [15]. Knowledge in TEAM is more practice based rather than ontologically based "Debates in Chi-nese medicine therefore are not concerned with the truth of a method but with its efficacy" [96:37], knowledge in ancient Chinese thinking was more "skill-knowledge" rather than "representational knowledge" [103:4] or "how-priority" knowledge rather than "what-priority" knowledge [44:149-150]. Thus the theories play a different role, they are seen by many as principally about giving guidelines to the selection of treatment [17, 19, 97]. On this basis I therefore make the important distinction between "explicit" and "implicit" [12, 15]. The textbooks describe theory and diagnosis in sufficient detail so that one can select and apply a treatment (the explicit aspects), but the actions and associated mechanisms required in order to implement that treatment are often not described (the implicit as-

pects) –or at least not in much detail. The distinction between the beginner, intermediate practitioner and advanced, experienced practitioner are at least in part about how one advances from using only explicitly described theory and methods to developing through practice implicitly engaged actions and mechanisms, some hints of which can be found in the literature.

127. "The earliest reference to sheng qi is the Lüshi Chunqiu in a passage describing the cycle of the seasons. In the last month of spring, we are told, 'sheng qi flourishes, and yang qi flows forth; shoots emerge, and buds unfold.' From this context it is apparent that the term means something like 'life giving energy'" [35].

128. "The presence of a person of virtue is what allows the resonance of tian's way" [31:326], the person of virtue alluded to here is the person in a higher state of development where, in my terms, yi operates as "awareness". The term "tian's way" or heaven's way can be interpreted to include "tianqi" "heaven's qi" or in other cosmological terms "yuanqi", original qi.

129. Although the term "tianqi" in the modern period has come to mean something like "weather", "air" (see chapter one above), the usage here is in the larger more traditional sense of the "qi of heaven", seen in a broader cosmological model as a source of much that exists. It is in the cosmological theories of a contrasting and mutually influencing "heaven-earth" that we see this larger meaning.

130. The yuanqi, original, basic or primal qi in literature on cosmology [78:83-84, 133:25-26], and internal alchemy [25:26] refers to something like the "extracorporeal qi of the cosmos" [25:26].

131. We ask the reader to bear in mind that our discussion of the three stages is only a set of labels applied to a continuum rather than three distinct stages.

132. Again a parallel can be seen in Le Blanc's analysis of the core messages of the Huainanzi, he describes a three-fold scheme where at the second level "simple resonance" operates and the third "total resonance" operates; he even portrays the role of "yuanqi" [原氣 ] to be lying at the second level [60:208-209].

133. Recall again the idea from the Mawangdui text the "Heyinyang" about the effects of the arrival of qi. This describes not only an improved and desirable (more ordered) condition, but seems to refer to something other than the physiological qi of the patient, something from somewhere else.

134. To understand how this might occur, it is helpful to recall Le Blanc's conclusions about how we might understand "ganying" [see chapter one above] ganying "may be defined, in the final analysis, as the power of things to affect and to be affected in such a way as **to bring about harmony**" (emphasis added) [60:209]. At the second stage where "relative" or "simple" resonance is utilised there will be a certain degree of increased regulation of things through the harmonising actions of ganying. In this third stage where

"total resonance" may be utilised, there will be an even greater degree of regulation brought about through a much larger harmonisation. The action of engaging "ganying" to work with qi in greater degrees will help bring about more "harmony" and restoration or maintenance of the more "natural" order.

135. I model this in detail elsewhere [12].

136. In his "Medicine in China: A history of ideas", Unschuld takes this as a central theme for the development of the medicine that emerged during the Han dynasty. Rather than being subject to the negative influences of demons and spirits (demonology, and ancestral spirits that need to be placated) or the ravages of the environment, the medical model suggested for the first time that one could control this through one's behavior, control of one's emotions, regulation of one's diet, living circumstances etc one could stay healthy and that one was responsible for the problems that result from improper activities [111].

137. This is clearly described by Chace in his analysis of Lingshu nine [23] and is seen in the next chapter by Chace and Bensky [24].

138. Which is the most common type of framework presented in textbooks on acupuncture, as they describe these ideas for the student or practitioner.

139. This idea is captured well in Lingshu chapter eight which states "the heaven in one is de [德] (virtue), the earth in one is qi. The de streams down and the qi rises up, subsequently there is life" [78:35].

140. Chapter two has discussions of this.

141. Order is returned in two ways. First supplementing what is weakened helps, by yin-yang logic, to counterbalance what is too strong. Internal counterbalancing mechanisms are employed; strengthening the lung channel can reduce its yang counterpart, the large intestine channel. Second, the extended cosmological correlations help import external order into the body.

142. As was discussed in the previous endnote since the jingmai and certain acupoints have five-phase correlations, treatment of them can start triggering counterbalancing effects that restore order. For example applying bu to the lung channel increases the lung channel, which then decreases the liver channel (metal controls wood) which in turn increases the spleen channel (reduced wood allows an increase of earth). The extended correspondences also help import order from the environment into the body.

143. The passage states "By meeting it and taking it away, how could one not achieve depletion (of the qi)? By pursuing and assisting it, how could one not achieve repletion (of the qi)?" [24]. See also footnote "i" in appendix two of the current chapter for further discussions of variations in how this Lingshu passage has been understood.

CHAPTER FIVE

# AN AXIS OF EFFICACY

## The Range of Meaning in Chapter One of the *Lingshu*[i]

Charles Chace, Dan Bensky[ii]

> From Chapter One of the Lingshu:
> Please tell me of the way [of needling].
> The essentials of the small needle are easy to explain but difficult to engage.
> The crude attend to the form, the superior attend to the spirit.
> Spirit oh spirit! There is a guest at the door.
> Without observing the disease, how can one know its origin?
> The subtleties of needling lie in its speed.
> The crude attend to the junctures and the superior attend to the dynamic.
> The movement in the dynamic is not separate from its empty spaces;
> The dynamic within this empty space is clear, still and subtle.
> Its coming cannot be met and its going cannot be pursued.
> Those who understand the way of the dynamic will not impede it and thus it manifests.
> Not understanding the way of the dynamic, one detains it and thus it fails to show itself.
> To understand its goings and comings, emphasize its periodicity.
> The crude are in the dark about this; sublime! Only practitioners have it.
> Going away from it is contrary, promoting its arrival is going with the flow.
> If one clearly understands the contrary and normal [flow of qi], then you can act correctly and without doubt or question.
> By meeting it and taking it away, how could one not achieve depletion [of the qi]?
> By pursuing and assisting it, how could one not achieve repletion [of the qi]?
> Whether meeting it or following it, by means of one's attention, one harmonizes it.
> This is all there is to say with regard to the way of needling.

Any serious effort to understand the approaches to needling described in the Huangdi Neijing 黃帝內經 (Yellow Emperor's Inner Classic, 3rd-2nd century BCE), demands a close examination of the first chapter of one of its compo-

i. This chapter was originally published in "The Lantern" as an article in two parts –2009:6(1):5-13; 2009:6(2):33-41. Special thanks to Steve Clavey for permission to reproduce the article here.
ii. We are grateful to professors Matthias and Antje Richter, Stephen Birch, Diane Sommers, Sharon Weizenbaum and Craig Mitchell for their helpful comments, questions and criticisms in the course of preparing this manuscript.

nent texts, the Lingshu 靈樞 (Divine Pivot). A book devoted largely to the practicalities of acupuncture practice, the first chapter of the Lingshu outlines the fundamental principles of needling that are developed and applied in different contexts throughout the text. Following an introductory preamble that establishes the chapter as part of the Huang Di lineage of medical texts [7:21-29],[1] this first chapter presents a short passage that stands by itself as an introductory overview of the most basic principles of needling. It is the foundation of all further discussion on needling within the chapter and arguably within the entire Neijing. This paper is an analysis of the first section of chapter one of the Lingshu and an assessment of its ramifications for the understanding of the needle techniques presented in that book. To make sense of how the passage in question relates to the rest of the treatise it is helpful to understand something about the structure and organization of the Neijing.

## Ancestral Texts

The two books of the Neijing, the Suwen 素問 (Basic Questions) and the Lingshu 靈樞 (Divine Pivot), referred to here as SW and LS respectively, are by no means a homogenous or consistent text. They constitute an anthology of many independent writings by many different authors that may or may not have any relation to one another. Each chapter may contain multiple subsections that constitute complete texts in their own right. For instance, the first two thirds of Lingshu chapter one, referred to here as LS-1.1 constitute a discrete text known variously as the Jiu Zhen 九針 (Nine Needles) the Xiao Zhen 小針 (Small Needles) or simply the Zhen 針 (Needles). This text is considered an "ancestral text" in that it most likely predates other texts in the Neijing that are effectively commentaries on it [7:208-209].[2] These later texts, known as "descendent texts," include but are not limited to the last section of the first chapter of the Lingshu, referred to here as LS-1.3, or first section of the 54th Chapter of the Suwen, referred to here as SW-54.1

Different descendent texts frequently posit different interpretations of an ancestral text [7:170-219]. For instance, the line 'xu er ji ze shi' 徐而疾則實in LS-1.1 is interpreted in LS-1.3 as "When one slowly inserts and quickly removes the needle this will make the qi replete."[3] SW-54.1 interprets the line differently. "When one slowly removes the needle and quickly presses the point [to prevent bleeding], this will make the qi replete." [3:v.2, 674].[4]

Other writings within the Neijing are also effectively commentaries on the *Nine Needles*. Descendent texts may appear in close proximity to their ancestral texts as does LS-1.3, or they may be scattered apparently randomly throughout the Neijing as is the case with SW-54.1. This raises a relevant point regarding the dating to the various texts within the Neijing. It is commonly believed that the Lingshu postdates the Suwen but in fact neither one, as a whole, is earlier or later than the other. SW-54.1 is clearly a descendent of LS-1.3, and LS-3, a distinct text in its own right known as the xiao zhen jie 小針解 (Explanation of the Small Needles) is also a descendent of LS-1.3 [7:208-209]. From all of this it is evident that even at the time of its compilation there were multiple lines of interpretation associated with the Neijing.

It is debatable whether this initial passage in the first chapter of the Lingshu, can be considered an independent text in its own right. Nevertheless, it is unquestionably a succinct précis of the core concepts that are subsequently developed later in LS-1 and throughout the Lingshu. However one chooses to label this passage, hereafter referred to as the Lingshu précis, it is worthy of critical examination. Its content bears directly on our fundamental understanding of what it means to perform acupuncture and the interpretation of this passage inevitably influences one's reading of the rest of the Lingshu.

The most common interpretations of the Lingshu précis, although plausible, coherent and informative, are not entirely satisfactory. A number of intriguing statements that form the core of the passage are either reduced to triviality by these standard interpretations or ignored entirely. We will examine this précis in detail and consider its possible range of meaning. In the process, we will demonstrate that the text contains at least two intertwined interpretive threads or layers, one of which has been largely overlooked in the commentary literature. The basis for this neglected interpretive thread is the text's use of the concept ji 機. We will examine this concept in some detail and consider its ramifications for our understanding of the passage and the chapter as a whole.

## A Pivotal Concept

The interpretation of Lingshu précis hinges on the word ji 機 and what it means that "the superior attend to ji" (shang shou ji 上守機). Most commentators take 'ji' in LS-1, to mean the "qi mechanism" or "qi dynamic" (qiji 氣機). This, of course, begs the question of what precisely a qi mechanism or dynamic is and how it pertains to the rest of this passage. The Lingshu suggests two interpretations, one narrow, and one broad.

1) LS-3 is among the most comprehensive and least ambiguous commentaries on LS-1, and it exemplifies the most common reading of ji 機. The qi mechanism is the dynamic between the correct and pathogenic qi. In practical terms, it is our awareness of and interaction with that dynamic that determines whether one will administer tonification or drainage techniques. This interpretation will be discussed in greater detail below. For the present it is sufficient to say that this straightforward explanation allows the Lingshu précis to be read as a basic discussion of excess and deficiency, correct and pathogenic qi, and tonification and drainage. That said, if one reads the text with an open mind, this simple equivalency leads to many questions. In this it is similar to another common interpretation that ji is a simple reference to the channel qi [18:277].

2) The Lingshu précis itself describes the qi mechanism as an expression of the pacing of the qi, its goings and comings (wang lai 往來). It stresses the importance of one's awareness of the "spaces" or intervals of stillness within the ji. From this perspective, one's attention to the relationship between the correct and pathogenic qi is the tip of an iceberg, a relatively minor aspect of a much larger scope of awareness that is essential to effective needling.

## The trigger of activity

The word ji 機 is an ancient term for the firing mechanism of a crossbow [15:93], and by extension, it is the crux or hinge of a thing. This root meaning of ji is especially apt when the word is used in the early acupuncture literature which often makes use of archery imagery. For instance LS-1 councils that at the moment the qi arrives, one must "withdraw [the needle] like [loosing an arrow] from a bowstring" (去如弦絕) [2:1.1]. Ji exerts its influence by virtue of its position at the beginning of things. For this reason, ji may be the trigger or cause of a disease as in SW-74, which states. "Carefully examine the appropriateness of the [seasonal] qi, and do not lose [sight] of the trigger [ji] of disease" (謹侯氣宜, 無失病機) [3:v.2, 1155].

Ji also refers to the articulations (guanji 關機) and may refer specifically to the acupuncture hole Circular Jump (huan tiao GB-30). SW-60 states: "What cleaves close to the hip is the ji" (俠髖為機) [3:v.2, 745]. The hip is, of course, a major hinge or pivot point in the body but it is also the initiator of movement through the lower extremities, harkening back to a more fundamental meaning of the word.

## Incipience

Ji is cognate with "incipience '(ji 幾), the "heavenly mechanism" (tianji 天機), the "divine mechanism" (shenji 神機). The Classic of Change (Yijing 易經, 9-7th centuries BCE) uses the word incipience (ji 幾) to denote an initial tendency toward change that is more minute than and precedes active transformation (hua 化). [17:207][5] According to the "Xici" 繫辭 (Great Commentary): "The Changes are the means by which the sages searched the profound and examined incipience. Only by the profound can one penetrate to the purpose under the heaven; only by incipience can one perfect the tasks under heaven." (夫易, 聖人之所以極深, 而研幾也, 唯深也, 故能通天下之志, 唯幾也, 故能成天下之務) [17:207].[6] The "Xici" also states:

> The Master said: Ah, to know the incipience, how divine! The gentleman in dealing with his betters does not flatter, in dealing with his inferiors is not rude for does he not know incipience? Incipience is the most minute aspect of movement and the first appearance of good fortune, the gentleman sees incipience and inaugurates; he does not wait until the ending of the day [17:207].[7] (子曰:知幾其神乎! 君子上交不諂,下交不瀆,其知幾乎,幾者動之微,吉之先見者也,君子見幾而作,不俟終日)

## The Expression of Natural Endowment

One's ji 機 is linked, at least to some extent, to one's relationship with the world at large. In the Zhuangzi, tianji 天機 is a natural endowment or disposition, and a capacity to be in accord with the universe. "Those whose desires are deep-seated will have a shallow natural endowment" (其耆欲深者其天機淺) [17:207].[8] In the Huainanzi 淮南子 (79-8 BCE), "the divine mechanism is hidden and closed. Its marks and imprints lack all trace, and it is subtlety of human ingenuity." (神機陰閉, 剞劂無跡, 人巧之妙也)[9]

Where shen and ji appear together in the Neijing it is often a general term for the life force, but SW-70 understands them as separate though inextricably related things. "Qi Bo said: The root at the center is called the spirit dynamic. When the spirit leaves then the dynamic ceases." (岐伯 曰: 根于中者, 命曰神機, 神去則機息) [3:v.2, 1008].

## The Wellspring at the Center of Things

Ji lies not only at the beginning of actions but at their center (shuji 樞機) insofar as it is the crux (guanjian 關鍵) of a thing. This use of the word appears in LS-69.1 which states: "the tongue is the key to speech," (舌者，音聲之機) [2:v.2, 259] and LS-75.5 which states: "the penis and testicles are the hinge of the body center" (莖垂者，身中之機) [2:v.2, 332]. Ji may also denote a specific situation or state of affairs (jishi 機勢), and by extension it denotes the opportunity inherent in a situation or disposition. Similarly, ji may be both an indicator of change and a source of change within something. According to the "Da Xue" 大學 (Great Learning) in the Liji 禮記 (Record of Rites, Han):

> From the benevolent example of one's family an entire state becomes benevolent, and from its courtesies an entire state becomes courteous, while from the ambition and perverseness of one man, an entire State may be led into rebellious disorder; its dynamic is such as this. (一家仁, 一國興仁, 一家讓, 一國興讓, 一人貪戾, 一國作亂, 其機如此)[10]

The Zhuangzi, expresses a similar sentiment. "The ten thousand things all come out from the wellsprings and all reenter the wellsprings." (萬物皆出於機，皆入於機) [9:173].[11] This translation by Victor Mair highlights the aspect of ji that lies at the source and is the "wellspring" of things.

Just as ji is situated at the center of events, Isabelle Robinet notes that "physiologically, ji is located in the center of the body which is in turn related to yi, intention and to the spleen, or it can be identified with the interval between breathing in and out, corresponding with the 'closing and opening of the world in the instant that preceded the movement of breath'" [13:536-537]. In this it is evident that even in its most material manifestations ji is associated with the empty spaces or intervals between phases of activity. Robinet also notes that ji is synonymous with the heart-mind (xin 心) and the spirit (shen 神). This association is central to the interpretation of the Lingshu précis where they are linked by the parallelism of its sentence structure. According to Robinet, those involved in internal cultivation aim at uniting their human ji with heavenly ji [13:536-537].

## An Axis of Quiescence

As a hinge or pivot, ji refers to a point of stillness around which effective intervention turns. It is equated with the "ultimateless infinite" (wuji 無幾), and the "great ultimate" (taiji 太極). It is "the wondrous movement that unites movement and quiescence, the true spring that moves spontaneously by itself (ziran 自然) and without intention (wuxin 無心) and acts without action and interference (wuwei 無為)" [13:536-537]. In light of this, it is worth mentioning that the book we are discussing is entitled the Divine Pivot. At least by the Tang when the text was given this title, it was clearly acknowledged that the needle itself is the pivot or axis of healing. The task of the acupuncturist is to make maximal use of this pivot or ji.

Synthesizing these layers of meaning, Robinet describes ji as the "spring of the world, its activating force... the extreme degree of quiescence and purity which is on the verge of changing into movement" [13:536-537]. The wealth of meanings associated with ji in the early literature of China suggests that whatever it is that that superior practitioner must attend to, it both includes and transcends the relatively mundane relationship between the correct and pathogenic qi, the state of qi in the channels. Ji is a reflection of the overall health or disposition of the patient; it determines whatever opportunities that might be available for improving the situation, it is closely associated with the spirit (shen 神) and according to Robinet, it subsequently came to be associated with source qi in the sense of a primordial breath (yuan qi 元氣) [12:105-120, 10:305-308].

From the discussion above it is apparent that no single English word does justice to ji's full scope of its meaning. For the present, however, we have provisionally translated ji as "dynamic" to amplify its' fundamental characteristic as the impetus of effective action, movement and transformation. That said, it is most productive to keep its full range of meanings in mind when contemplating the Lingshu precis. When approached from this perspective the focus of this passage shifts significantly. One's engagement with ji is clearly the overall topic of the passage. It is through the ji that one harmonizes the excesses or deficiencies in the states of the correct (zheng 正) and pathogenic (xie 邪) qi, and it frames the way in which one approaches tonification and drainage.

What follows is a translation of the Lingshu précis accompanied by an overview of representative commentaries including those appearing within the descendent texts of the Neijing itself. This essay will illustrate how the concept of ji as described above establishes a coherent train of meaning throughout the entire passage that both complements and deepens the importance of the established commentaries. It is not so much an alternative interpretation of the material as a subtle but significant shift in emphasis. We have omitted the introductory paragraphs to LS-1.1 that do not bear directly on the content of the chapter and numbered the lines for easy reference.

## The *Lingshu* précis: Translation and Commentaries

請言其道. 小針之要, 易陳而難入. [1]
**Please tell me of the way [of needling]. The essentials of the small[12] needle are easy to explain but difficult to engage.**

What are the essentials of needling? They are apparently easy enough to describe, a simple idea that is difficult to implement. According to LS-3.1, "what is referred to as easy to explain, means that it is easy to talk about," (所謂易陳者, 易言也) and "difficult to engage means difficult to apply to people." (難入者, 難著于人也) [2:v.1, 66]. Whatever this means, it is unlikely that it is a mere needle technique. As Ma Shi 馬蒔 articulates below in his Huangdi Neijing lingshu zhuzheng fawei 黃帝內經靈樞注証發微 (Commenting on the Evidence and Explicating the Details Yellow Emperor's Inner Classic, Divine Pivot, 1586), mere needle techniques are an expression of "the crude attending to the form" [8].

粗守形, 上守神. [2]
**The crude attend to the form, the superior attend to the spirit.**

The word shou 守 means, to guard or protect, and by extension, to attend to. Its use here suggests that the physician must not just protect the integrity of the form and the spirit, but must also attend to and somehow engage it.

### *The Crude and Superior*

The distinction between the crude and the superior is central to the structure of the passage.[13] Appearing again in line 6, the crude and the superior frames two sets of related ideas, and the parallelism it creates links the notions of form (xing 形) to the junctures (guan 關), and the spirit (shen 神) to the dynamic (ji 機). It will become apparent that the essentials of needling transcend the mechanics of its forms.

According to LS-3.1, "That the crude attend to the form means that they attend to the methods of needling." (粗守形者, 守刺法也) [2:v.1, 67]. Zhang Zhicong's 張志聰 Lingshu jizhu 靈樞集注 (Collected Commentaries on the Lingshu, 1670) interprets form not in terms of needle technique but as the corporeal body of the patient. He explains that "When needling, the crude attend to the skin, vessels, flesh, sinew, and bone." (粗守形者，守皮脈肉筋骨之刺) [20:3].

## *Shen as Qi And Blood*

Most commentators and the descendent texts within the Neijing itself interpret spirit in terms of the qi and blood or the correct (zheng 正) qi. LS-3.1 states "The spirit is the way of qi and blood." (神者，氣血法也) [2:v.1, 67]. This rather ambiguous statement is clarified with the explanation, "That the superior attend to the spirit means that they attend to a patient's surplus or insufficiency of qi and blood, and this enables them to tonify or drain." (上守神者，守人之血氣有餘不足，可補瀉也) [2:v.1, 67]. Where LS-1.3 identifies the spirit as the correct qi [2:v.1, 67], LS-18 links the spirit to the blood. "The blood is the spirit qi." (血者，神氣也) [2:v.1,359].

The descendent texts within the Lingshu inform us that needle techniques are useless without an appreciation of the state of the qi and blood. Yet, if we take LS-3, and LS-18 seriously, then spirit in this context is nothing more than the qi and blood itself, or more specifically, the overall state of excess or deficiency of the qi and blood. From this perspective, the message of line 2 is that one must attend to the state of qi and blood rather than the physical form or the mechanics of needle technique.

## *Shen and the Focus of One's Mind*

The rather circumscribed interpretation of spirit propounded in LS-3.1 and LS-18 is by no means definitive. The following lines from later in LS-1.1 itself clearly adopt a broader understanding of the spirit. "The spirit resides in an autumn hair." (神在秋毫) [2:v.1, 11]. This line is generally understood to mean that the practitioner must focus his/her attention on the tip of the needle. The successive lines in LS-1.1 clarify the role of the practitioner's spirit at least to the extent that one must be highly focused and concentrated. "Those who would examine disease must calm their minds when gazing upon a patient, looking neither left nor right." (審視病者，靜志觀病人，無左右視也) [2:v.1, 11]. This focused and concentrated state allows the practitioner to comprehend the spirit within the patient and make a diagnostic assessment. According to Zhang Zhicong, "If when needling, one attains it [spirit] in the heart-mind, then when the spirit connects to those who are sick, one will know whether the patient will survive or perish." (方刺之時，得之于心，則神屬於病者，而知病之存亡矣) [20:5].[14]

The spirit here includes but clearly transcends a simple awareness of the state of a patient's qi and blood. It is the way in which one is aware of the patient's condition.

Line 2 can then be summarized as meaning that while the inferior practitioner attends to the external mechanics of his/her needle technique, the superior practitioner quite literally attends to the spirit within themselves as well as that of the patient. It will be come apparent in the lines below that spirit in this sense is intimately related to one's appreciation of and interaction with the ji-dynamic introduced in line 8.

## *Shen as a Knack or Capacity for Efficacy*

Finally, shen may refer to something or someone with a remarkable capacity for efficacy. Its defining characteristic is that it is somehow more than simply an expression of consummate skill. One story in Fan Ye's 范曄 (398-455) Histories of the Latter Han (Houhanshu 後漢書) illustrates this use of the word specifically as it relates to acupuncture. When Emperor He 和帝 (fl. 89-105) called upon the physician Guo Yu 郭玉 to describe his approach to needling, Guo explained,

> As for doctors talking about intention, the interstices and pores have extremely subtle divisions, so to follow the qi requires skill. When inserting needles and the stone [probes] between them, being a hair off means failure. The knack exists in the connection between the heart-mind and hand. It can be understood, but it cannot be spoken of. (醫之為言意也，腠理至微，隨氣用巧，針石之間，毫芒即乖。神存於心手之際，可得解而不可得言也)[15]

The language of this passage bears some remarkable similarities to that used in the Lingshu, and it makes a crucial point regarding the nature of needling. Shen here resides in the subtle relationship between the mind and the hand, which both includes and transcends mere skill and technique. It is a "knack" insofar as it is particular skill that can be learned but is often innate or intuitive. That is why "it can be understood but not spoken of." In line 2, the crude attend to the forms of needle technique but the superior go beyond this to make use of a subtle knack that is necessarily grounded in technique. This understanding of shen amplifies the shadings of the word discussed above. The knack for needling that is so difficult to talk about hinges on the quality of one's attention and one's capacity to utilize it when needling. This is something one must ultimately discover for oneself.

神乎神.客在門. [3]
**Spirit oh spirit , there is a guest at the door.**

Most commentaries read this line as a statement regarding the correct and pathogenic qi . LS-3 contains three statements to this effect.

> The 'spirit and guest' is the conjoining of the correct and pathogenic qi.(神客者, 正邪共會也)
> The 'spirit' is the correct qi. The 'guest' is the pathogenic qi. (神者, 正氣也, 客者, 邪氣也)
> At the door' means that the pathogenic [qi] travels along the exits and entries of the correct qi. (在門者, 邪循正氣之所出入也) [2:v.1, 67]

LS-32 corroborates this interpretation of spirit, emphasizing its physiological basis.

> Therefore, the spirit, is the essence qi of the water and grains. (故神者, 水谷之精氣) [2:v.1, 509]. Ma Shi adopts a similar perspective, defining the "door" as an afflicted channel. "An affliction by pathogenic qi is at times like the periodic coming and going of a guest, so it is called by the name 'guest.' The guest at the door is the pathogenic guest [qi] at the gate of each channel." (邪氣之所感, 有時如客之往來有期, 名之曰客, 客在門者, 邪客于各經之門戶也) [8].

Yet, SW-26 uses the phrase "Spirit oh spirit," in quite a different context that again suggests it is something more and perhaps more subtle than simply the correct qi.

> Spirit oh spirit! Although my ears cannot hear it, if my eyes are keen, the heart-mind open and the will luminous, then I will be the only one to be conscious of it. The mouth cannot speak of it, and many look at it, but I alone perceive it. Although it is appropriately obscure, it is clear to me alone, like the wind blowing the clouds. For this reason it is called the spirit." (神乎神, 耳不聞, 目明心開, 而志先, 慧然獨悟, 口弗能言, 俱視獨見, 適若昏, 昭然獨明, 若風吹雲, 故曰神) [3:v.1, 364-365]

As already mentioned above, ji and shen are nearly synonymous in many contexts. Central to the appreciation of both is a state of open awareness that is itself spirit. It is this state of awareness that is emphasized in line 3. Where line 2 contrasts a spirit of attention with a preoccupation with external forms, line 3 may be understood as emphasizing the importance of a certain quality of attention in assessing states of health and disease.

未睹其疾, 惡知其原. [4]
**Without observing the disease, how can you know its origin?**

In interpreting this line, LS-3.1 emphasizes the importance of examining the state of correct and pathogenic qi within the channels prior to treatment. "Without observing the disease' means that one must first know about the pathogenic and correct and in which channels there is disease... how can one know its origins, means that one must first know how to identify the location of the diseased channels." (未睹其疾者, 先知邪正何經之疾也... 惡知其原者, 先知何經之病所取之處也) [2:v.1, 67].

Following this interpretive thread through these first four lines we learn that one must assess the state of the qi and blood prior to actually needling. This is fine as far as it goes, however, we have already established that there is another layer of meaning imbedded in this rather self-evident message. The preceding lines of the Lingshu précis first clarify that not only must one observe a disease to identify its cause, one must do so in a very particular way; with concentration, focus and attention to the spirit. Later in LS-1.1 we are informed that the "the spirit resides in an autumn hair," [2:v.1, 11] suggesting that the focus, concentration, or spirit one brings to the diagnostic process must be maintained through the needling process. As already mentioned, "autumn hair" may be understood as both the quality of one's attention in needling and as the needle itself. This makes perfect sense in that the process of diagnosis and treatment are inextricably intertwined. One's attention to what is happening around the needle in the course of treatment becomes a means by which one assesses the state of the qi and blood in the channels. Only once we have grasped this can we turn our attention to the mechanics of needle technique.

刺之微在遲速. [5]
**The subtleties of needling lie in its speed.**

According to LS-3.1, "That the subtleties of the needling lie in its speed, means slow or fast [needle manipulation]." (刺之微在(數) [速] 遲者, 徐疾之意也) [2:v.1, 68].

If it is the crude who attend to the mechanics of needle technique, then how is it that "the subtleties of the needling lie in its speed." This is a relative statement, predicated upon the sensibilities established in the first four lines.

It is not that technique is unimportant, only that it is useless without the proper level and quality of attention.

The first five lines establish that the superior way to practice is to develop a relationship with spirit that is played out through one's engagement with the patient's qi, blood and corporeal form, and is also expressed in one's application of needle technique. The text now presents a new dichotomy, one that echoes the formulation described in line 2 that "the crude attend to the form, the superior attend to the spirit."

粗守關上守機. [6]
**The crude attend to the junctures and the superior attend to the dynamic.**

This line is the crux of the passage. LS-3.1 explains,

> That the crude attend to the junctures means that they attend to the four extremities and do not understand the departure and arrival of the correct and pathogenic [influences] within the qi and blood. That the superior attend to the dynamic means that they know how to attend to the qi. (粗守關者, 守四肢, 而不知血氣正邪之往來也, 上守機者知守氣也) [2:v.1, 68]

Zhang Jiebin 張介賓 comments on this line in his Leijing 類經 (Classified Classic, 1624) saying: "That the superior protect the dynamic, means that one must examine the movement and quiescence of the arrival of qi." (上守機, 察氣至之動靜也) [19:v.2, 627]. For Zhang, ji is primarily a reflection of the activity of the qi. At this point in the discussion, the state of the correct or pathogenic qi, its excess or deficiency is secondary to more general appreciation of the qi's comings and goings, a mode of perception that is defined by the focused concentration of the spirit within one's self. One attends to the ji by means of one's spirit and one's attention.

It is no accident that the superior practitioner attends both to the spirit and to the dynamic. As already discussed, they are two sides of the same coin. The dynamic is the way the spirit expresses itself and the way to truly engage the spirit is through the dynamic. The two words are closely linked in the Neijing, when they appear together they refer to the overall life activity (生命活動的概括) [1:433]. According to SW-70, "What is at the center, is called the spirit-dynamic; if the spirit departs then the dynamic ceases." (根于中者, 命日神機, 神去則機息) [3:v.2, 1008]. Zhang Jiebin explains this as: "What is at the center of things takes the spirit as primary, and one's conscious activity is the expression of the spirit-dynamic. For this reason, if the spirit departs, then the dynamic also follows and ceases." (物之根于中者，以神為之主，而其知覺運動，即神機所發也，故神去，則機亦隨而息矣) [19:v.2, 887].

One might equally say that the superior attend to the situation or disposition (shi 勢). As Zhang Jiebin points out, this is not a static state of affairs, but a fluid ebb and flow of circumstance that is played out in the qi. The job of the physician is to discern the precise moment, place and manner to intervene. Perhaps the most important characteristic of this intervention is that it too, will issue from the spaces between phases of activity, a place of stillness.

> 機之動不離其空 空中之機，清靜而微. [7]
> **The movement in the dynamic is not separate from its empty spaces; The dynamic within this empty space is clear, still and subtle.**

LS-3.1 continues its interpretive thread in reading this line both as a simple statement of one's understanding of deficiency and excess, while also acknowledging the deeper thread that the quality of one's intention is pivotal to the efficacy of one's needling.

> That the movement in the dynamic is not separate from its empty spaces means that one understands the state of deficiency or excess within the qi, and the speed with which to wield the needle. That the dynamic within this empty space is clear, still and subtle means that when needling to obtain the qi one must be extremely focused, attending to the qi so as not to lose it. (機之動不離其空中者，知氣之虛實，用針之徐疾也. 空中之機清靜以微者，針以得氣，密意守氣勿失也) [2:v.1, 68]

Zhang Jiebin endorses the interpretation of the second passage. "This means that one must examine [the patient] with detail and circumspection." (言察宜詳慎也) [19:v.2, 628]. The modern commentator Guo Tian 郭湉 similarly emphasizes the state of mind essential to a careful examination. "The physician must maintain a high degree of concentration and quietude." (醫生高度集中安靜) [1:433].

## *The Dynamic is Defined by Space and Emptiness*

The crux issue, however, as the next line makes clear, is that the ji is defined by the space or emptiness around which all this activity hinges. It is *the axis of quiescence from which activity springs*. This is the reason why one must quiet oneself in order to perceive it. On one hand, ji is the overall state of the qi and blood, and relative balance of healthy and pathogenic qi. As such, it is the disposition or propensity (shi勢) of the situation.[16] An appreciation of the initial propensity of a situation allows one to act effectively. Of equal importance, it allows one to intervene at the beginning of things when they are still nascent or incipient (ji 幾) so that it appears to be effortless (wuwei 無為).[17]

Then again, ji resides in the spaces between activities. It is the quiescence between phases of activity, and it is from here that one's intervention must be based. On another level, ji is the incipient point of stillness from which health arises and it is the job of the physician to discover that within the patient. Even the most materialistic commentaries acknowledge that because ji resides in "empty spaces," its' engagement requires a certain kind of attention.[18] Therefore, physicians must themselves be clear, quiet, and focused to competently assess the stillness of the dynamic that also expresses itself in the empty spaces within the matrix of qi. Such a perspective encompasses the viewpoints of existing commentaries, even as it lends continuity to the entire passage.

其來不可逢, 其往不可追. [8]
**Its coming cannot be met, and its going cannot be pursued.**

Line 8 is another pivotal line in the interpretation of this text. LS-3.1 reads the line as an expression of the well known axiom that one must not drain an deficiency or supplement an excess. "That its arrival cannot be met means that the qi is brimming and cannot be tonified" (其來不可逢者, 氣盛不可補也)... and "that it's departure cannot be pursued means that the qi is deficient and cannot be drained." (其往不可追者, 氣虛不可瀉也) [2:v.1, 68]

There is some debate as to just what kind of qi is being referred to here. Zhang Zhicong interprets the unspoken topic of line 8 to be specifically pathogenic qi. "If this qi has just arrived, then the pathogenic qi will become properly exuberant. If the pathogenic qi is exuberant then the correct qi is greatly deficient. If one cannot avail one self of the qi's arrival then one should meet and tonify it." (如其氣方來, 乃邪氣正盛. 邪氣盛, 則正氣大虛. 不可乘其氣來, 即迎而補之) [20:v.1, 3].

Line 8 introduces another aspect of ji relating to the timing of one's intervention.

It is, of course, ill-advised to tonify excesses and drain deficiencies, but the manner and timing with which one acts is equally important. This emphasis is apparent in the explanation provided in SW-27.3.

> If one awaits the pathogenic qi and does not examine it until the great [pathogenic] qi has already passed, and then drains it, the true qi will collapse. If it collapses, it will not recover. The pathogenic qi will return again and the disease will worsen. This is why 'its going cannot be pursued'. (俟邪不審, 大氣已過, 瀉之, 則真氣脫, 脫則不復, 邪氣復至, 而病益蓄, 故曰, 其往不可追, 此之謂) [3:v.1, 371].[19]

Zhang Zhicong also stresses one's awareness of the "the subtleties of both coming and going."

> One cannot avail one's self of the [correct] qi's departure, but [still] pursues and drains it, the concern is that one may damage [the patient's] correct qi. The crux is in the subtleties of it nascent coming and going. (不可乘其氣往, 追而瀉之, 恐傷其正氣, 在於方來方去之微, 而發其機也) [20:3]

Ji lies in the spaces of quiescence between things which in this context are the comings and goings of the qi. When one works from the ji and one's action becomes effortless (wu wei 無為) and even the most subtle influence has a significant impact. Once again, the state of one's mind or spirit is a crucial part of the equation. According to Zhang Zhicong, "[One must] calmly attend to the intervals between the comings and goings [of the dynamic] and tonify or drain it. Even the slightest error of a hair's breadth and it will be lost!" (靜守于來往之間, 而補瀉之, 少差毫發之間, 則失矣) [20:3].

One's attention to the periodicity of the qi and its relation to the dynamic is an important thread in the Lingshu précis that is reiterated in line 11. Before one can hope to execute any needle technique one must attune oneself with the timing of the qi itself. One must neither go rushing to meet, nor chasing after the qi, but remain instead with the dynamic. The superior practitioner executes the techniques of tonification and drainage from the within the empty spaces between the comings and goings of the qi in a calm and focused state of mind. The idea is to stay out of the way of the healthy functioning of the qi. This principle is then stated explicitly in the following line.

> 知機之道者, 不可掛以發 [9]
> **Those who understand the way of the dynamic, will not impede it and thus it manifests.**[20]

LS-3.1 states: "That one cannot impede it and thus it manifests, means that the qi is easily lost." (不可掛以發者, 言氣易失也) [2:v.1, 67]. Subsequent commentators link the ji, the subtle interval between the comings and goings of the qi to the goal of its overall unification. Ma Shi, in particular, emphasizes the single pointed-nature of ji. "For those who know the way of the dynamic, there is only this unifying qi, and it is as if it cannot be impeded by so much as the space of a single hair's breadth." (知機之道者, 唯此一氣, 而已猶不可掛一髮以間之) [8]. In interacting with it, one must match the subtlety of the dynamic as the incipient initiator of activity.

**不知機道, 扣之不發.[21] [10]**
**Not understanding the way of the dynamic, one detains it and it thus fails to show itself.**

Those who comprehend the dynamic do not impede it. By impeding the dynamic it fails to manifest itself. If the dynamic and consequently the qi fails to manifest itself, one cannot even begin to comprehend the intricacies of tonification and drainage. This is the central message of the LS-3 commentary. "One detains it, and thus it fails to show itself means that one has know knowledge of the meaning of tonification and drainage. Once the qi and blood are exhausted, the qi cannot be directed downward." (扣之不發者, 言不知補瀉之意也. 血氣已盡, 而氣不下也) [2:v.1, 68].[22] This is what happens when one is too aggressive in one's intervention, or even one's intention. By perturbing the dynamic, one creates unfavorable circumstances for its expression. How does one allow the dynamic to express itself? The following line explains the way in which one must attend to the intervals of its comings and goings.

**知其往來, 要與之期. [11]**
**To understand its goings and comings, emphasize its periodicity.**

This and the next 4 lines concern the concept of goings and comings (wanglai 往來) that define the qi dynamic and its relationship to meeting and following (yingsui 迎隨). LS-3.1 picks up its interpretive thread reading line 11 in terms of flow and counterflow, excess and deficiency. "To understand its goings and comings means that one knows the qi's states of contrary and normal [movement] and whether it is brimming or deficient." (知其往來者, 知氣之逆順, 盛虛也) [2:v.1, 68]. Yet even this text acknowledges that such considerations are dependent on one's attunement to the periodicity of the qi. "One who emphasizes its periodicity knows the opportune moment when the qi can be taken." (要與之期者, 知氣之可取之時也) [2:v.1, 68].

Zhang Jiebin emphasizes proper timing in accordance with the comings and goings of the qi even as he articulates the mechanical details of tonification and drainage techniques. "One should tonify and one should drain according to the opportune moment in the instant when one meets the qi." (當補當瀉, 用有其時, 在氣會之頃) [19:v.2, 641].

LS-8.2 directly links one's attunement to ji to various aspects of the spirit. "What follows the coming and going of the spirit is called the ethereal soul and essence. That which goes out and in together with the essence is called the corporeal soul." (隨神往來者, 謂之魂並精, 而出入者謂之魄) [2:v.1, 174]. Such a reading broadens the scope of possible meanings considerably.

The topic of line 8.2 is still the ji. There is no question that the goings and comings of the qi are nothing more than an expression of ji, which is what Isabelle Robinet describes as "the dynamic aspect of the Way" [13:536-537]. The Neiye 內業 (Inner Workings) chapter of the Guanzi 官子 (late fourth century BCE), an early text of Chinese mysticism describes the goings and comings of the Way in terms that presage the language used in the Lingshu précis and elsewhere in the Neijing.[23]

Where the Neiye asserts, "The way is what fills the body, yet people are unable to fix it in place. It goes forth but does not return. It comes back but does not stay." (夫道者所以充形也, 而人不能固, 其往不復, 其來不舍)[24] SW-15 echoes this sentiment in asserting that, "the spirit changes and does not revert, if it reverts it cannot change, and so loses its, ji." (神轉不回, 回則不轉, 乃失其機) [3:v.1, 190]. The expression of ji is necessarily in a constant state of flux even as it remains still within itself. The Neiye repeatedly identifies tranquility as a prerequisite for the appearance of this essential vitality. Moreover, it fixes the qi both within the heart-mind and within the corporeal body.

| | |
|---|---|
| There is a spirit naturally residing in the body, | 有神自在身 |
| One moment it goes, the next it comes, | 一往一來 |
| And no one is able to conceive of it. | 莫之能思 |
| If you lose it you are inevitably disordered. | 失之必亂 |
| If you attain it you are inevitably well ordered. | 得之必治 |
| Diligently clean out its lodging place | 敬除其舍 |
| And its vital essence will naturally arrive. | 精將自來.[25] |

| | |
|---|---|
| That miraculous qi within the mind | 靈氣在心 |
| One moment it arrives, the next it departs | 一來一逝 |
| So fine there is nothing within it, | 其細無內 |
| So vast there is nothing outside it, | 其大無外 |
| We lose it | 所以失之 |
| Because of the harm caused by mental agitation, | 以躁為害 |
| When the mind can hold on to tranquility, | 心能執靜 |
| The way will become naturally stabilized. | 道將自定.[26] |

In practicing acupuncture, physicians must certainly attend to the relatively mechanical goings and comings of the qi, its pacing and its intervals. But it is essential to remember that this is the most superficial expression of a much deeper dynamic playing itself out in the interaction between one's patients and oneself.

**粗之暗乎. 妙哉! 工獨有之. [12]**
**The crude are in the dark about this. How sublime! Only [skilled] practitioners have it.**

The topic of this line is the goings and comings of the qi dynamic that are essential to effective needling. Yet in light of the broader perspective on ji detailed above, it is not surprising that the author of the LS-1.1 would consider the principles he has presented to be sublime. According to LS-3.1, "That the crude are in the dark means that they are benighted and do not understand the subtleties of the qi. That it is sublime and practitioners alone have it means that they have an exhaustive knowledge of the implications of needling." (粗之暗者, 冥冥不知氣之微密也. 妙哉工獨有之者, 盡知針意也) [2:v.1, 69]. SW-26.2 uses remarkably similar language in pointing out that it is not the outward appearance that one must attend to. "Examination by the benighted means that the circulation of qi, nutritive, and defensive is not manifested externally and [superior] practitioners alone know it." (觀于冥冥者, 言行氣營衛之不形于外, 工獨知之) [3:v.1, 360].

Up to this point the Lingshu précis has established that one must attend to the ji by means of the spirit. The ji is characterized as an empty space and as a place of quiescence between the intervals of activity. Attention to these intervals is the key to an effective needle technique. These are the true essentials of needling. Here the two interpretive threads begin to merge. The focus of the discussion now shifts to address more specifically the way in which one should interact with the movement aspect of the qi.

**往者為逆來者為順 [13]**
**Going away from it is contrary, promoting its arrival is going with the flow.**

Line 13 introduces the opposing concepts of ni 逆 and shun 順, which are defined in relation to the departure and arrival of the qi. Ni here does not necessarily suggest a state of "counterflow" or a going against the "normal" (shun 順) flow of things. LS-3.1 suggests that ni refers to the normal ebbing of the qi as it departs. The qi is ni in that it relatively deficient during this phase of its cycle. "That going away from it is contrary, refers to the qi's deficiency and its frailness. To be 'frail' is contrary" (往者為逆者, 言氣之虛而小. 小者, 逆也) and "promoting its arrival is going with the flow, refers to a balanced state of the form qi . 'Balanced' is going with the flow" (來者為順者, 言形氣之平. 平者順也) [2:v.1, 70]. The emphasis here is that one must act in accordance with the normal cycles in the flow of qi.

明知逆順, 正行無疑問. [14]
**If one clearly understands the contrary and normal [flow of qi], then one can act correctly and without doubt or question.**

One's appreciation of the ebb and flow of qi is crucial to effective needling. LS-3 makes the interesting point that such an understanding informs one's selection of acupuncture holes, as well as the timing and the needle technique one will use. "If one clearly understands the contrary and normal [flow of qi] one can act correctly and without errors, means that one knows how to select the place [for needling]." (明知逆順, 正行無間者. 言知所取之處也) [2:v.1, 70]. The Lingshu précis goes on to make two much more general statements as to how such an understanding promotes effective intervention.

迎而奪之, 惡得無虛?[15]
追而濟之, 惡得無實?[27] [16]
**By meeting it and taking it away, how could one not achieve depletion [of the qi]?**
**By pursuing and assisting it, how could one not achieve repletion [of the qi]?**

The descendent texts in the Neijing and the commentary literature are fairly clear as to the meaning of these lines. LS-3.1 succinctly states: "Meeting and taking it away is drainage," (迎而奪之者, 瀉也) and "Pursuing and assisting it is tonification" (追而濟之者, 補也) [2:v.1, 67].[28] Only if you follow and assist the qi, acting as a midwife to the qi, will you make the qi flourish.[29]

迎之隨之, 以意和之. [17]
**Whether meeting it or following it, by means of one's attention, one harmonizes it.**

The crux of line 17 is yi 意, generally translated as intention, denoting an expression of volition or purposefulness that is closely linked to will (zhi 志). The Mengzi, 孟子, Mencius states: "The will is the general of the qi; qi is what fills the body. When the will arrives, qi follows. Thus it is said; "Maintain your will and do not violence to your qi." (夫志, 氣之帥也: 氣體之充也. 夫志至焉, 氣次焉. 故曰: 其志, 無暴其氣)[30]

Mencius' point is that people should be governed by their will and not their qi, but his statement has resonance for those involved in medical practice as well. For some physicians, intention is the key to regulating the qi and it is brought into harmony by the force of their willpower. This reading of yi works but it is at least somewhat at odds with the principles laid out previously in the précis.

Before yi becomes *intention*, it is first an awareness or an attention in the sense already described above. This use of the word is prominent in the Neiye which asserts the primal nature of yi in no uncertain terms.[31]

| | |
|---|---|
| That mind within the mind: | 彼心之心 |
| It is an awareness that precedes speech. | 意以先言 |
| Only after there is an awareness does it take shape; | 意然後形 |
| Only after it takes shape is there a word. | 形然後言 |
| Only after there is a word is it implemented; | 言然後使 |
| Only after it is implemented is there order. | 使然後治 |
| Without order you will always be chaotic. | 不治必亂 |
| If chaotic, you die. | 亂乃死.[32] |

Yi is what occurs before one thinks in words. Before one forms an intention one first becomes aware. Prior to exercising one's intention in needling, one must first refine one's attention. In contrast to Mengzi, (Mencius), the author of the Neiye asserts that qi is not so much governed as it is stabilized, and this is accomplished not by the force of one's willpower but by the stabilization and attentive awareness of one's consciousness.

| | |
|---|---|
| Once the qi is attended to and apprehended, | 氣意得 |
| The sub celestial realm will submit. | 而天下服 |
| And once the mind's attention is stabilized, | 心意定 |
| The sub celestial realm will listen. | 而天下聽.[33] |

Using language that is remarkably similar to that used in the Lingshu précis, the Neiye explains that the qi cannot be bent to one's will using force of any kind,

| | |
|---|---|
| Therefore, as for this qi, | 是故此氣也 |
| it cannot be halted by force, | 不可止以力 |
| and yet it can be calmed by virtue, | 而可安以德 |
| It cannot be called by sound, | 不可呼以聲 |
| but it can be met with attention. | 而可迎以意.[34] |

One's capacity for efficacy resides in effortless activity and the influence of one's consciousness resides in quiescence.

| | |
|---|---|
| Relaxed and unwound, yet benevolent, | 寬舒而仁 |
| In solitude you delight in your own person. | 獨樂其身 |

This is called "revolving the qi": 是謂雲氣
One's attention and actions seem heavenly. 意行似天.[35]

Finally, the text even outlines the means by which we attain this tranquility.

When the four limbs are aligned, 四體既正
and the blood and qi are tranquil, 血氣既靜
One may unify one's attention, and concentrate one's mind. 一意摶心
One's eyes and ears will not be sullied. 耳目不淫
[To attain this,] though it seems distant, it is close at hand. 雖遠若近.[36]

Anyone who has ever practiced acupuncture will appreciate the truth of this statement. Form matters; in the process of needling one cannot be sloppy in one's structural alignment. This an essential means for unifying one's mind, and thereby one's own qi and blood. It allows one to place oneself in the optimal position to appreciate the ji of the patient and to act both effortlessly and efficiently.

For all its subtlety, ji is fundamentally grounded in substance. That may well be why subsequent Lingshu commentators have tended to focus on its most materialistic attributes; they are the easiest to talk about. Be that as it may, when all is said and done, regardless of whether one is meeting or following, tonifying or draining, whether one is working with qi, blood, the channels, or the subtleties of one's needle technique, the harmonization of the qi is depends on one's attention to the ji.

針道畢矣. [18]
**This is all there is to say with regard to the way of needling.**

## Conclusion

The final line of the précis may be taken quite literally. That really is all there is to say about the art of acupuncture. The rest of the Lingshu is exegesis. The importance of this initial passage has less to do with the mechanics of excesses and deficiencies, tonification and drainage than it does with the fundamental sensibility with which they must be engaged. This sensibility is intimately connected to the resonance between one's spirit and the dynamic. Whatever else the notion of spirit may encompass, it most certainly involves focused quiescence on the part of the practitioner. At the core of the concept of ji is a state of quiescence occurring between the comings and goings of qi. Ji is the pivot around which the qi organizes itself. By attuning oneself to the ji one can most profitably assess and exploit the disposition of a situation. From here, one need do very little to exert a profound influence, and for this reason, ones intervention becomes very subtle. "Going to meet" or "following after" the qi is not a headlong thrust in one direction or another so much as a nod or a wink at just the right moment and in just the right way. In moving from the ji, it is not only the needle that becomes the Lingshu 靈樞, the divine pivot, but the practitioner.

## Bibliography

Classical texts translated from the original are taken in the following archive: Lau DC, Chen FC. (eds). The ICS Ancient Chinese Texts Concordance Series. Hong Kong; Commercial Press, 1996-2004.

**Book Title Abbreviations**

| | |
|---|---|
| Guanzi zhu zi suo yin 管子逐字索引 | GZSY |
| Huainanzi zhu zi suo yin 淮南子逐字索引 | HNZSY |
| Liezi zhu zi suo yin 列子逐字索引 | LZSY |
| Liji zhu zi suo yin 禮記逐字索引 | LJSY |
| Mengzi zhu zi suo yin 孟子逐字索引 | MZSY |
| Zhouyi zhu zi suo yin 周易逐字索引 | ZYSY |

1- Guo T. *Neijing jiangyi* 内经講義, Beijing; Renmin weisheng chubanshe 人民衛生出版社. 1984.
2- *Huang di Neijng lingshu jiaoshi* 黃帝內經靈樞校釋 . Beijing: Renmin weisheng chubanshe 人民衛生出版社, 1980.
3- *Huang di Neijng suwen jiaoshi* 黃帝內經素問校釋). Beijing: Renmin weisheng chubanshe 人民衛生出版社, 1980.
4- *Houhanshu jizhu shizong he yinde* 後漢書及注釋綜合引得. Taipei: Chinese Materials and Research Aids Service Center/ Harvard Yenching Institute, 1966.
5- Jullien F. *The Propensity of Things, Toward a History of Efficacy in China*, trans. Janet Lloyd. New York; Zone Books, 1995.
6- Jullien F. *A Treatise on Efficacy, Between Western and Chinese Thinking*, trans. Janet Llyod. Honolulu; University of Hawaii Press, 2004.
7- Keegan, J. *The Huang-ti nei-ching: the Structure of the Compilation; the Significance of the Structure*, doctoral diss. Berkeley; University of California, 1988.

8- Ma Shi. *Lingshu zhuzheng fawei* 靈樞注證發微 in Zhonghua yidian中華醫典, section 3. CD-ROM. Changsha; CD-ROM. Changsha; Hunan Dianzi yin-xiang chubanshe 湖南電子音像出版社 2004. [Hereafter LSZZFW]
9- Mair V, trans. *Wandering on the Way, Early Taoist Tales and Parables of Chuang Tzu*, New York; Bantam Books, 1994.
10- Qing XT. *Zhongguo dao jiao* 中國道教. Shanghai; 知识出版社 1994.
11- Rickett, AW. *Guanzi, Political, Economic, and Philosophical Essays from Early China, A Study and Translation*. Princeton New Jersey; Princeton University Press, 1998.
12- Robinet I. *Introduction a l'alchemie interieure taoiste; De l'unite et de la multiplicite*. Paris; Les Editions Du Cerf 1995:105-120.
13- Robinet I. in Pregadio F. (ed). *Encyclopedia of Taoism*, Oxford; Rutledge: 2008:536-37.
14- Roth H. *Original Dao, Inward Training and the Foundations of Taoist Mysticism*, New York; Columbia University Press, 1999.
15- Schuessler A. *ABC Etymological Dictionary of Old Chinese*, Honolulu; University of Hawaii Press 2007.
16- Slingerland E. *Effortless Action, Wu-wei As Conceptual Metaphor and Spiritual Ideal in Early China*, Oxford; Oxford University Press, 2003.
17- Zhang DN. *Key concepts in Chinese philosophy*, trans. Ryden E. New Haven, Conn; Yale University Press, 2002.
18- Zhang DB, Wu CC, (eds). *Neijing cidian* 內經詞典, Beijing; Renmin weishen chubanshe 人民衛生出版社 1990.
19- Zhang Jiebin 張介賓. *Leijing* 類經 v. 2. Beijing; Renmin weisheng chubanshe 人民衛生出版社 1964.
20- Zhang Zhicong 張志聰. *Huangdi Neijing Lingshu jizhu* 黃帝內經靈樞集注 in Cao DZ. ed, Zhongguo yixue dacheng 中國醫學大成, vol. 2. Shanghai; Shang hai kexue jishu chubanshe 上海科學技術出版社 1988.

## Endnotes

1. Joseph Keegan identifies the Huang Di lineage of medical texts as an "assemblage of a group of texts composed, exchanged and transmitted among a group which perceives itself to have some common interests and identity." Most of the other texts in this tradition have since been lost but they included one fifth of the medical texts recorded in the Hanshu漢書 (History of the Han, 1st century) bibliography. Despite its identification with the Huang Di lineage, the Neijing itself refers to few of these texts.

2. This collection of texts was not titled the Lingshu until the Tang.

3. The edition used for references to the Lingshu is Huangdi Neijng lingshu jiaoshì 黃帝內經靈樞校釋.

4. The edition used for references to the Suwen is Huangdi Neijing suwen jiaoshi 黃帝內經素問校釋.

5. Translation by Zhang Dainan and Edmund Ryden. Unless otherwise noted, all references to classic texts are keyed to the *ICS Concordance Series*. See the bibliography for a table of title abbreviations. ZYSY: 66/79/22.

6. ZYSY: 66/79/22.

7. ZYSY: 66/83/13-14.

8. ZZSY: 6/16/3.

9. HNZSY: 11/101/25.

10. LJSY: 43.2/165/25.

11. ZZSY: 18/49/17. A similar passage also appears in the Liezi. LZSY: 1/3/1.

12. Xiao 小 (small) is generally understood to mean 微 (fine).

13. Editor's note: This distinction is discussed in detail in previous chapters especially chapter three by Dianne Sommers 'How to become a shang yi or 'superior physician' An exploration on the influence of the practitioner in early China.'

14. Alternately, this may be read as "one will know whether the disease will persist or resolve." [20:5].

15. 4:112 下/5b-6b.

16. For two excellent discussions of the concept of shi 勢 in Chinese culture, see [5, 6].

17. For an excellent discussion of wuwei see Slingerland [16].

18. Ma Shi is a holdout who is content to interpret the "empty spaces" in very concrete terms. "The Suwen has a 'Discourse on the Bone Boles' (Chapter 60) that indicates this means the empty spaces along each channel (素問有骨空論, 指各經之穴言.)" [8].

19. In many editions si 俟 is hou 候.

20. An alternate translation might be "The way of knowing the dynamic, is that it cannot be impeded and thus it is expressed."

21. Kou 扣 is alternately be read as kou 叩 "to knock." "One knocks [on its door] but it does not show itself."

22. The implication is that the qi cannot be directed downward, lest it counterflow upward regardless of the practitioner's intention.

23. The Neiye appears as a chapter in the Guanzi 管子, however, it is generally considered an independent text in its own right.

24. Translations of the Neiye are our own, with reference to Harold Roth [14] and W. Allyn Rickett [11]. GZSY: 16.1/115/26.

25. GZSY: 16.1/116/14.

26. GZSY: 16.1/117/29.

27. In other editions ying 迎 is ni 逆. and zhui 追 is sui 隨. The meaning is the same.

28. The reading of these lines here is based on the version that appears in the Systematic Classic, the Zhenjiu Jiayijing, 鍼灸甲乙經 (circa 282 CE).

29. Editor's note: these two lines are frequently interpreted to mean to needle against the flow of the jingmai for drainage and with the flow of the jingmai for tonification. See discussions of this in the last chapter, chapter four, 'The jingmai and qi –acupuncture perspectives'.

30. MZSY: 3.2/15/20.

31. Editor's note: the authors have argued for a different sequencing of the terms 'intention', 'attention' and 'awareness' from that promoted in earlier chapters, see chapter one and chapter four in particular.

32. GZSY: 16.1/116/20-25.

33. GZSY: 16.1/117/3-4. Alternately, Rickett translates this passage as "When qi's attention is apprehended, the subcelestial realm is served, When the mind's attention is fixed, the sub celestial realm is heard." [11:51].

34. GZSY: 16.1/115/18-19. Here attention (yi 意) is an alternate reading for yin音.

35. GZSY: 16.1/117/25.

36. Both Harold Roth and W. Allyn Rickett translate yi 意 as awareness. GZSY: 16.1/117/10.

CHAPTER SIX

# QI, JINGMAI, YAOYI

## A study of their relationships[i]

Manuel Rodríguez Cuadras

## Introduction

Chinese herbal medicine is an important part of the whole Chinese healing tradition, and, as such, is intimately tied with the major classic Chinese paradigms, like the need for harmonious flux in the Universe or the pervasive influence and activity of qi[1]. Unfortunately, the qi concept and its related theories and therapies had, during the history of herbalism, a very different expression of what has allowed acumoxa, the other main branch of Chinese therapies, to more explicitly rely on them. Typically a herb or a formula are described in terms of its effects upon the human body or in terms of its functional or therapeutic effect, thus leading easily to the –wrong– conclusion that herbal medicine was an empiric discipline which paid only lip service to the socially dominant thought paradigms of its time. This way of thinking only too easily leads to focusing the bulk of the modern research to "rescue" herbalism in the purest Aristotelian sense, i.e. identifying the "active principle" or the molecules that in the terms of Western medicine make sense in relation to the already well known effects of the herb as it was traditionally presented. For reasons which will be developed below, I perceive that as fundamentally wrong, and the purpose of this chapter is to open the way to demonstrate that Chinese Herbal Medicine was, and still is, a field of Chinese healing craft which during its history, and especially after the second half of the eleventh century was closely related with the concepts making Chinese Medicine what it is, showing that qi, jingluo, zangfu, etc. were and are as fundamental to herbalism as they are to acumoxa, although they were used in rather different and distinctive ways.

Chinese Medicine has historically developed along two separate traditions, which although apparently sharing some theories and concepts, revolve around two very different therapeutic methods: acupuncture and drugs[2]. While the

i. I would like to thank and acknowledge Charles Chace, Stephen Birch and Emmanuel Moreno for their valuable comments, help and feedback during the writing of this chapter.

relationship between acupuncture and the basic Chinese cosmological and medical classical theories is well established, herbal medicine does not seem to show a consistent, structured, relationship with what has become one of the main concepts of Chinese Medicine, qi, its movements and pathways. The main theories defining the usage of herbs are more about functional systems and fluids, which by their own nature are more vulnerable than the qi concepts to the frequent confusion between the "explanatory models" that are common in the West, and the "practical descriptive models" more akin to the Eastern cosmological vision [4]. Also a good part of the herbal medicine literature consists of prescriptions presented side-by-side with some illness or symptom, without ever mentioning any possible relationship between prescription and illness through models employing the qi concept as their basis.[3] The conceptual vulnerability of the zangfu theories and the existence of a huge body of "recipes" with only empirical justification has made Chinese herbal medicine many times during its history a simple compilation of illnesses, symptoms and prescriptions. But, notwithstanding the importance of empiricism in herbal medicine, there is documentary evidence showing that there was a theoretical nucleus in the main body of herbs and formula design, prescription and usage. It could be useful to remark that most physicians in China were and are mainly herbalists, and it seems only a very remote possibility that such close ties between culture, medicine and plants could have been sustained along the centuries without intimately sharing the most common concepts of Chinese culture, like the concept of qi, ideas about causality, or the preference for practical models to act upon the world. Also, the same history of medicine shows that herbal-related concepts have heavily influenced the whole craft of medicine, including acupuncture, and this could not have been done without a deep commonality of the basic paradigms. We know that herbal doctors use many of the same categories as their acupuncturist colleagues,[4] but their different usage of these concepts make it sometimes difficult to clearly identify explicit connections between herbal therapy and the concepts presented and developed in the ancient classics of systematic correspondences.

Handicapped by its own practicality and by its easy assimilation to Western causal thinking, and widely documented as what can be easily understood as "recipe books", Chinese herbal medicine risks being reduced to a series of handbooks, or, in a complementary scenario, to being abridged to the bio-chemically recognizable molecules, which are only a part of its complex nature and therapeutic properties. But this is not an unavoidable fate, because herbal medicine has in its own history and development the visible proof being that its effectiveness was based not only in empirically accumulated knowledge, but also in an original, distinctive and comprehensive way to perceive and interact with the world thorough the same medical concepts that are so visible in the field of acupuncture. It is very probable that concepts like qi, jingluo, etc. were for the herbalist physicians thought tools used differently that in the systems of acumoxa therapy, but, as I hope to demonstrate, there can be no doubt that they were consistently using them. I strongly support the concept that, to be faithful to itself, herbal medicine should revisit its relationship with the deep and fruitful concepts of Eastern thinking, it should update its function in relation to these ideas and, in a nutshell, it needs to do work similarly to what is being done in some areas of acupuncture. This is a very ambitious proposal, and while I am not a sufficient scholar to accomplish this I can sound a bell on the subject. I will briefly explore the several paths historically followed by herbal medicine, trying to understand and expose what were the different relationships between herbs and qi-related paradigms. I shall offer here some raw ideas about the whole, in the hope that someone more able than me will take and adequately develop them to put Chinese herbal medicine back home, well into the rich Chinese models and concepts and far away from the danger of the short-sighted, narrow, bio-chemical interpretations of the modern period.[5]

To this purpose, we shall briefly examine the history of herbal medicine following with more detail its two best documented traditions (the Bencao and the Shanghanlun) highlighting the coincidence and divergence points showed by those traditions with what was termed as the "medicine of systematic correspondence" and succinctly explore what could be the herbal reflections of the ancient, structuring concepts like qi [氣], jing [經], or jingmai [經脈].

## *1. In and around*

Drugs and the use of drug remedies seem to have been a part of the common culture since ancient times. We find documentary mention in the Mawangdui scripts, Wushier Bingfang, [五十二病方] Prescriptions against fifty-two illnesses, [18], but it seems obvious that the scripts there refer to a common and older body of knowledge [41, 45]. A rubbing from a Han tomb shows a shaman offering or preparing a potion to a mounted gentleman, [49:66], establishing a relationship among shamanism and herbs, thus linking the usage of drugs with the oldest Chinese traditions, including shamanic healing.

Due to the broad spectrum of drugs and drug use, and the antiquity and variety of its usage, it is necessary to adopt some orderly criteria to explore its origins. For this purpose, the history of drug use could be considered as coming formally from two separate traditions: the purely empirical and the more structured one.[6] The oldest tradition is the empirical, and it probably started simultaneously with the shamanic origins of the healing arts. The second broad line of tradition, first documented with the Shanghanlun, [傷寒論] is solidly rooted in Chinese cosmology, and consistently uses cosmologically influenced basic concepts –like qi [氣], zangfu [臟腑], jingluo [經絡], etc.– to describe the pathological processes and its remedies. This current, although strongly influential in the development of Chinese medicine, has had some dark periods up to the Song Dynasty (960-1200 CE)[7] when its exegesis, analysis and commentaries explode in a flood of literature continuing up to this day, with a special flourishing during the Jin-Yuan period of medicine theory renovation. The commonality of some names and concepts used in this current with the set of structures becoming what is called "systematic correspondences" has led some experts [40:169] to describe this current as an attempt to relate drugs and drug therapy with the conceptual world of systematic correspondences.

I shall separately analyse these two main currents, the cosmologically ordered –as represented by the Shanghanlun– and the –apparently– more empirical one, which, for pure exposition convenience, following Unschuld's idea [41:3 and following] can be ordered in three main subsets:

1. Private writings. This group is formed by a collection of highly diverse works, quite varied in extension, scholarship and contents, and written down by a great variety of authors. Since pharmaceutics was historically part of a general education,[8] and everybody able to write had the authority to publish their experiences [41:5], a broad group of heterogeneous authors, including practicing physicians, travelling high officials, Daoist hermits, even educated common citizens, recorded and privately published their findings. As a rule, the works of this group are just descriptions of drugs or prescriptions along with symptoms or illnesses to be treated with them. Usually no consistently structured theories are found in these books, which we can consider as a kind of "recipe books" [經方] although they tend to reflect the paradigms common in their cultural milieu at their times of publication.

2. Encyclopedic works. A group of massive works, many of them the result of imperial commissions. Starting with the Shennong Bencao Jing [神農本草經] (author/authors unknown), tentatively dated around the East Han Dynasty (202 BCE–220 CE), or, for short, the Bencao Jing [本草經] or Benjing [本經], these books not only describe a number of drugs, their properties and uses, but also try, in some instances to give herbalism a theoretical backbone, or, at least, a sense of organisation. Among the most notorious we find the Shennong Bencao Jing

(or Shennong Bencao Jing Jizhu) by Tao Hongjing [陶弘景] (456-536 CE). Following this there are a number of works commissioned by the Emperors from the Song up to the Ming dynasties, and there is, of course, Li Shizhen's [李時珍] monumental Bencao Gangmu [本草綱目]. Together these texts compose a collection of well preserved and documented works, constituting the theoretical reference for what can be named the "Bencao [本草] tradition". In accordance with the times and the evolution of scientific knowledge, these books show a progressive sophistication in taxonomy, classification and order of the materia medica, and frequently refer to what sometimes appear as the "qi" of the plants. Most of the later authors show a deep familiarity with this paradigm and its derived concepts –like the jingluo-, but in general they fail to construct a theory tying together qi, herbs, jingluo and zangfu, just presenting the qi-related issues as a collection of empirical facts, like the thermal effect of plants on the human organism or their preference for a specific jingluo or zangfu.[9]

3. Handbooks. The remaining works of the first group are of a very irregular quality, and the ones of the second are in many aspects (size, price, drugs classification) unpractical for everyday clinical practice. Thus, a third group of pharmaceutical literature emerged: the works structured in a clinical way, smaller both in size and scope than the "encyclopaedias" and written by recognized medical experts. Coming from totally eclectic and pragmatic clinical traditions and practices, they have been somewhat neglected by historians, although many "handbooks" [手冊] from the Ming and Qing eras are still in use in the non-continental Chinese communities.

Among these three types of documents, I shall first follow the evolution of the second kind, the ones itemized as "Bencao tradition", because these are the ones within this empirical tradition which, as far as I know, show from time to time a theoretical intention of marrying the herbal traditions with the theories and practice of the medicine of systematic correspondences, i.e. explicitly considering qi, xue [血] or jingmai [經脈] as a part of the same theory supporting the selection and use of herbs.

## *2. Pathfinding*

### Before the Bencao jing

The legend of herbalism starts with Shennong [神農], one of the four fundamental benefactors of humanity, reputedly the founder and teacher of agriculture and drug therapy and the inspirer of the first herbal medicine text, the Shennong Bencao Jing [神農本草經]. The name of Shennong appears for the first time connected to pharmacy in the Huainanzi [淮南子] (Liu An, circa 122 BCE). Since then, the name of this mythological figure is tied to drugs, and mostly cited in works of Daoist character or bias. Several of the first books on herbalism (mentioned by Tao Hongjing) tied the names of both, Shennong and Bencao, with the pharmaceutic discipline or activity[10] originating what is known as the Bencao tradition and literature. Before the publication of the first "Bencao Jing", around the East Han dynasty (202 BCE–220 CE), we have documented references to drug treatments in at least two sources:

1. "Mawangdui"[馬王堆] . The Mawangdui's found text "Wushier bingfang" (Prescriptions against fifty-two illnesses)[11] presents one hundred and seventy prescriptions along with various other therapeutic techniques (surgery, pressure with stones, cupping, steaming, spells), comprising two hundred and seventy four drugs. There are no explicit references to theoretical foundations of the use of specific drugs against particular illnesses; from the context it is possible to deduce that the selection of substances had been determined largely by magical correspondences or demonologic beliefs [18].

2. "Wuwei" [武威]. A Han grave found in Wuwei County, Kansu, 1972 contained some herbal texts. These were apparently written in the early East Han period (202 BCE–220 CE). Ninety-two bamboo strips were found describing one hundred drugs, with therapeutic indications closer to the indications and spirit of the Bencao Jing.

One can safely state that, although the documented history of drug therapy starts with the publication of the first Bencao Jing in the Han Dynasty, drugs and drug therapy already had by that time a long history, probably rooted in the shamanic origins of the medicine itself. It is already well know and documented that preparation and use of potions were since before recorded history part of the primitive shamanic armoury, together with a set of other healing tools, like dancing, chanting or spitting [40]. Also it is known that throughout history some shamans evolved into or specialized as healers,[12] as is well represented by the changes suffered by the Hanzi "yi"[毉, 醫], its radical evolving from "gong" [工] (work, common with "wu" [巫] or "shaman") to "jiu" [酉], a representation of a bottle with some liquid inside.[13] There is no structured documentary history of this evolution, but we know that, at least initially, the potions (or other pharmaceutical forms, like spirits or fumes) were considered mainly as the vehicle for the real healing agents, which were fundamentally of magic nature [40:40]. The appearance of the Bencao Jing represents the first documented evidence in the herbal tradition of the acknowledgement of the intrinsic efficacy of the drugs themselves. This marks an important turning point from magic to medicine. However, having said that, this view of the drug as vehicle rather than as an active healing agent by itself, or as an intimate collaborator of purely magical practices, can be traced almost continuously throughout the history of medicine in China, at least, being conservative, up to the Tang´s physician Sun Simiao [孫思邈].[14]

## The main tradition of the Bencao literature

We can note several steps in this drug tradition, defined either by the appearance of a very influential scholar or doctor, or by the publishing of some seminal work, as important landmarks, many times coincidental. In this somewhat artificial way, we can better follow the on-going sophistication in understanding the effects of drugs, including the continuous improvement of the knowledge of their nature, and the structuring of their classification. Periodically we find appearing some isolated links between the purely empirical recommendations of drug use and other paradigms and theories, like qi and the jingluo, more akin to what Unschuld calls "the medicine of systematic correspondences" [40].

We shall first review the poorly documented times before the appearance of the first copies of the Bencao Jing, examine some possibilities around the publishing of this book, and then plunge in more detail into better documented areas, starting with the works of Tao Hongjing [陶弘景] (456-536 CE), bringing us well into the last part of the Song Dynasty.

### *a) Before Tao Hongjing. From the dawn of times to the first Century CE*

We already mentioned that potions[15] and other drug administration forms that appear closely related with the shamanic practices were so old as to be far out the reach of literary evidence. Potions and their components were referred to, or represented in, numerous texts and pictures dedicated to various other subjects, like history, rituals or simply decoration.

By the time of the Warring States the practitioners of the healing and divinatory arts were already a kind of well-established group of professionals [41:13], but there is still no literary evidence of drugs being considered separately from magic. The name of the mythological Shennong, which was to be closely related to pharmaceutics from the Han times, appears already in the fourth century BCE,[16] but his connection with pharmaceutics does not appear in an explicit form before the publishing of the Huainanzi, a compilation made by scholars of the circle of Liu An, who died in 122 BCE [41:11]. An additional reference to this legendary hero and his healing arts was recorded later, in the Shennong Huangdi Shijin, [神農黃帝食禁] a part of a book on the history of the Western Han dynasty.[17] Since the Huainanzi, anyway, the name of Shennong appears frequently related with one or another usage of herbs, but the documentary evidence of books having the title or partial title of "Shennong Bencao", is not found until the much later work of Tao Hongjing (452-536 CE) [41:17].

The name "Bencao" itself appears also for first time in the Hanshu [漢書] circa 110 CE, in relationship with unsuccessful attempts to achieve immortality. The way it is mentioned clearly indicates the existence of herbalists, which were called "Bencao officials". It is not clear in this reference what was the relationship between those "Bencao officials" and the "prescription masters", presumably another kind or school of herb-using physicians, which are mentioned separately. [41:13]

The old tradition of healing with herbs is mostly undocumented up to Mawangdui scripts, dated before 168 BCE, the date of the burial,[18] but it seems obvious that the scripts there refer to a common and older body of knowledge, for the most part closely related with shamanic concepts, like demonology and magic correspondences.[19]

It seems to be the Eastern Han Dynasty (202 BCE–220 CE) the times when the first book titled Shennong Bencao Jing appears –at least, this was the view of its first documented compiler, Tao Hongjing. It should be mentioned here that, although the historical records are still unsure about the evidence of the materiality of a specific original work entitled Shennong Bencao Jing, there is no doubt about the existence and influence of a herbal tradition which, wearing this or other drug-related names, has been built around the notion of Bencao and the name of Shennong.[20] The origins of this tradition can be traced up to around the first century CE, when the first Shennong Bencao Jing is supposed to have been published.[21]

Around the time of compilation of the Bencao Jing [本草經] (or, in brief, Benjing [本經]), at least three paradigms tried to explain in the healing traditions the origins of illness and the basis for therapeutic intervention: the concepts of demonology, of magical correspondence, and of systematic correspondences.[22] Of those three, the third one, the paradigm of the systematic correspondences which was so well developed in the acupuncture tradition by this time, was almost completely missing in the evolving herbal tradition, or, at least, its influence doesn't appear explicitly in its foundational text. These paradigms don't appear either in another set of time-related documents, the ones found in the bamboo strips unearthed in a Han grave in Wuwei County [武威漢代醫簡武威] in 1972. These scripts, believed to have been written during the early Eastern Han period (202 BCE-220 CE), and buried in the first century CE,[23] don't mention the Benjing as such, but the therapeutic indications they give about drugs are mostly free of magic. This shows the influence of a turn towards a more methodical approach to medicine that the healing arts were experimenting with during Han times, a turn marked in herbal therapies by the appearance of the Bencao Jing. The Wuwei texts are closer than the Mawangdui's to the methodical spirit of the Bencao Jing, but they do not mention anything allowing us to relate the proposed drug therapies with the already codified paradigm of systematic correspondence.

Four hundred years later, by the time of Tao Hongjing, history records eight different works named Shennong Bencao Jing, or variants of this name [41:18]. Some of them might simply be rearrangements of the original, believed to have been published in the later Han dynasty, compiled by an unknown author or authors. This Shennong Bencao Jing consists of four chapters describing three hundred and sixty five drugs and, although the term qi appears in it (in relationship with illness, "xieqi" [邪氣], and as part of a description of the drugs), there is not mention of the jingluo system, nor is there any reference to what could be considered to be part of a systematic approach to medicine. The drugs are classified following a cosmological criteria (Heaven, Man, Earth), and then the prescription is explained in terms of several categories, like yin-yang, child-mother, part of the plant, etc. But these explanations do not relate with any structured abstract theory, being more determined by some material effects or observable features of the substances described.[24] There is nothing about the possible plant-jingluo relationships, and what is presented as "qi" of the plant has a character exclusively related with its effects on the body expressed in thermal terms: hot, cold, warm, and cool.[25] Some five phase correspondences can be traced to the study of the tastes (wei [味]) [37:182-183], but there is no explicit reference to the five phases theory.

The Huangdi Neijing Suwen [黃帝內經素問] reflects some attempts to include drugs into the theoretical framework of systematic correspondences. Several chapters (twelve, nineteen, twenty-four, seventy-six) deal with drugs and its preferred uses, sometimes as the only desirable therapy (generally to fight against internal or long-standing illnesses), sometimes together with acupuncture. Following the "qi" conceptual guide the book proposes, the use of drugs are also mentioned as, for instance, to "regulate the qi" (chapter seventy-four). But when talking of the drugs themselves, the Suwen focuses on its taste (wei, [味]), does not mention any specific drugs, and seems to have a preference for using foods –rather than drugs– as a substance-related therapeutic method. Altogether, although drugs, qi and jingluo are mentioned in the same text, it would be most unsafe to assert that the drug therapy contemplated in the Suwen constitutes the slightest bond between the herbal tradition and the new paradigm of systematic correspondence. Also it should be considered that many of the references to drug therapy are in the "seven comprehensive discourses", (chapters sixty-six to seventy-four), added by Wang Bing [王冰] in his eighth century edition of the Suwen [43], so might not have been part of the Suwen when originally written. On the other hand, it can be said that the concepts about drugs appearing in the Suwen match almost one-to-one with those proposed in the Benjing, believed to have been published about the same time, so we can assume a certain degree of mutual basic knowledge.[26]

The lack of cross references between those two books can maybe be ascribed to their different implicit purposes. While the Bencao Jing is more about looking to natural substances and trying to order them with a pragmatic goal, the Suwen links the human body, its ailments and its possible therapies with a mostly abstract theory, offering – or hoping to offer - the possibility to better understand the medical aspects of human reality, so as to be, in short, more effective in healing. The relevant fact for this paper is that, even though these two books are close contemporary works, there are not in the Bencao Jing any reasonably solid ties with the theories of systematic correspondences expounded in the Suwen.

## *b) Tao Hongjing [陶弘景] (456- 536 CE)*

Tao Hongjing was born in 456 CE into a family of respected status and learning, and after attaining the level of a high scholar and serving in various prestigious official positions, developed an active interest in alchemy, ending his life retiring to the Mao Shan [茅山], where his works were so important as to be considered by some as "the virtual founder of the Mao Shan Daoism".[27] Among his works, he compiled and published two seminal books on herbalism, the Shennong Bencao Jing and the Shennong Bencao Jing Jizhu [神農本草經集註]. Actually these two titles are the same book, distributed first in three (the Shennong Bencao Jing) and then in seven chapters (the Shennong Bencao Jing Jizhu). Tao Hongjing explains in the first chapter of both books his methods and sources, among which he chose to adhere mainly to the first Bencao Jing. In this first chapter he mentions "testing the pulse" [診脈] as a necessary ability to be a good physician. He also, mentions "qi" several times in what we can assume were at the time common cultural concepts (xieqi, qi), and mentioned the jingluo as a system which could pick up the xieqi and lead them to the zangfu.[28] Also the concepts of "xu" [虛] and "shi" [實], vacuity/depletion and repletion, are mentioned as pathological conditions. Following the first Bencao Jing, he continues mentioning the sort of thermal qi this book uses when describing a drug, but there is no relationship of this thermal nature with more abstract theories about the intrinsic nature of the drug or its uses.

In a nutshell, Tao Hongjing made a systematic compilation of the several texts on herbalism available to him at his time, and he appears to have made no use of any other books (or at least does not make explicit use of them),[29] like the Suwen, the Nanjing [難經], or even the Shanghanlun [傷寒論], which were probably well known in his time by medically oriented scholars. In his books he made a detailed description of seven hundred and thirty different drugs, their synergies and incompatibilities. He gave detailed instructions on how and when to use them, and constructed an index of drugs listed according to illnesses, which can be considered as the first "Guide of Drug Usage". Undoubtedly a great piece of work, but, once more, without any explicit or implicit relationship with the theories of qi or jingluo (or any other, for that matter) which helped to explain the properties of the drugs in function of their "qi", if we are to understand "qi" in the broad sense that the term had already acquired in other traditions since the Suwen and Nanjing.[30]

### *c) Symbolic syncretism: the Bencao yenyi [本草衍義] and the Chen qunang (Jin-Yuan Dynasty 金元)*

The Song attempted to unify some previously divergent worldviews and launched a kind of reviewed version of "rujia" [儒家], which is termed "Neoconfucianism". This new set of state-supported eclectic theories also affected medicine. In the words of Unschuld:

> If the intellectual expansion that took place during the first phase produced an interest in sources that, at least officially, were not exactly closely associated with Confucians, Chinese medical writers in the second half of the 11th century began to produce works that conscientiously combined –at the beginning in almost symbolic manner– Daoist and Buddhist, as well as Confucian elements. This process represented the first period in the transfer of Neoconfucian syncretism to the field of medicine [41:85].

Throughout the subsequent period, many books appeared wearing in their title either the words Bencao and/or Shennong, and, although they usually refer to the still common categories of qi, jingluo, etc, none of them presented a real advance in the coordination of the two main healing traditions, herbs and acupuncture.[31] A representative work of this period is the Bencao Yanyi [本草衍義] (Elucidation of the meaning of Pharmaceutics), by Kou Zhongshi [寇宗奭], published in 1116 CE. Kou Zhongshi attained his pharmaceutical knowledge by extensive travel, and his scholarship and critical spirit allowed him to work with this information towards a very ambitious goal: to integrate the hitherto rather pragmatic use of drugs into the theories of systematic correspondence [41]. He expressly mentions "qi" as an object of treatment, and gives high importance to the emotional states and qi states. For the first time in an herbal therapy text, the drugs are not arranged just in relation to the illnesses to be treated, but rather the characteristics of the drugs themselves stand for principles of effect that Kou then tried to standardize. This attempt to systematically assign principles of effect to drugs in accordance with drug qualities is the first attempt to create a real theoretical base for their successful use. Kou Zhongshi recognizes the physiological effects of the five qi, (climatic factors) and the corresponding therapeutic effects of the five tastes (following the Suwen's drug use suggestions). He states that the qi and wei (taste, flavour) complement each other, and proposes general guidelines for the use of both to fight the xieqi. Also, when talking about the "eight important points to treat illness", he mentioned the quality of the movement in the jingluo. He even tried to clarify the meaning of qi in the original Bencao Jing, concluding that there was just a mistaken use of the term, "xing" [性] (nature, natural tendency) being a word more consistent with the actual concepts used in the Benjing. So, all in all, it is clear that Kou Zhongshi was familiar with the ideas of qi, five phases, jingluo, etc., but notwithstanding his valiant attempt, he was unable to relate the properties of the drugs to their use employing this theoretical model. A more solid approach to fuse the two dominant medical paths was done by Zhang Yuansu [張元素], also known as Zhang Haogu [張潔古] [41:102].

Zhang Yuansu (probably 1130–1210 CE) devoted himself to the study of medicine after an unsuccessful attempt at a career as a Confucian official. A contemporary of Liu Wansu [刘完素 ] and teacher of Li Gao [李杲], he was considered by Li Shizhen to be the real originator of the so-called Jin-Yuan Medicine [41:101]. Besides promoting a revolutionary, non-traditional way of practicing medicine, he wrote a small treatise (the Zhenzhunang, [珍珠囊] "Bag of Pearls", known as "Essence of the Method of Experience") where, quoting Li Shizhen:

> He distinguished the qualities of the drugs according to their qi and wei, their yin-yang affiliation, their strength or weakness [of qi and wei], their [ability] to rise or descend [in the body], to float or to dive, to replenish depletions or drain repletion, according to [their relations to the] Liu qi and [their ability] **to penetrate the Twelve conduits** (emphasis added). In addition, [he differentiated] the process of drug use according to symptoms. [On the basis of these conceptions] he created the `Secret Instructions for Treatment with the Main Therapeutic Effects" in connection with the "Essence of the Method of experience" and called his work Zhenzhunang... [41: 102].

In Zhang Yuansu's Qin dynasty biography are examples of how he used the ideas related to the twelve jingmai or channels [41:102]. Zhang Yuansu, then was revolutionary not only because his idea of treating different people suffering the same illness differently, but also in his ways of evaluating the patient's condition (which he did using the paradigm of systematic correspondences) and in composing his prescriptions on the basis of the characteristics of the drugs, including their ability to penetrate the twelve channels. He is, then, considered the first to have placed drug knowledge into a theoretical framework, including in his theory the systematic correspondences, the qi and the jingluo. After him, concepts like jingluo, yin-yang or qi were found –together with the older zangfu concepts and the purely empiric drug usages– in pharmaceutical works. Not all the jingluo, though, have "its" drug (in the Zhenzhunang there is a list of the twelve channels with some drugs which have a preference to go to them), and he never explained why a specific drug has a preference for a specific channel. Nevertheless, the seeds of his thinking will directly flourish on two of his students, who come to be known as two of the Four Great masters of the Medicine of the Jin-Yuan period: one was Li Gao, also known as Li Dongyuan [李東垣], style name Mingzhi.

Following his master, and maybe in close collaboration with him, Li Gao, in the Zhenzhunang Buyi Yaoxing Fu [珍珠囊補遺藥性賦] (The Bag of Pearls expanded and made easily understood. [combined with] verses on the properties of drugs)[32] theorizes about the yin- or yang- related attributes to drugs, their effects on the five zang, odour penetrations of the five zang, presenting a table of correlations among the five phases, five colours, five tastes and five zang, as well as the parts of the organism mastered by the five zang. Additionally this table included dietetic prohibitions related to illnesses of the five zang, together with a list of drugs for the reduction of fire-evil in all channels, among other lists and, of course, drug enumeration and description.

Li Gao, a well established Confucian scholar, wrote a number of books, always expanding the central ideas he got from his teacher Zhang Yuansu. In all of them he kept insisting on the need for careful assessment of the patients condition, on the importance of tailoring the remedy to it and on the significance of the internal irritants as cause of illness. Titles like Neiwai shangbian huolun [內外傷辨惑論] (Treatise on solving confusion in discriminating internal and external damages) or Yixue faming [醫學發明] (Medical theory made clear), or even Yong yao faxiang [用藥法象] (Methods and approaches to using medicines), all revolve around those nuclear ideas. However, the core work of Li Gao, where he reunited and condensed all his concepts and knowledge, is the Piweilun [脾胃論] (Treatise on the Spleen and Stomach), probably the last work he wrote before dying at the age of seventy one. In this seminal book he not only expounded his central theory about the primary significance of the stomach-spleen system, but also stressed the importance of the internal causes of illness –thus complementing the Shanghanlun, which dealt mainly with external aetiologies. He also presented the idea of yin fire, so rich in the interpretation and healing of many chronic illnesses. The theoretical core of the Piweilun was a real innovation in herbal medicine, exhaustively referring to the Neijing as its basis, but offering an original and intelligent interpretation of the old classic in the light of the already well developed theories of systematic correspondences.[33] In this work, Li Gao not only smoothly incorporated those basic theories, but also related them to both herbal and acupuncture treatments, thus making an important contribution in linking needle and drug therapies and greatly enriching both healing systems.[34]

He, for instance, decided which medicines have to be used in relation to the function of the five phases principles (Book I, Chapter 3); he distinguished in a formula which medicines enter into some channels and which do not (Book III, Chapter 2); he composed formulae in relation to the function of the channels (Book I, Chapter 6); he insisted on the necessity of identifying the channels involved in a pathology to administer medication (Book I, Chapter 8); and he discussed the qi of the herbs (Book I, Chapter 5), although there he alludes to the qi in the usual herbal concept - their thermal nature. Concerning acupuncture, the concepts and treatment approaches he presented in the Piweilun are important enough to be called "Dongyuan's acupuncture method" by Gao Wu in his Zhenjiu Juying [鍼灸聚英] (The gathering of the blossoms of acupuncture, 1529) and have attracted the attention of some scholars up to today [11].

The Tangye Bencao [湯液本草] (Medications to be administered as decoction) by Wang Haoku [王好古] (a disciple of Li Gao, and initially also a student of Zhang Yuansu) continues the line of combining ancient empirical wisdom of herbal medicine with the intellectually dominant paradigms of the Confucian and Neo-confucian medicine of systematic correspondences. He always presented his works as a reaction to a false development, as a "return to the origins." This is an aspect typical of medicine in the Jin-Yuan period with striking similarities in other areas of literature. The Neo-confucians, like Han Yu (768-824), Li Ao (768-844), and Chu Xi (1130-1200) always referred to a "tradition" in which they saw that the transmission of the true principles continued only as far as Mencius [孟子] (372-289 BCE), claiming themselves to be the renewed continuation of this genuine tradition. This way of presenting the new as a true continuation of "the ancient wisdom" has a longstanding tradition in China, and allows its adherents to get away with a not small number of true innovations.[35]

In the Song Dynasty, as a part of the movement to systematize and dignify the Medicine, and probably confronted with the presence of at least three major ways of practice (The Bencao, the Neijing, Nanjing and the Shanghanlun) whose theories were not very compatible, some important works tried to coordinate them. This was a gradual process, marked by the following works:

–Bencao Yanyi [本草衍義] (Dilatations on Materia Medica) by Kou Zhongshi [寇宗奭]. Published in 1119 shows an intention of coordinate the existing knowledge about the materia medica with the theories of what Goldschmitdt tems "Classical Medicine." It is "the first materia medica collection to discuss the doctrines of Classical Medicine" [15:122]. For instance, "Kou draws a direct connection between the five sapors (wu wei) of drugs and the climatic environment and its qi [15:178], advocated applying the classical categorization of the Eight Rubrics and the Four Methods… and he was the first to use the term 'Channel Tropism' (guijing, [歸經])" [15:179]. Nonetheless, although he proposed connections between drugs and its physiological effects in the context of the theories of Classical Medicine, he failed to establish clear theoretical reports between the drug and its effects.

–Zhenghe Shengji Zonglu [政和聖濟總錄] (Medical Encyclopaedia: A Sagely Benefaction of the Zhenghe Reign Period), prefaced by the emperor Huizong [徽宗], it is an exhaustive collection of materia medica and formulae, but also includes "specific acupoints and circulation tracts, incantations, and amulets" [15:182]. Its importance lies, not only in its intrinsic contents, but also in being paired[36] by the same Huizhong with a book he authored, the Sheng Ji jing [聖濟經] (Canon of Sagely Benefaction) which "stressed the importance of the classical cosmological and medical doctrines" [15:181]. It discusses the classical doctrines of the Huangdi Neijing in relation with contemporary Neo-Confucian perceptions of nature [15:185], and also attends to the clinical aspects of medicine. In some instances he clearly ties drug treatment with fundamental doctrines of Classical Medicine, like the Five Phases or Yin-Yang.[37]

–Suwen Rushi Yunqi Lun'ao [素問入式運氣論奥] (Profound Discussions on Models of Yunqi Doctrine Received from the Suwen) was submitted to the throne in 1099. This book was written by Liu Wenshu [劉溫舒] elaborating on the Yunqi [運氣] theory and explains by illustrations of circles its application in physiology, pathology, diagnosis, and therapy, predominantly drug therapy.[38]

The previous works by Huizhong and Kou Zhongshi [寇宗奭] don't really integrate the drug therapy with the Classical doctrines; rather the authors mixed them in their writing while stressing the importance of classical doctrine without providing specific means to use them in drug therapy [15:188]. About one generation later, Xu Shuwei [許叔微] wrote his innovative formulary which represents another phase in the integration of classical doctrines into drug therapy, with an attempt to use the classical theories into the process of diagnosis and prescription. Leizheng Puji Ben Shi Fang [類証普劑本事方] (Original Formulary of Classified Manifestation Types for Popular Relief) probably from around 1144. "Xu integrated classical doctrines into his discussion of formulas in every aspect, from the basic description of the formula to the elaborate case histories" [15:189]. Of note is that he presents the effect of drugs on the channels and their adjoining viscera, although there is no mention of a nuclear theory supporting his choices, the link between drug traits and their physiological effects remaining purely empirical.

Yixue Qiyuan [醫學啟源] (Expounding the Origins of Medical Studies) and Zhenzhu Nang (Bag of Pearls) [珍珠囊] are two of the nine books written by Zhang Yuansu [張元素] (ap.1120–1200), a highly praised physician of his time. In the first one, starting with a discussion of the Neijing, he reviews the classical doctrines of physiology and pathology, and then describes the suitable formulas for the pathological conditions, presenting those formulas classified by six common manifestation types. When in the last chapter he presents some simple drugs, he classifies them after five major categories which are in accordance with the five phases. He also add more features to be considered in a drug, like "penetrating or superficial" (hou bo) [厚薄], and the methods of "rising and descending" (sheng jiang) [升降], "floating and sinking" (fu chen) [浮沈], supplementing and draining (bu xie) [補寫], "ruling and governing" (zhu zhi) [主治], thus adding considerable sophistication to the selection process for drugs and formulae altogether.[39] Notwithstanding the interest of this sophistication, the essential contribution of Zhang was to associate each drug with an organ and with a specific jingmai. This established a nexus with the acumoxa therapy, creating a systematic medical system based on common doctrinal bases. This is probably Zhang's most significant contribution.[40]

All in all, we can say that "by the end of the twelfth century, drug therapy literature was transformed" [15:198] but, there is one issue still open to discussion, namely what was the impact of these transformations in the real practice of herbalism, especially in the Southern Song dominated area. At least the information recorded in Chen Yan's [陳言] formulary Sanyin Yiji Bingzhang Fanlun [三因極一病證方論] (The Three Causes Epitomized and Unified: Discussions on Medical Disorders) compiled in 1174 shows an appreciation of the classical doctrines, but never integrates them into the discussion of specific formulas.[41]

So we can see that by the end of the Jin-Yuan period especially in Northern China, under the Jurchen-Jin dynasty there was a sort of pharmacology of systematic correspondence.

This included an innovative doctrine concerning the effects of drugs on the organism based both in the nature of the drugs and in an understanding of the physiology following some aspects of the theory of systematic correspondences, (namely qi, zangfu and jingluo). But there is still a lack of a structured theory consistently linking herbal therapy with qi and qi-related paradigms. There were two main problems making it difficult to completely fuse the two traditions: the standardization of drugs and the complexity of the diagnosis. The first had no real solution at the time; without chemical analysis or similar techniques, the drug position with respect to yin-yang or the five phases has to be and was determined solely in relation to human perceptions (i.e. they were subjective). While this was a system that was generally useful, it showed inconsistent results in some instances, for example, when a drug with strong taste or a spectacular appearance had only a minor, mild effect on the body.[42] A second crucial problem was in the way of diagnosis. Following the "new" theories, the patient's condition must be evaluated primarily by examining the movement of the vessels (i.e., the pulses), and this can be extraordinarily difficult. Even today experienced practitioners of herbal medicine often rely more on other aspects of the diagnostic process (like colours, symptoms, tongue, etc.) than on channel or pulse assessment, so that the whole diagnostic process remains a highly subjective one. Even though the establishment of a systematic medical theory was a vast improvement over the former empiricism, the practice of this kind of herbalism continued by and large to be based mainly on the experience and drug classifications arising out of the purely empirically presented works.[43]

### *d) Herb organization: Li Shizhen and the Bencao Ganmu*

Li Shizhen's [李時珍] (1518-1593) grandfather was a "bell physician" (lingyi) [鈴醫], a wandering medicine practitioner, a class socially considered well below the Confucian medical scholars (ruyi) [儒醫]. His father achieved a degree in the state exams, and thus he could avoid selling his medical skills, although he continued practising and even was employed for a time as an official in the Imperial Medical Office. He was recognized not only because of his medical skills, but also because he wrote several medical works, of which we know five. Among them there is one about diagnosis techniques and another on the doctrine of the pulse.

Li Shizhen himself was unable to pass the state exams, and after three unsuccessful attempts, devoted himself –with his father's consent– exclusively to the study of medicine. A dedicated student, he became a well-known physician, and was called to the Court and put in charge of the temple of ancestors, obtaining afterwards a position in the Imperial Medical Office. When he was less than 30 years old, he started on his own an enormous task, the compilation and organization of the pharmaceutical knowledge of his time. He worked for about 40 years, compiling and comparing books (he took 30 years only to do this part), travelling extensively, and studying the imperial collections already at his disposal. The result was the Bencao Gangmu [本草綱目], an encyclopaedic work he himself failed to see published.

This is not the place to analyze the significance of the Bencao Gangmu, probably the single most influential work –together with the Shanghanlun– among the classics of herbal medicine. I should only mention that Li Shizhen not only did a massive compilation work, but he also organized the drugs in groups and subgroups, starting then each drug monograph with the name of the drug under which its early description appeared, a system still in use today for certain scientific nomenclatures, such as in zoology and botany. In the monographs themselves, he introduced the taste of the drug, its yin-yang nature, and its "thermal" characteristics, for which he employed the term "xing" [性] –nature, character– and not the term "qi" as was used in the Bencao Jing. He apparently reserved the term "qi" in reference to herbs only when he needed to contrast the more subtle qualities of the studied substance with its more substantial features, its "wei" [味].[44] He wrote about qi and jingluo when describing the uses and effects of drugs even quoted the Suwen on the mutual inter-influence between drugs and the climatic factors,[45] but, once more, no effort was made to deduce the drugs properties from its intrinsic nature, contemplated from the standpoint of the theory of systematic correspondences.

It is relevant to remember that Li Shizhen was also describing the "qijingbamai" (eight extraordinary vessels) in his Qijingbamai kao [奇經八脈考], and even described their pulse diagnosis (maizhen [脈診]), so we must assume he was well acquainted with all the existing theories and paradigms around the concepts of qi and jingluo. We can conclude then, that even having a wonderfully organized mind and a treasure of knowledge including both drugs and systematic correspondence theories, including qi, mai and jingluo, he was unable –or unwilling– to establish a real systematic correspondences pharmacology, where the effects of the drugs could be related to their intrinsic nature contemplated after these correspondences, paradigms and rules.[46]

### *e) The evolution of the Bencao tradition. Xu Dachun [徐大椿]*

Throughout medical history, this way of relating drugs with illness was being refined and enlarged, sometimes elaborating in an attempt at drug classification, but always failing to introduce in the core of the classifying concepts the ideas of qi or jingluo. The most common ways to order the use of herbs and prescriptions was by ordering their metabolic effects in different groups. This system was already present on the Bencao Jing[47] and evolved into more specific methods of drug therapy, which themselves kept evolving over time, from the initial "eight basic methods of drug therapy" systematized in Cheng Guopeng's [程國彭] Yixue Xinwu [醫學心悟] (The awakening of the mind in medical studies, 1732) up to twenty-one presented by Wang Ang [汪昂] in his Yifang Jixie [醫方集解] (Collected explanations of medical prescriptions) [37:185-193], without ever reaching the status of real standards. Eight or twenty one, and more or less accepted in their own time, these classifications were always relating drugs to disorders, and sometimes mentioning qi or jingluo, but without giving these concepts the leading role accorded to them by the acupuncture tradition.

One good example of the use of qi-jingluo concepts in this tradition is the work of Xu Dachun (1693-1771). This scholar and physician, one of the foremost advocates of the movement called Hanxue Pai [漢學派] ("school of Han learning", revindicating the validity of the concepts developed during that era) explicitly discussed qi and jingluo,[48] but in his extensive revision of the medical practices of his time [42], he always presented drug therapy as related both to illness, patterns and patient's condition, without consistently using the concepts of the systematic correspondences, either in diagnosis or treatment.

### *f) The selection and use of drugs: a parallel history*

Although the more intimate structure of plants seems not to have been determinative of their use, and although the relationship with the herbal medicine with the theories of the systematic correspondences is very thin and irregular, the fundamental paradigms of the Chinese craft of healing were present in the thinking and acting of relevant herbalist physicians. Sun Simiao, for instance, stated that medicine is "yi" [意]. He wrote 醫者意也, 善於用意，即為良醫. "Medicine is yi. Those who are proficient at using yi are good doctors."[49] Dealing with how to correctly select between different modes of administering medicines, he repeats that only 能參合而行之者，可以為上工。... 故曰醫者意也: "... those who can match [the correct type of medicine with the appropriate condition]... can be considered superior craftsmen. So it is said, "Medicine is yi."[50]

Also, although it is usual to relate drug therapy mostly with zangfu concepts and theories, an anecdote about the famous Tang physician Xu Yinzong [許胤宗] clearly underlines the importance of the pulse and pulse reading when selecting medicines. In refusing to write about his medical skills, he said:

> 醫者，意也，在人思慮。又脈候幽微，苦其難別，意之所解，口莫能宣。且古之名手，唯是別脈，脈既精別，然後識病。夫病之於藥，有正相當者，唯須單用一味， 直攻彼病，藥力既純，病即立愈。今人不能別脈，莫識病源，以情臆度，多安藥味，譬之於獵，未知兔所，多發人馬，空地遮圍，或冀一人偶然逢也。如此療疾，不 亦疏乎！假令一藥偶然當病，複共他味相和，君臣相制，氣勢不行，所以難差，諒由於此。脈之深趣，即不可言，虛設經方，豈加於舊。吾思之久矣，故不能著述 耳
> Medicine is signification (yi); it is in one's thoughts and deliberations. Moreover, the indicators of the pulse are murky and subtle and the difficulty in distinguish them is distressing. That which is understood by intention cannot be disseminated by the mouth.[51] All of the famous practitioners of antiquity are so only [because of the abilities] to differentiate pulses. Once the pulse is clearly differentiated, one recognises the disease. As for the disease's relation to the medicine, it is one of appropriate matching... If one has one medicinal that happens to match the disease and other ingredients are added to "harmonize" it, the chiefs and the ministers will restrict each other's [effect] so that the force of qi does not proceed ... The profundity of the pulse cannot be spoken of ... I have thought about this for a long time and am not able to write anything.[52]

A Ming dynasty physician, Zhao Xuemin [趙學敏], reiterates several hundred years later:

> 醫者意也，用藥不如用意，治有未效，必以意求
> Medicine is yi. It is not as good to use medicinals as to use yi. Whether or not a treatment works is based on yi.[53]

Yi was an important concept in the craft of healing,[54] and not only in acupuncture. As shown in the examples, herbalists made consistent use of this concept when trying to explain the subtleties of their craft. And yi is not a purely empirical concept; its use, the explicit mention of its importance, implies a certain model of reality where qi is always present, if not central. The important place of yi in the writings of some relevant physicians throughout history, together with the consistency of the use of words like qi or jingluo, provide evidence that the qi paradigm was not alien to herbalists. At the same time though, they were either reluctant to extend it to the structure marked by the systematic correspondences, or they did not feel the strict metaphors usually tied to this specific structure conveniently reflected the function of qi in the reality of drug use.

**In consequence, from the review of this pragmatic tradition, we can say that...**

–Although from very early times (Suwen, Bencao Jing) there are some characteristics of drugs which appear to be ordered following yin-yang and/or five phases rules, their correlations bear more relationship with the observed effects of the drugs on the body (including jingluo and zangfu) than with the theory of systematic correspondences itself.

–Although the paradigms and concepts of qi, jingluo, etc. are mentioned extensively in the pharmaceutical literature, there is no real theoretical connection between the empiricism of drug uses and the more abstract theories involving those concepts. Specifically, the development of herbal-related ideas and healing methods did not follow closely the structure of the so called "medicine of systematic correspondence," or, at least did not follow it as closely as acupuncture did.

–The essential paradigm of qi is mentioned since early times in the herbal literature, but it is usually described in terms of thermal properties. This opens up the idea that for the Bencao herbalist, qi had a character mostly experiential, intimately related to the interaction plant-person (or, in other words, Earth-Man) whilst the Suwen and Shanghanlun traditions tended to consider qi phenomena in terms of importing the celestial order to the human body, i.e., were centred on qi as agent of the Heaven-Man relationship. This difference also reflects the different consideration of the Man-Nature relationship present in what we schematize as Daoist and Confucian cosmovisions.[55]

This apparently loose relationship with the main medical and some systematic models did not mean that herbal medicine was only materially empirical. The emphasis on yi showed by some prominent physicians, as well as the repeated references to qi, jingluo, etc., clearly indicates that there were some features in herbal healing that transcend the simple accumulation of empirical illness-plant relationships, it reveals the existence of some healing paths and methods conceptually sound, but maybe so subtle as even to escape the possibility of putting them into words.[56]

In the main drug tradition and literature, with only the exceptions of the Suwen and the Shanghanlun, almost no mention is made of acupuncture general theories and/or treatments up to the Song dynasty. Even after those times, drug therapy and acupuncture seem to have evolved mostly separately, even when –as in the case of Li Shizhen– they were studied by the same individual.

## But there it was the Shanghanlun...

The main body of the big pharmaceutical traditions, including both the Bencao and the eclectic, were concerned with the properties of drugs and the details of the illnesses and symptoms they were useful for. But there is a completely separate approach, which, starting in the East Han era (202 BCE-220 CE), seems to try to contemplate the illness mechanisms in relation to a sort of "energetic" physiology[57] –directly relating channels[58] with zangfu– and to propose adequate remedies in the form of sophisticated, elaborate prescriptions. The first document we have received related to this vision of herbal medicine is the Shanghanlun [傷寒論], the work of Zhang Zhongjing [張仲景].

Zhangji [張機] (style name Zhongjing) lived from around 150 to 219 CE. We do not have documentary records about him or his medical training from his own time, although several legends tell us about his medical skills and scholarly works. We also ignore the real personal motives of Zhang Zhongjing to write his Shanghan Zabing Lun [傷寒雜病論] –his original work– although in its not fully authenticated preface, Zhang Zhongjing says he lost two thirds of his family to the continuous epidemics that were occurring in the country as a consequence of the continual war and strife associated with the politics of his time. The descriptions of the externally contracted illnesses –the subject of the book– and their treatment reflect a deep theoretical understanding of the Huangdi Neijing, the Nanjing and the Bencao Jing [31], but the texts he studied or that were actually available to him are not yet fully known.[59]

No matter which texts Zhang Zhongjing used to base his Shanghanlun, his strong influence in herbal medicine, as well as the often claimed idea of being the first attempt to tie herbal medicine with the medicine of systematic correspondence, make it necessary for us to examine this work in some detail, even if that means we have to go back to the last years of the Han Dynasty.

### *a) One book, many versions, strong influence*[60]

The original work, the Shanghan Zabing Lun covered a broad area, including the interpretation of pulse presentations, the damages caused by cold, the theory of six stages[61] pattern identification[62] and the treatment of a series of miscellaneous diseases, including the specific ailments afflicting women and children and even dietary contraindications [31]. It represents a major advance in the integration of theoretical knowledge with clinical observation and practice. Its focus was on the study of the attack of external pathogens –most notably wind and cold– through the channels and network vessels triggering disturbances of the bodily functions that can be recognized by distinct groups of signs and symptoms known as "patterns." It is then considered as the basis of diagnosis and treatment rooted in some kind of pattern identification, a way of medical thinking which, promoted since the Qing dynasty, becomes more and more important, and is now considered as the quintessence of Chinese medical genius.

The complete text of the Shanghan Zabing Lun didn't survive the turbulence of the period of the Three Kingdoms (220-265 BCE), but in the Western Jin period, an Imperial physician, Wang Shuhe [王叔和], besides including some elements of the Shanghanlun in his own Mai Jing [脈經] (Classic on the pulse),[63] collected, edited and collated Zhang Zhongjing's work. It is believed he organized the texts he could rescue in two books: the Shanghanlun [傷寒論] (Discussion of the damages caused by cold) (150-219), in which he put all that concerns the attack by external pathogens, and the Jingui Yaolue [金匱要略] (Prescriptions from the golden chest), in which he put what he could recover regarding the diagnosis and treatment of miscellaneous diseases.

The text of the Shanghanlun was not widely available in the Eastern Jin (256-479 CE) and Northern and Southern dynasties (479-581 CE).[64] In the

Tang dynasty (618-906 CE), Sun Simiao drew from it in his Beijiqianjin Yaofang [備急千金要方] (Prescriptions [more valuable] than thousand pieces of gold) (652 CE), but apparently the complete text was not available to him until later. When compiling the Qianjin yifang [千金翼方] (Wings to the Thousand Gold Pieces Prescriptions) probably around 682 CE, towards the end of his life, he included most of the text, and this therefore constitutes the earliest known version of the Shanghanlun.

Wang Tao [王燾] (707-772 CE) of the Tang dynasty, writing in his Waitai Miyao [外臺秘要] (Essentials secrets from outside the metropolis) quotes over 200 lines from the Shanghanlun and presents several pre-Tang writings discussing it. Both from Wang Tao's own words and by inference, we can see that the Shanghanlun continued influencing at least a certain group of medical practitioners and scholars.

In the Song dynasty (960-1179 CE), a Shanghanlun version supervised by Lin Yi [林億] was published by the Song's Medical Literature Editing Bureau, and taking advantage of the invention of the wood printing blocks, is supposed to have been diffused, at least among the more scholarly of the medical practitioners. Unfortunately, no copy of this first printing survives, and the earliest available is a Ming reprint of a text claimed to date from 1056, which, nonetheless, is believed to be identical. The term "Song version" now refers to this Ming reprinted version. This Song-Ming printed version is larger than most modern versions of the Shanghanlun, and some Ming scholars argued that the first four and last seven fascicles should be discarded because they contained matter that either did not relate to externally contracted illness, or that they are really more representative of Wangshuhe's thought than Zhang Zhongjing's [31].

### *b) The book itself*

In his original preface, Zhang Zhongjing mentioned a number of books he had studied. Of these, only the Suwen and the Nanjing have arrived to us, so the complete set of theories and works upon which Zhang Zhongjing built his own is not entirely clear. There are clearly concomitant passages in the Suwen showing that even heat diseases were there considered as provoked by cold (chapters five and thirty-one)[66] and considering the disease as progressing thorough the six channels (chapter fifty-two). Moreover, both books ascribe specific sets of symptoms to the disease of each of the (jing) stages or channels,[67] even if in the Shanghanlun the scope of the externally contracted illness is envisaged as having a much larger dimension. The Shanghanlun can be considered in this aspect even more rigorous than the Suwen, because, in associating heat and repletion patterns with the three yang stages and cold and vacuity signs with the three yin, it does a more systematic application of yin-yang theory. But there are some differences in the associations between jingmai and symptoms. For example, the signs given in the Suwen for a taiyang [太陽] disease are located in the corresponding channels pathway, but those given in the Shanghanlun are predominantly general exterior signs. Such differences prompted Mei Chunhua to comment, "One cannot use the six channels... of the Suwen to explain the six channels of Shanghanlun"[68] [31].

Also the timing and ways of passage of the pathogen thorough the channels are different, the ones given in the Shanghanlun more flexible and complex, probably because the concept of jing as stage is in itself broader than the Suwen's idea of jingluo. It is possible to think that, while the Suwen statements represent a neat theoretical scheme, Zhang Zhongjing worked from clinical observation [31] and wrote consequently. All in all, it is reasonable to conclude for instance, in the words of Wiseman, that, "although similarities do exist between the Shanghanlun and Suwen, they are only partial, and that however much Zhang Zhongjing drew on the Suwen, the Shanghanlun represents a thorough reworking of ideas contained in it" [31:7].

Of course, all that is without mentioning a major difference in the treatment methods. The Neijing provided more detail on needle therapy than on drugs, while the Shanghanlun proposed medicinal remedies almost exclusively, which is why we are dealing with the book here.

### *c) The Shanghanlun tradition*

Even before the Song edition, the Shanghanlun was repeatedly stated to be a very important work by influential figures in the development of Chinese medicine, although the book itself –if we are to believe Sun Simiao's statements– was jealously guarded by those who possessed copies[69] [31], or, in any case, wasn't largely distributed and known by the majority of practising physicians [15:11].[70]

In any case, after its printed publication, the Shanghanlun and its scholars made concerted efforts in the Song-Jin-Yuan dynasties to apply the yin-yang and five phases doctrines in the analysis of drug actions, so that Zhang Zhongjing was universally recognized as the "first to combine the use of drug therapy with the theory of systematic correspondence" [40:168].[71]

Even admitting this "revolutionary" character, it is probable that its revival in the Song dynasty was due to its being the only classical book dealing with epidemics [15:145]. Besides this specific feature, several ideas make the Shanghanlun a work well worth its reputation: the in-depth insights in cold damage, the diagnosis and treatment established in function of pattern identification (the six-stages pattern identification –which some understand as the precursors of the eight principle pattern identification, and zangfu pattern identification) and the treatment addressed to specific pathomechanisms rather than to the symptoms. We shall briefly review them.

**Shang han.** The concept of shang han ("damage by cold", or "cold damage") can be understood both in broad and narrow meanings. The Suwen already stated "now all heat diseases are of the cold damage kind". The fifty-eighth difficulty of the Nanjing stated, "There are five damages due to cold. They are wind stroke, damage by cold, damp warmth, heat disease, and warm disease". According to Zhang Zihe [張子和] (1156-1228 A.D), "all qi that is not right qi is called cold damage" [31]. Thus, the broad meaning of cold damage encompasses all the externally contracted diseases; the narrow meaning is just the external attack by wind-cold and the resultant diseases. The Shanghanlun provided considerable detail for everything related with the externally contracted wind-cold, but, more importantly, it dealt with cold damage in its broadest sense, discussing the six excesses as the cause of disease and combining internal and external factors in the analysis of pathomechanisms, symptoms and treatments.

The six-stages pattern identification and system. Zhang Zhongjing elaborated upon the astronomically derived system of six stages[72] (which he denominated as "jing"[經]) in a way which, sometimes appears coincident with the elaborate descriptions of the Suwen for the main twelve channels (termed "jingmai" [經脈]). He uses these terms to suggest a system in the human body which will be consistent, at least in name, with the more universal categories of taiyang, yangming, etc. In studying these categories as manifested in the human body, he takes them and gives each of them specific features, reactions and correspondences, which are sometimes coincident which the ones appearing in the Suwen, but differ from them also in many aspects. For instance, in Zhang Zhongjing's presentation, the taiyang "great yang" stage (which he denominates differently from the Suwen) controls the construction and defence and governs the exterior of the body, serving as the body's most external barrier. Thus, in the Shanghanlun model, the external pathogens usually attack first this taiyang stage or level [31]. Some, especially modern TCM books, have considered because of the use of the label "taiyang" that this can be seen in relation to the "taiyang" channels, the arm and leg taiyang channels (small intestine and bladder channels). Zhang Zhongjing elaborated in different ways how this protective level can be altered (wind damage, cold damage, transmuted patterns) studying the effects of the pathological changes first on the functional, qi level (pain, breathing, stiffness), and then on a more metabolic level, the zangfu tied with those channels, describing more material symptoms and patterns, like water amassment (taiyang xushui [太陽蓄水]) and blood amassment (taiyang xuxue [太陽蓄血]). The first stages of a taiyang disease are usually referred to as exterior repletion, but the irregular developments (transmuted patterns, bianzheng [變證]) and concurrent patterns, such as "exterior vacuity with concurrent water-rheum", are a mix of external and internal causes. For all of them Zhang Zhongjing gave adequate treatment, mostly based on herbal formulae, many of them still in use up to the present times. He then described with the same sort of detail the features of the other five stages, as well as their illnesses, symptoms and treatments.[73]

In brief, Zhang Zhongjing, while still partially following the Suwen in the admission of the existence of some sort of almost abstract human structure, uses it in a more flexible approach. Without explicitly stating which this structure is, he, nonetheless proposed that an externally contracted illness tends to follow a specific pathway in its attack on the body, and that the "typical" pathogenic penetration will probably follow an order (taiyang-yangming-shaoyang- taiyin- shaoyin- jueyin [太陽 - 陽明 - 少陽 - 太陰 - 少陰 - 厥陰]) determined by the different aspects or functions of qi ("energetic levels or stages") in the body. After his theoretical construction, we can see in an ordered, useful way, the interplay of the different pathogens (external and internal) and how they interact with the different systems and substances of the whole body.

Notwithstanding the differences with the Suwen, the structure of the Shanghanlun is more akin to what Goldschmidt terms "Classical Medicine" than any of the works of the Bencao tradition. Maybe this proximity was one of the factors favouring first its selection by the Song's Bureau for Revising Medical Texts, and later on, being the subject to the progressively deep intention of integrating herbal medicine with the Classical Medicine theories.[74]

**Eight principles pattern identification.** (Bagang bianzheng, [八綱辯證]) The notion of eight principles was not formalized until much later in history, but it is sometimes considered as already implicit in the Shanghanlun [31].[75] The six-stages pattern identification system provides a way to understand the development, consequences and signs of an external attack, but underlying the whole theory, the notions of exterior-interior, cold-heat, vacuity-repletion, in short, yin-yang relationships, are always present. Broadly speaking, the diseases of the three yang stages are characterized by the strong body resistance (strong zhengqi [正氣]) and exuberance of the pathogen (xieqi [邪氣]), and takes the form of heat excess, which following the eight principles will be considered a yang disease. By contrast, disease of the deeper three yin stages are characterized by debilitation of the zhengqi with the continuing presence of xieqi, and tend to show aspects of cold and vacuity, which on the eight principles will be characterized as yin disease. In the Shanghanlun special attention is given to adequately distinguish between the exterior-interior, cold-heat and vacuity-repletion couples, giving the clear indication that, although the eight principles are never mentioned as such, at least part of the theory they represent, with some of its implications, correlations, and abstractions, were already well know and considered by Zhang Zhongjing, who also succeed in integrating it with specific pharmacological methods of treatment.

This said, it is necessary to admit that the presence of the eight principles in the Shanghanlun is a controversial subject. The facts are, by one side, that the ba gang [八綱] did not appear explicitly until the twelfth century when it was first described by Xu Shuwei [15:163-166] and was then popularised by the Yixue Xinwu [醫學心悟] in 1732 [37:330]. But, on the other hand, it is clear that the concepts summarized in the ba gang (yin-yang, cold-heat, external-internal, excess-vacuity) are extensively used in the Shanghanlun, although they were never explicitly recognized, nor stated by Zhang Zhongjing in relation to the "ba gang". Even one of his much later commentators, Xu Shuwei, considered that the correct categories of the invasion by cold should not be the Six Stages, but the Eight Principles [15:166]. Besides this "ba gang controversy", the historical fact of the much later appearance of its codification does not negate the idea of the Shanghanlun representing a fundamental step in the rationalisation of herbal medicine, as well as in relating this form of healing with concepts like qi or jing understood as cosmological structures projected on the body, a clear difference from the concept of qi as human experience more related with the Bencao tradition. This change could be considered as a path to integrating the herbal medicine with the sophisticated classical postulates, in some ways pushing the theories of herbal medicine one level further beyond the more pragmatic herb-to-illness procedures of the Bencao approaches.

**Zangfu pattern identification** (zangfu bianzheng [臟腑辨證]). Like the eight principles pattern identification, the notion of viscera and bowel patterns and pattern identification was not developed until later in the evolution of Chinese medicine [31]. Yet it is a key feature of the Shanghanlun, which intimately relates the stages and their diseases with their corresponding "organs" and their dysfunctions. Once more, Zhang Zhongjing not only clearly refers the body functioning to a coordinated function of stages and "organs", but he states specific sets of signs and symptoms related to the whole, and proposes sophisticated herbal treatments for them.

**Treatment in relation to the pathogenic mechanism and pattern identification.** Another revolutionary medical idea of the Shanghanlun was the approach to treatment. Recognizing the difficulty of a successful treatment based on the variety of symptoms usually present in real clinical practice, Zhang Zhongjing not only established diagnosis processes allowing them to be grouped into more abstract patterns, but also, based on this conceptual integration, he also proposed treating the whole, the pattern, instead of the multiplicity of signs or symptoms [31]. By integrating any specific sign –like the floating pulse, for instance– into a larger group of signs and symptoms, he was able to differentiate its diagnostic value, and by designing a treatment of the whole pattern, he was able to establish treatment methods that not only aimed to address the core of the problem, but also to relieve in a very efficient manner the majority of the simultaneously present symptoms.

The Shanghanlun is fundamentally a drug based medical book. Although it makes reference to several different forms of treatment, including acupuncture, moxibustion, and steaming, the work is mainly and above all, about drug therapy. Only occasionally does Zhang Zhongjing suggest acupuncture, and several times he mentioned it as a treatment which a patient received previously with no results, or even with negative results.

The medicinal therapy applied by Zhang Zhongjing is based on the notion that each drug has specific properties, including its thermal nature and its preference for a concrete organ or stage that affect the body in a specific way [31]. The basic treatment, addressed to the pathomechanism and pattern, is then tailored to suit the majority of or the more important symptoms. As another seminal concept in herbalism, concomitant with what is expressed in the Nanjing, the stress of Zhang Zhongjing treatments was always placed on enhancing the body's power to dispel xieqi, evil qi; even in the diseases of the three yang stages the treatment is mostly directed to adjust the bodily functions so they become able to release or expel the pathogenic evil [31]. There are also other special features in the theories presented by Zhang Zhongjing, like the use of the terms yin and yang, the definition of prescriptions based on the pulse characteristics, or how the book approaches the subject of "jaundice" [31], but this is not the place for a more detailed analysis of the contents of the Shanghanlun and its" significance. The purpose of the current discussion is only to underscore the fact that there was already in the last part of the Han dynasty at least one great work linking drug therapies with some of the theories of systematic correspondences and its qi paradigm, although they were interpreted in a way which was basically more suitable to drug use than to manipulation of the channels or jingmai.

## A second set of conclusions

Taking into account the Shanghanlun, and its approach to illness and drug usage, both in large part very different to those presented in the Bencao, we can conclude the following:

a) In recognizing and using –although in a different way– concepts and theories of the medicine of systematic correspondences and relating them to pharmaceutical remedies, the Shanghanlun is the first received book to actually relate drug therapy with the qi concept in a detailed and practical way. This opened a way to a new herbal medicine, which being kept mostly discreet up to the Song dynasty, was afterwards expanded and manifested with great force, receiving a definitive bill-of-health thorough the Jin-Yuan period [40:168-169]. But either in the hands of a scholarly elite, or more largely diffused among some drug-using physicians, this line of thought didn't interact –or did it only barely– with the mainstream works on herbs, which for the most part continued revolving around the more empirically based traditions.

b) Although we don't really have any solid argument on why the Shanghanlun didn't have any strong influence in the practice of medicine before the mid-eleventh century, it is possible that this relatively low influence in the herbalism represented by the Bencao tradition and works were related to the possible resistance of this later tradition to anything resembling a formal –or perhaps perceived as too rigid– structure. This points to the fact that all the subsequent works in what –following Unschuld– I shall name "the Shanghanlun tradition" were written or mentioned by more or less state-related physicians, i.e., probably Confucian or Neoconfucian scholars.

c) The water and political metaphors, so cherished by the Confucians and their followers, were more applicable to the tradition of acupuncture and moxibustion than to the herbal therapies. The official body of scholars was by and large more dedicated to developing the qi concept and its theories in the field of acupuncture and moxibustion rather than in drugs therapy, which then became commonly the area of expertise for less structure-loving people. It remains a possibility that in the mind of the most enlightened among them, the goal of a rational use of drugs was closer to that of achieving a sort of mystical identification with the drugs themselves than to the projection of a suspicious structure upon the natural object. This offers a possible explanation why all efforts were focused on putting order in what they found,[76] rather than investigating any possible "intellectual" or subjacent structure. That would also explain why, although familiar as they were with all the usual ideas –qi included– found in the medical schools that employed the theory of systematic correspondences, they preferred to use them in a purely functional terms, presenting the channels as a regulatory and communications system, and talking about qi mostly by its functions.

## How does Chinese drug therapy relates with the qi paradigm and its theories?

After reading through the texts and history of Chinese Medicine in general and specifically on Chinese herbal therapy (or, more precisely, Chinese drug therapy), and comparing them with the evolution of the basic qi paradigms and theories in acupuncture, we can advance some ideas on the qi and herbs relationships.

Qi and qi-related concepts were –and are– extensively used in the definition and prescription of drugs, but these ideas seem to be employed there in a rather different way than in acupuncture. For example, acupuncture incorporates common cosmological models, and the idea of qi thus remains as some undefined characteristic or even a kind of immaterial fluid or substance, while in drugs therapy, the idea of "qi" tends to either define the effects of an interaction (the qi or the xing of the plants) or a relatively well defined set of functions in the body. However, this difference does not represent a theoretical inconsistency; following Birch and others [5:87-89, 49], we can understand "qi" as a general word broadly used throughout Chinese culture to refer to many different realities, a way to verbalise many different more or less abstract categories, functions or implications. We can safely say that both the acupuncture and herbal practitioner used the idea of qi, but they were using it in different ways, revealing here once more the very Chinese way of adapting a concept to the practicality of its use in a strongly syncretistic manner. Qi for the herbalists was very important, and they used this concept mostly in relationship with observable phenomena related to the human body. A good example of this concept is what is repeatedly presented as the qi of the plants, which is many times interchanged with the character "xing" [性] (nature, natural tendency). This qi-xing is described in thermal terms, but the thermometer used to make the classification is not a characteristic intrinsic to the plant itself, but rather a description of the reaction it provokes in the human body once the plant is ingested [37]. This understanding of qi in relation to human experience and thus consciousness was discussed in chapter one [4].

One of the forms in which the herbalist considered qi was as a way to conceptualise functions. There is nothing tangible in, for instance, piqi [脾氣] (spleen qi), but the term is a way of referring to a set of clearly defined metabolic actions and processes. As is usual in Chinese medicine, this does not represent a definition of 'pi", spleen metabolism, but offers a logic, a useful path to act upon its failure. The definition of qi, or the concept of qi of any zangfu, never appears as an independent category, being always linked to some symptom or sign which will offer a possibility of action. Here we must be careful in to remember the active nature of the Chinese functional models and be alert to avoid confounding these descriptions with explanatory models.[77] The Chinese models were not intended to build a physiology comparable to that of Western medicine, no more than they were defining an organ only by its weight or its anatomical position. When the scholar-physicians were grouping a specific set of bodily functions under the term of 'qi of this or that zangfu", what they were doing was just framing and focusing the possibilities and means of treatment.

The same goes for the jingluo. Although herbalists were familiar with this concept since the start of documented Chinese medicine, the way of evaluating their symptoms and signs, and, naturally, the way of treating their illnesses, was quite particular. Even Zhang Zhongjing, the pioneer of linking herbs and a kind of theory of energetic pathophysiology used the labels taiyang, shaoyang etc. in different ways than his acupuncturist colleagues. Remember the comment of Mei Chunhua when talking about this subject: "One cannot use the six channels ... of the Suwen to explain the six channels (levels) of the Shanghanlun" [31] and the comments in this same chapter about "jing" versus "jingmai".

If we link the idea of different concepts about qi and channels with the idea of relating drugs and humans, and add that the herbalist doctor does not usually interact physically with their patients like other therapists who place their hands to feel the body, locate the points etc, we might understand better why the concept of the channels is so different for the herbalist and the acupuncturist. The herbalist will palpate and evaluate the channels, but he won't attempt and thus be able to generally act directly upon them.[78] The channels, then, would be conceptualised by the herbalist basically along two ideas: as a kind of regulatory system, susceptible to suffer their own illnesses, and as communications pathways running to the interior of the body from its exterior and vice versa, able to both communicate the internal with the external and to reflect a common state of the interior and the surface. The literature starting with the Shanghanlun strongly points us to the first idea, while the books coming mainly from the Jin-Yuan period show a strong tendency to use the second concept. But, and this is very important, these two ideas were never in conflict. We find in many important books, like the Piweilun of Li Dongyuan, a consistent use of both concepts: jingluo as system and jingluo as passageways.[79]

Taking into account the strength and efficacy of the empirical tradition of drug therapy, why was it so important for the scholar-physicians to use the qi paradigm and its closely related notions? Why did they need to refer to these notions at all? This is, I think an interesting question, and one that I shouldn't like to see answered only in terms of cultural environment. Of course it is clear that, except for some "hard-nosed" herbalist, at least a part of the medicine of systematic correspondence was seeping into the drug therapists, offering in many cases better ways to design their treatments, or even to somewhat explain themselves to their customers.[80] Taking for this purpose concepts that were at the time part of even the layman's culture, the literature shows us in many instances an insistence on using concepts like qi and the jingluo which cannot be explained as just simple cultural or inter-technical contamination. The consistency of the use of these concepts, especially visible in authors like Li Gao and Li Shizhen, not to mention the same Zhang Zhongjing, must have been based on some assumptions about qi which they didn't bother to expose.[81]

I feel that finding a good answer to these questions is crucial for the survival of a genuine practice of Chinese Herbal Medicine. Based on all the above, I shall suggest some ideas as a way to advance in this path:

The qi of plants are of different nature -or have different characteristics, or represent different manifestations– than the qi of humans. One of the more visible differences is that "it" is slower, but basically both, humans and plants, participate in, are made of, manifest, qi. On this basis, the herbalist's thinking could have been: "plants and humans interact, and being of a different nature, their interactions might still be explained by the qi paradigm. If we can refine our understanding of qi interactions, we will surely have the possibility of improving the therapeutic value of drugs, improve the efficacy of herbs and drug prescriptions".

Medical history shows and underscores that the good use of herbs will always be depending upon yi [意], and its selection and effects will be many times difficult to explain, or, if explained, will appear as totally unrelated with common bio-chemical or even formal parameters.[82] Unfortunately, this way of using drugs would be, by its nature, the privilege of only a few enlightened practitioners. Medicine must be a craft, open for practice by craftsmen of different levels, and not reduced to an "esoteric" art accessible only to a few very special individuals. It was necessary then to look for a relatively down-to-earth way of selecting plants, of matching illness and remedy, a way which, being conceptually and technologically accessible, allowed the powerful healing possibilities of the natural world to be used by people less endowed than "the chosen few".

The theories of systematic correspondences and the reflection in the human body of some cosmological structuring concepts –like "jing"– will offer at least a working framework to meet the above. Admitting qi, zangfu, jingluo ideas, etc., and applying these concepts of plant-human interaction, the qi of plants could be described in terms of their "natural tendency" (xing), an inherent vital quality which would be manifest only when resonating with a more rapid or visible manifestation of qi, in this case, the human qi. The human qi will get the impulse of the plant's qi and integrate it into its own mechanisms, "accelerate" this plant's qi, making it more visible and manifest its influence as a change in its own functions. The interaction mechanism could be compared with the phenomenon of harmonics in physics, familiar to musicians, where a vibration of a specific frequency can awake, or reinforce vibrations in other frequencies to which there is some close relationships. In other terms, then, plants and humans will have the possibility of "resonating", and do it selectively, some plants resonating better than others with some specific parts of the human body. And what about the channels? The channels would represent to the herbalist a kind of carrier wave system (a carrier wave is both transported and transporter, like the fixed frequency of a radio station), the idea of the *locus* where this qi interaction will take place, the part of the human system more able to perceive and resonate with the qi of external stimuli, qi-xing of plants included.

None of this could have been known and expressed by the classics of herbal medicine, but it is a reasonable possibility that their insistence on using the rather complicated model offered by the cosmology or by theories of systematic correspondences could have been influenced by a common intuition about resonances –in itself an already known phenomenon at the times.[83] Then qi and the jingmai offered the best functional model to further investigate plant-human interactions, but it should be constructed and used in very different way that it was and is used in acupuncture. The herbalist should always consider a tangible Universe much larger than his acupuncturist colleague. He cannot so heavily prioritize the qi of the human body, but always has to consider it in intimate relationship with the larger reality of the surrounding matter/energy and its changes and tendencies. Qi and jing will be for the herbalist very broad categories, uniting by its commonality the man and the universe and allowing their interaction. This model or way of thinking about how herbal drug substances may have been thought about in terms of qi employs an idea that we saw in chapter one, that of resonance, "ganying" [感應]. It was argued that "ganying", resonance, is an important concept for how to understand the way that qi can manifest and act in the world [4]. I suggest here that the herbal therapist focuses on trying to establish a strong and appropriate "ganying", resonance between the patient, its illness, and herbal substances. This allows us a reasonable way for understanding the relationship of the herbs to the concept of qi, or at least how the concept of qi was used in herbal medicine thinking.[84]

## Conclusion

Drug usage has been historically proven by its effects, and especially in the West, has been considered mostly an empirical healing discipline. Nonetheless, there is in China an important body of knowledge which, starting with the Shanghanlun, structured the drug usage around a mostly cosmologically-based structure and its reflection within the human body, this reflection being many times coincident –at least terminologically– with the corresponding structures and functions clearly expressed in the evolving acupuncture theories.[85] On the whole, herbal medicine makes extensive use of the same basic concepts of Chinese medicine, but its more broad use and its expression thorough a material substance easily hide them. The West, already comfortable with herbal medicine when the contacts with China started, overlooked this theoretical substrate, applying to the Chinese herbs the same category of empiricism that were already being used in the classification of the therapeutic effects of its own herbal medicine. In the West herbal medicine evolved in a medicine of extracts, and the study of those extracts was the start of the modern synthetic medicines, so it was only logical that when the Chinese herbal medicine started to be diffused in the West, their proponents by and large used the same approach: the detailed examination of the Chinese herbs looking to identify and isolate the "active principle."[86] Even most of the present efforts of Chinese Medicine look to what is called the "integrated approach", which from a scientific point of view is simply a kind of recombining idea: trying to mix some Chinese plants with already accepted Western Pharmacology molecules, and see if we can have better medicines.[87] Of course, this cocktail medicine has some technical potential –and surely has a lot of commercial possibilities– but it continues to be based in the reductionist aspects of the older Newtonian- biophysics.[88]

This approach can be problematic. Chinese drug therapies, with their long and varied history, their extended uses and proven efficacy, were never subjected to chemical or biochemical analysis. But now we have these tools at our disposal, and the temptation to use –or overuse– them is great. However, before breaking apart the herbs in search of the Western-cherished "pharmacologic active principle", before freely taking out the "non-useful' components of classic formulae, let's stop for a moment and consider the possibilities opened by fresh, scientifically updated research in the less visible relationships we have with the rest of the universe. This is not a call for esotericism; chemical medicine works because its molecules chemically interact with similar, or in any case, closely related, molecules already present in the human body, which in itself is a good example of resonance. But there is much evidence that within us there are a lot of other systems which, although related to the biochemical manifestations, are of different natures, like electromagnetic processes, just to mention one already acknowledged in the West. A very important area of science, physics, is deeply questioning the validity of the currently dominant mechanistic models of the body, promoting other models that might fit better with older Chinese concepts:

> A look into the history of biology and biophysics shows that there have been alternative traditions to the molecular-reductionistic approach now dominant in these fields. In biology, during some periods, e.g. in the first half of this century –holistic or organismic approaches have been far from marginal, in some disciplines, such as developmental biology, even constituting the dominant trend [7:1].

Scientists working in this direction often don't accept the usual pragmatic molecular biology –and its technical derivative– biopharmacy –as science, rather they qualify molecular biology as "engineering, not science" (Primas, Hans, mentioned and referenced in [7]), and, admitting the unavoidable insufficiency of any description of nature and its phenomena, propose the framework of quantum physics for the study of the living organisms and life phenomena in what has been called "Holistic Biophysics."[89]

If we can admit the effects of a chemical drug, or of an electrical impulse, if, as many scientist start to do, we admit that life, illness, and even being-to-being interactions are in fact a lot more complex that a simple action of one molecule upon another, why could we not investigate other mechanisms and take advantage of the immense treasure we have at our disposal due to the work of the hundreds and thousands of scholars, physicians and laymen who worked with Chinese drug therapy through the centuries?

Chinese drug therapy was never based on the detailed analysis of chemical components; its proven efficacy came both from a long history of empirical findings and from a deep understanding of the commonality of the phenomena of life, the last expressed thorough a very useful paradigm, the qi, and a set of related practical models, including the jingluo, zangfu and fundamental fluids. If Chinese herbal therapy has to progress, and especially, if it doesn't want to be reduced to another kind of biochemical medicine, it has to go back to its basic paradigms, and update them following the best that modern science and technology can offer.[90] Meantime, let's just be careful...

## Bibliography

1- Berlanger CA. *The Chinese Herb Selection Guide*, Richmond, Ca. Phytotec, Databased Publishing Co., 1997.
2- Birch S. Chapter four: The Jingmai and qi –acupuncture perspectives. In this volume.
3- Birch S, Bovey M. Chapter eight: Qi, Jingmai –Scientific investigation of concepts based in traditional East Asian medicine: challenges to cross-paradigm research. In this volume.
4- Birch S, Cabrer Mir MA, Rodriguez M. Chapter one: Qi and the mind –explorations of the links between qi, the mind, mental and emotional states. In this volume.
5- Birch S, Felt R. *Understanding Acupuncture*, London, Churchill Livingstone, 1999.
6- Birch S, Rodriguez M, Cabrer Mir MA. Chapter two: The jingmai –a summary of their development and nature. In this volume.
7- Bischof M. *Field concepts and the emergence of a Holistic Biophysics.* in Belossov LV, Popp FA, Voeikov VL, Van Wijk R (eds.) Biophotonics and coherent systems, Moscow University Press, Moscow 2000, pp. 1-25.
8- Brooks NR. Hope Springs Eternal Biotech Firm Wants to Grow Herbal Medicine Business. See http://www.aegis.com/news/Lt/1997/LT970108.html.
9- Buriani A, Garcia-Bermejo ML, Bosisio E, Xu QH, Li HG, Dong XB, Simmonds MSJ, Carrara M, Tejedor M, Lucio- Cazana J, Hylands PJ. Omic techniques in systems biology approaches to traditional Chinese medicine research: Present and future. *Journal of Ethnopharmacology* 2012;140:535–544.
10- Cabrer Mir MA. Chapter seven: Qi and stillness –Taijiquan, qigong and acupuncture. In this volume.

11- Chace C. Wild at Heart. Dongyuan's Acupuncture Model for Treating Complex Conditions. Unpublished, 2008.
12- Chace C, Bensky D. Chapter five: An axis of efficacy. The range of meaning in chapter one of the Lingshu. In this volume.
13- Dai JY, Sun SJ, Cao HJ, Zheng NN, Wang WY, Gou XJ, Su SB, Zhang YY. Applications of New Technologies and New Methods in ZHENG Differentiation. *Evidence-Based Complementary and Alternative Medicine Volume* 2012, Article ID 298014, 8 pages.
14- Farmer S, Henderson JB, Witzel M. *Neurobiology, Layered Texts, and correlative Cosmologies: A Cross-Cultural Framework for Premodern History*. Bulletin of the Museum of Far East Antiquities 72 2000 [2002] 48-90.
15- Goldshmidt, A. *The Evolution of Chinese Medicine*. Song Dynasty, 960-1200. Abingdon, Routledge, 2009.
16- Hamburg MA, Collins FS. The Path to Personalized Medicine. *New Engl J Med* 2010;363(4):301-304.
17- Harper D. *The "Wu Shih Erh Ping Fang": Translation and Prolegomena*. PhD Thesis, Berkeley, University of California, 1982.
18- Harper D. *Early Chinese Literature. The Mawangdui Medical Manuscripts,* New York, Columbia University Press, 1998.
19- Holloway KW. *Guodian*, Oxford University Press, New York, 2009.
20- Jiang M, Lu C, Zhang C, Yang J, Tan Y, Lu AP, Chan K. Syndrome differentiation in modern research of traditional Chinese medicine. *Journal of Ethnopharmacology* 2012;140:634–642.
21- Jiang M, Zhang C, Zheng G, Guo HT, Li L, Yang J, Lu C, Jia W, Lu AP. Traditional Chinese Medicine Zheng in the Era of Evidence-Based Medicine: A Literature Analysis. *Evidence-Based Complementary and Alternative Medicine* Volume 2012, Article ID 409568, 9 pages.
22- Jullien F. *The propensity of things*, Urzone Inc., New York, 1995
23- Le Blanc C. *Huai-nan Tzu. The Idea of Resonance (Kan-Ying)* With a Transltion and Analysis of Chapter Six. Hong Kong University Press, Hong Kong, 1985.
24- Levi J, Galvany A. *Elogio de la anarquía por dos excéntricos chinos*, Pepitas de calabaza Ed., Logroño (Spain) 2009.
25- Lewin R. *Complexity: Life at the Edge of Chaos*, London, Phoenix, 2003.
26- Li Dongyuan. *Treatise on the Spleen and Stomach*. Translated by Yang Shouzhong. Boulder, Blue Poppy Press, 1997.
27- Li JW, Lin SS. Zhongguo Yixue Tongshi. Gudaijuan. Zhongguo Renmin Weisheng Chubanshe, 2000.
28- Lin LL, Wang YH, Lai CY, Chau CL, Su GC, Yang CY, Lou SY, Chen SK, Hsu KH, Lai YL, Wu WM, Huang JL, Liao CH, Juan HF. Systems biology of meridians, acupoints, and chinese herbs in disease. *eCAM*. 2012;2012:372670
29- Lu AP. *Science*, Vol 338, 21 Dec.2012, pages 1653-1654.
30- Lu X, *Selected Works*. Foreign Languages Press, Beijing 1956.
31- Mitchell C, Feng Y, Wiseman N. Shanghanlun, *On Cold Damage*, Brookline, Paradigm Publications, 1999.

32- Nicholson JK. Global systems biology, personalized medicine and molecular epidemiology. *Molecular Systems Biology* 3 October, 2006; 6 pages. doi:10.1038/msb4100095.
33- Rosenthal MM. *Health Care in the People's Republic of China*. Boulder, Westview Press, 1987.
34- Rubin VA. I*ndividual and State in Ancient China*, New York, Columbia University Press, 1976.
35- Scheid V. *Patterns, syndromes, types: who should we be and shat should we do?* Eur J Oriental Med. 2013;7(3):10-21.
36- Scheid V, Bensky D. Medicine as signification. *European J Orien Med*, 1999:2, 6:32-40.
37- Sivin N. *Traditional Medicine in Contemporary China*, Ann Arbor, Center for Chinese Studies, University of Michigan, 1987.
38- Sommers D. Chapter three: How to become a shang yi or "superior physician," An exploration on the influence of the practitioner in early China. In this volume.
39- Tsutani K. *The evaluation of herbal medicines: an East Asian perspective*. In Lewith GT, Aldridge D. (eds). Clinical Research Methodology for Complementary Therapies. London, Hodder and Stoughton, 1993, pp.365-393.
40- Unschuld PU. *Medicine in China, A History of Ideas*. Berkeley, University of California Press, 1985.
41- Unschuld PU. *Medicine in China, A History of Pharmaceutics*. Berkeley, University of California Press, 1986.
42- Unschuld PU. *Forgotten traditions of Ancient Chinese Medicine*, Paradigm Publications, Brookline, MA, 1990.
43- Unschuld PU. *Huang Di Nei Jing Su Wen –nature, knowledge, imagery in an ancient Chinese medical text*. Berkeley, University of California Press, 2003.
44- Unschuld PU. *La sabiduría de curación china*, Barcelona, La liebre de Marzo, 2004.
45- Wang ZG, Chen P, Xie PP. *History and development of Traditional Chinese Medicine*, Beijing, Science Press, 1999.
46- Wu XF. (editor), *Traditional Chinese Diagnostics*, China Chinese Medicine and Pharmacology Press, (Zhongyi Zhentuanxue, Wu Xiufen (editor), Zhongguo Zhongyiyao Chubanshe), Beijing, 1994].
47- Yang SZ. *The Pulse Classic*. A translation of the Mai Jing by Wang Shuhe. Blue Poppy Press, Boulder, CO, 1997
48- Yin HH, Shuai XZ. *Fundamentals of Traditional Chinese Medicine*, Foreign Languages Press, Beijing, 1992
49- Zhang YH, Rose K. *A Brief History of Qi*. Brookline, Paradigm Publications, 2001.
50- Zhang Zhongji, *Shanghanlun*, Renmin weisheng chubanshe, Beijing,1985

# Endnotes

1. I am perfectly aware that in using those words I am just projecting some pure modern Western concepts into the multifaceted and varied old Chinese ways of thought, but a detailed discussion of Chinese "real" thought processes versus modern Eastern projections of them would be now irrelevant to the main purpose of this chapter.

2. Although the Chinese Pharmacopoeia includes mineral and animal substances, the bulk of Chinese material medica is of a vegetal origin, and this is probably the reason why, even since classic times, it is usual to refer to the whole Chinese pharmaceutical panoply as "herbs". I shall, then, use here both terms, "drugs" and "herbs", interchangeably.

3. A good modern example of this tendency is the book of Charles Berlanguer [1]. Also Unschuld suggest a strong current of undiluted pragmatism in the use of pharmacological remedies [44: 80 and following].

4. Just think of the continuous reference to the Neijing made by the masters of the Four Great Schools in the Jin-Yuan period

5. In the modern period economic and political forces are driving the agenda with regards how Chinese herbal medicine is viewed. In the late 1800s in Japan as the country went through the Meiji Restoration, herbal medicine was placed solely under the domain of Western trained medical doctors [5:40], a law changed later just to include people trained in Western pharmacy. Starting in 1976 many traditional herbal prescriptions were grandfathered so that they became reimbursable within the national health care system in Japan if appropriately prescribed [39:377]. Thus herbal medicine in Japan (Kampo) falls mostly within the domains of the pharmaceutical industry and Western medical system and is commonly prescribed and utilized [39]. While the political process in China has been different, by the mid 1980s the export of herbal medicine had become a significant *export trade* for China [33:159-161]. Since China's economic revitalization initiated by Deng Xiaoping, it has slipped back considerably in terms of its import value. However, possibly as a compensation for this, the Chinese government has been investing heavily in research to investigate and develop patentable herbal products or herb derived products that can be sold on the international market. In the 1990s they invested in the WHO sponsored research into the "pharmaprinting" method [8]. The Chinese government like the Japanese before them, are essentially stripping the unique conceptual and historical values out of the medicines so that they can be widely employed and made profitable within a predominantly Western medical framework.

6. The distinction (which I took from Unschuld, see [41:5 and on]) although useful for this study, is formal and purely artificial. As we will see, the herbal tradition is one of interweaving theories, methods and knowledge, so there is always some structure even in the most empirical manuals and a lot of purely empirical knowledge reflected into the most sophisticated works of the structuring tradition.

7. See [15:11+ 14+ 18+ 70+ 72+ 92+ 141].

8. This is mostly true from the second half of Song Dynasty and on. Before that time, medicine tended to be considered as a low class activity. See, for instance, [15:20], although the whole Part I of this same Goldschmidt book is entirely dedicated to this subject.

9. We have some brilliant examples that, at least some of them were using fundamentally the concept of "yi" [意], instead of theories more related to timing or to hydraulic metaphors, less convenient to herbalism than to acupuncture. See below, in this same chapter.

10. The name of this first book (Bencao, which could be translated now as "[Compendia of] roots and herbs") for reasons still unclear, become also a common name for the generic for at least some styles of herbal medicine activity, as well as for pharmacy and drug based methods of prolonging life and fighting illness.

11. This text was first translated by Donald Harper as his doctoral thesis [17] and then published in his text on the Mawangdui medical texts (see in bibliography [18].

12. For more detailed explanations about the evolution of Chinese healing arts, see, for instance Unschuld [41, 44], or Sivin, [37].

13. The historiographic references don't allow us to exactly confirm when those two characters originated, although we know that "毉" appears already in oracular writings, which is not the case of "醫." Both characters appear in texts before the Qin era, and although it is supposed they have a common origin, gradually they acquired different connotations. This evolution towards differentiation seems more marked since the Warring States period, and the difference of meanings appears already clear over the Qin and Han Dynasties: The Liji [禮記] gives to the physician the right to use medicinal substances: "you must not ingest medicinal substances from a doctor which has not been [at least] practising by three generations. The Zhouli [周禮] also refers the use of toxic substances by the physicians [醫]. Also the Guanzi [管子] says the doctors [醫] do some divinatory practices [27:62]. Xushen incorporates both signs in his Shuowen Jiezi, [說文解字] defining [醫] as "the craftsman treating illnesses" [Xushen. Shuowen Jiezi. Zhonghua Shuju: 313].

14. In fact, we know that at least at a popular level, healing concoctions might include purely magic components even in 20th Century China, as illustrated by Lu Xun's short history "Medicine" [30].

15. Shamans used drugs in several forms: potions, vapours, fumes, pills, pastes, liquids, talismans, etc. As the distinction between diverse pharmaceutical forms is not useful for the purpose of this paper, I shall use the term "potions" implying not only the potions in its material sense, but including any other form of drug preparation.

16. See Mencius and the Daquan Yijing [大全易經] (Great Commentary on the Book of Changes), as mentioned by Unschuld [41].

17. The book mentioned, the Shennong Huangdi Shijin appears only in a section of bibliography of the Hanshu, a book of Han history. The contents are unknown, but it might have been a manual on dietetics. [41].

18. "Most of the manuscripts are thought to have been copied nearer to 200 BCE. than to the date of burial" [38].

19. For a complete and commented transcription of Mawangdui's findings, see Harper [38].

20. For a more detailed history of this part of the Chinese Pharmaceutical tradition, see Unschuld [41].

21. Goldschmidt put the publication of this first Bencao Jing in the late first or the second century CE, although also stating that the original text did not survive. [15:105].

22. To avoid confusion between cosmological models and systematic correspondences models, I chose here to temporarily ignore the first ones, which will be more explicit in the other broad herbal tradition, the one documented with the Shanghanlun as its starting point.

23. See Sivin [37:178] and Unschuld, [41:15].

24. "The paradigm of systematic correspondence is almost completely missing in the Benjing. … the drugs are brought into relation to yin and yang in a brief section of the first chapter. This categorization, however, was probably based upon primary observations rather than upon an abstract theory…" [41:26].

25. Sivin states that in these descriptions "It is obvious that something more than sense impressions are involved" [37:182]. However, although Sivin's arguments has its merits, the fact remains that there are not in the Shennong any attempt of deducing or relating any properties of the drugs with its "qi", whatever the grade of abstraction we want to understand the Bencao implies with this word.

26. With the data currently available, we can hypothesize then that both, the Bencao Jing and the Suwen, were most likely compiled around the same time, which, having in mind the contemporary social structure, also make probable –or at least possible– that the compilers of one of them were familiar with the theories expounded in the other. Why then the "Bencao gentlemen" –as the herbal physicians were known– chose to ignore the new medical paradigms? Why the Suwen compilers "tended a hand" to their herbal colleagues –and possible competitors? Maybe the inconsistence of the medical literature is a reflection of the already old "state/Confucian versus individual/Daoist" conflicting ways of seeing the world (Weltanschauung) considered by some as so characteristic of that time in China [34]. We can only speculate.

27. See Unschuld, [41].

28. This is a model that is clearly articulated in the Suwen (chapter sixty-three) where is describes the penetration of xieqi into the body through the skin, into the sunluomai then the luomai then the jingmai then to the organs [43:171], see also chapter two above [6].

29. See the previous note which suggests that his description of how the jingluo were affected by pathogens to affect the organs is very similar to that of the Suwen.

30. If we choose to support the idea of two conflicting cosmovisions –very schematically, Daoism and Confucianism- and their rather different metaphors and social proposals, we could imagine that maybe the Daoist tendencies of Tao Hongjing make him disdain the sort of state/Confucian metaphors and concepts sometimes implied by these works. Also, in considering the qi of the plants in terms of thermal properties, he also pointed to "qi" as an experiential phenomenon, describing the effect, the feeling, the user will get out of the ingestion of the plant, and not considering "qi" as an intrinsic feature of the herb, iso-lated from the rest of the Universe . This idea of qi will also be consistent with the Daoist tendencies of Tao Hongjing.

31. Here is not the place to delve into these books or detailing its contents. For more details, see Unschuld [41].

32. The authorship of this book is not yet firmly established. See Unschuld [41:106].

33. For a translation of the text see Li [26].

34. Chace considers that "the acupuncture material in the Piwei lun must be understood both as a theoretical basis for herbal practice as well as an incisive strategy for treating complex conditions with acupuncture" [11].

35. For example the Huangdi Neijing corpus is attributed by name to the mythical "Huangdi" of many centuries before. The "Nanjing" is attributed to Bianque a famous physician of questionable origins, in any case placed several centuries earlier. This manner of attributing authority to the ideas through historical references can be seen to have a long-standing tradition in the medical literature.

36. See Goldschmidt [15:181].

37. See Goldschmidt [15:185-188].

38. Goldschmidt [15:184].

39. Goldschmidt [15:195].

40. Goldschmidt [15:196].

41. Goldschmidt [15:198].

42. Chapter one developed the evidence showing that in its early uses as the medical literature was being developed, qi was often seen in relation to different sensory experiences [4]. It was thus natural that this way of thinking about qi would be found in relation to early herbal medical descriptions, and also natural in a way that it would prove insufficient to understand the effects of the herbs, many of which lie outside sensory experiences or at least classifiable sensory experiences.

43. As we will see below, this empiricism were not only about historically collected information; in the assessment of the patient's condition and in the definition of the adequate drug, the use of "yi" [意], a subtle category tied with concepts such as shen, qi, signification, etc. was signalled to be essential for the healing practice by physicians as significant as Sun Simiao and Xu Yinzong (see [35:14]).

44. See the categories listed in each monograph, one of which is "qi wei" [41].

45. Mutual inter-influence meaning that drugs can be influenced by climatic factors, and also they can influence the climatic factors when they act as xieqi.

46. This apparent contradiction suggest an interesting question, the core of which could be the consideration that herbalism and acupuncture were using the same words and basically the same conceptual framework, but they were using them in their own, different, way. For instance, what an herbalist understood as "qi" could have been a very large and multifacetic group of features identifying a specific matter, including its intrinsic nature –mineral, animal, or plant, for instance, but also its *locus* in the universe (or, in a specific use, the effect it can cause when interacting with the human body). The qi of the herbal medicine would be a complete definition of a specific piece of matter in the universe, including its intimate nature and its relationships (the effect of the plant in the body will be then part of this plant's qi), and this concept will match only marginally the acupuncturist's use of the concept, not to mention their restricted –although useful– ideas of "channels" or their repeated hydro-metaphors.

47. The Bencao Jing already classified the drugs in three main groups, mainly taking into account their toxicity: the ones of the higher sort, without any toxicity, the ones of the middle sort, which can be toxic or not, and the ones of the lower sort, which are mostly toxic [37:181].

48. Unschuld translated Xu Dachun's "Yixue Yuan Liulun", where Xu Dachun discussed qi as one of the foundations of life [42:8] and discussed the channels [42:59-60].

49. See Scheid and Bensky [36:35].

50. Qianjin yaofang [千金要方] (Thousand Ducat Formulas), Sun Simiao, 652 CE, juan 1.4, zhen hou ("Diagnosing and reflecting). Edition used is Li Jing Rong et al. (editors), Qianjin yaofangjiashi 1998. Beijing; Renmin weisheng chubanshe, 5. 5. Mentioned in [36:35].

51. Xu Yinzong incidentally offers here and in the conclusion of his paragraph one possible reason why we do not have many theoretical studies about herbal medicine. There seems to have existed among the herbalist a line of thought considering that the real subtleties of the craft of healing were not approachable by words, a concept which is very consistent with Daoist ideas, as shown in Zhuangzi [A.C. Graham, Chuang-tzu: The seven inner chapters and other writings from the book "Chuang-tzu".1981. London: Allen & Unwin, 48 f.], and therefore writing about it would not be useful and could even be misleading.

52. Jiu Tang shu: Xu Yinzong chuan ("History of the former Tang: Xu Yinzong"), cited in Ma Boying, 1993, 779, Mentioned in [36:36].

53. Chuanya neibian [串雅內編] ("Connecting elegance: core section") Zhao Xuemin [趙學敏]. 18th cent. Zhulun ("Introduction"). Edition used is He Yuan (editor), Chuanya quanshu.1998, Beijing Chuanya quanshu, 1988. Beijing; Zhongguo Zhongyiyao chubanshe, 5. Mentioned in [36:35].

54. For more extensive discussion on yi and Chinese medicine, see the paper by Scheid and Bensky [36] and chapters one, three, four and five [2, 4, 12, 38].

55. The idea of two separate schools of thought under the name or theories of "Daoism" and "Confucianism" is only an artifact of Western way of classify the things. In fact current evidence points to the complementarity of both trains of thought. As a simple example, the Neiye, considered a very Daoist text, is a set of advices and admonitions to a ruler to be more fair and efficient, a typical "Confucianist" endeavour, while the books of Kong Zi continually remind the reader the need for reaching and practising the Dao. See, for instance Jullien [22:179 and note 9 of Chapter 9], see also [19:5-8]. Nevertheless, we have documented evidence of controversies confronting two largely different sociophilosophic standpoints, one supporting structure, hierarchies and a kind of imposed order, and the other defending the return to a "Golden Age" where no authority or State was needed [24:10].

56. The consideration of the study and practice of medicine changed clearly during the Song period. Adding to the revolutionary intent of making herbal practice cohere with the Classical doctrines, and possibly due to the personal involvement of some Song Emperors, not only did medicine become a respectable craft, but also the physician acquired the level of what Sivin says "amateur ideal", i.e., someone whose skills and goals were subordinate to a way of life. The requirements of the physician thus involved not only technical skills and knowledge, but also a good deal of self-cultivation. On this period, Sivin writes: "Only a moral (and to be sure, social) paragon for whom medicine was a facet of self-cultivation could fully comprehend the unity of body, mind, ambiance and moral life that constituted true health" (Sivin, N. Ailment and Cure in Traditional China, unpublished manuscript) see [15:182]. Clearly, this emphasis on self-cultivation will contextualize some of the more subtle aspects of medicine, namely, the cultivation and use of mental-spiritual abilities, like shen and yi.

57. I want to clarify that this term does not mean any affirmation or opinion about the "energetic" nature of qi and channels, but that I employed it just to underline the difference between Chinese physiology –which take into account categories like qi, shen or jingluo– with any organ-and-fluids-only physiology, like the one currently taught in Western medicine.

58. See note 61 on the term "jing" "channels". The "jing" in the Shanghanlun very probably are more related with astronomical and cosmological concepts that the jingmai or jingluo appearing in the Suwen, the first book in which this cosmological category (jing) is expressed in terms of and in relationship with a previously known human physio-anatomical element, the "mai."

59. One possible source for Zhongjing could have been the Tangye Bencao [湯液本草] of Wang Haogu [王好古], a partially reconstructed work which some people now think was the basis for Zhang's thought [Chace, personal communication, 2009].

60. It is important to remember that this influence was only real after the compilation and diffusion of Zhang's work starting in the mid-eleventh century. The reasons why those texts (there were three versions of it by the time of its compilation) and the history of its promotion and diffusion are the subject of chapters 3 and 5 in Goldschmidt's book on the evolution of Chinese Medicine in the Song dynasty [15].

61. There is a discussion about what term should be used here. Zhang Zhongjing himself always wrote "jing"[經] in reference to these six aspects (see [50]). Mitchell, Fengye and Wiseman choose to translate this "jing" as "channel" [31], but the meaning of "jing" in the Shanghanlun cannot be directly assimilated with other meanings of the word in other medical texts, like the Suwen or the Nanjing, even if it was only because the term in these texts usually refers either to the jingmai or jingluo. The origin of the idea of the six "X" (jing) is rooted in astronomical concepts, and is not very closely related with other theories more akin to acupuncture, like five phases or jingmai. In studying modern TCM, I had been told about "the six levels", but the texts of Chinese origin also translate "jing" as "meridians" (see, for instance: [48] and [46]). Sivin translates the Shanghanlun's "jing" as "warps" [37:80], directly relating them with the textile metaphor, thus giving to the term a sense of static structure which I do not completely feel adequate to the Zhongji's dynamic concepts, so we also discarded this option. Trying to escape from the trap of identifying the Shanhanlun's "jing" with the Neijing-Nanjing's "jing", we discussed at length with Stephen Birch which term should I use. Other than "channels" or "meridians", which we agree to avoid for the above reasons, we evaluate "level" and "stage", finally deciding for "stage" because, when using the word "jing", Zhongji is always talking about an evolving situation, like the progression of an illness, and is not defining a static structure or speculating about a kind of "energetic anatomy", like the term "level" seems to suggest. For a more detailed discussion in the origin and meaning of this six "X", see Sivin [37:80-87].

62. As we will see it is debatable as to whether Zhangji's choice of terms like "taiyang", "shaoyang", etc can be understood in relation to the Neijing's adoption of these terms with reference to the channels (e.g. "shou taiyang", "zu shaoyang", etc) [37]. See below for further discussion.

63. The date varies after different historians: some time in the second century CE, after Yang Shouzhong version [47], circa 280 after Sivin [37:87]. For a translation of the text see Yang [47].

64. Goldschmidt states that none of the "Great Classics", i.e. the Huangdi Neijing, the Nanjing or the same Shanghanlun, were easily available before the Song times. [15:26].

65. For a more detailed discussion in how the Shanghanlun become rescued, compiled and diffused in the Song dynasty, see Goldschmidt, A. [15], especially chapters 3 and 6.

66. This comes from the section 31, Relun [熱論] (Discussion of Heat disorders) describing the development of acute febrile diseases as the external pathogen enters the body [15: 95]. For larger discussion on the relationship between the Suwen and the Shanghanlun, see Mitchell et al. [31].

67. See previous notes on the use of the term "channels" in the context of the Shanghanlun.

68. Maybe the same texts gives us a clue: while the Shanghanlun always use the term "jing", the Suwen uses frequently the term "jingmai", uniting for the first time the cosmological "jing" with the human "mai" (see chapter two in this book). Before the Suwen the term "mai" was always used in a clearly human anatomy context, whilst the term "jing" is more ancient and used in esoteric and cosmological texts, so it is highly probable that the jingmai of the Suwen (an innovation in itself) and the jing of the Shanghanlun were actually different concepts, although presenting numerous coincidences due both of its common origins and to the commonality of the ground of its application: the human body. See chapter two and four for further discussions [2, 6].

69. We do not really know the reasons of this lack of diffusion. Maybe it was because its more advanced vision gave the physicians using the Shanghanlun a competitive advantage over the physicians of the Bencao tradition.

70. It seems some different opinions exist about the influence of the Shanghanlun in the period between the Han and the Song dynasties. As Mitchell and Wiseman say that during this period it was already appreciated as a very important work [31], Goldschmidt repeatedly states that the book was then practically unknown by the vast majority of physicians: "It seems that most physicians during the centuries following the third century CE until the eleventh century were not familiar with the Treatise. Even when medical authors mentioned Cold Damage Disorders they failed to cite Zhang Zhongjing or his book" [15:97] even stating that it was recorded as a lost book in the history of the Sui dynasty [15:97].

71. This point is open to controversy. Although Zhang Zhongjing mentions in the preface of the Shanghanlun that he studied the Suwen –from which we can assume he was familiar with concepts such as the five phases– the truth is that in his book he ignored many of the theories presented there. Sivin cites Otsuka Keisetsu (a deep scholar of the Shanghanlun) that the Shanghanlun "not only ignores the circulation tracts and the visceral systems of function, but does not even refer to the Five Phases" [37:87]. This does not

mean that Zhang Zhongjing did not think in terms conceptually similar to the ones collected in the Suwen; Otsuka, after studying all the surviving fragments of the author's other writings, also concludes "Zhang was a physician in the tradition of the Inner Cannon who acknowledges [in his preface] the importance he accorded to the world-view –absent from the text of the Treatise– of which the Five Phases theory, the visceral systems of function, and the circulation tract systems form parts" (Otsuka cited by Sivin [37:88]).

72. See chapter two for some discussion of this [6].

73. For more on the six stages, see Mitchell et al. [31].

74. This integration was a progressive advance. Some landmarks are:
–Zhu Gong. (died 1108) Nanyang Huoren Shu [南陽活人書] (The Book for Saving Lives as at Nanyang), 1108. He states by the first time during the Song dynasty a definite connection between the twelve tracts and the pathology of Cold Damage Disorders [15:159]. It can be considered as the first attempt to integrate the classical doctrines with Cold Damage doctrines [15:163].
–Xu Shuwei (1079-1154). Wrote several books mentioning and suggesting clinical uses of the Shanghanlun. We can highlight the Shanghan bai zheng ge [傷寒百證歌] (One Hundred Mnemonic Verses on Cold Damage Manifestations), which has the merit of being "the first attempt, although perfunctory, to annotate the Song Treatise by using classical canons" [15:164].
–Cheng Wuji. Zhu jie shanghanlun [注解傷寒論] (Annotations on the Treatise of Cold Damage), 1172 With extensive references to the Huangdi Neijing and to the Nanjing, it seems he regarded these classical texts as the doctrinal base explaining Cold Damage Disorders [15:168].

75. The eight principles were first described as such by Xu Shuwei in the twelfth century [15:163-166] and were popularized by Cheng Guopeng [程國彭] in the Yixue Xinwu [醫學心悟] of 1732 [37:330]. The idea of its appearance in the Shanghanlun is probably just a projection of the admiration this work receives.

76. See discussions in chapters one, two, three and four [2, 4, 6, 38].

77. The difficulty of ascribing "explanatory" functions to Chinese models is discussed in Chapters one and eight [3, 4].

78. I am excluding here the application of drugs directly on the skin, which represents only a minor, rather specialized, part of herbal medicine.

79. This concept of the "passageways" needs to be clarified. There is nothing allowing us to suppose the Chinese thought of zangfu and related jingluo as separate realities. On the contrary, all evidence points to the idea of the zangfu and jingluo were considered just different manifestations of the same system, both being closely related to qi (or qi in one of its many as-needed definitions). The concept allows a unification of the more material

and internal aspects of human functions with its more subtle and superficial aspects. The different uses and meanings of the jingmai are discussed in chapters two and four [2, 6].

80. Today in the West it would be almost impossible to prescribe anything to a patient without offering him/her a kind of explanation. Curiously enough, it seems that any type of explanation will do: "energies", five phases, whatever. Probably this has to do, among other things, with establishing a confidence relationship between the patient and the therapist, to give the former the idea that the latter understands his/hers problems, even if he/she fails to follow the therapist" logic. Patients need to confide in the therapist. If we imagine that need being present also in some of the better educated patients of doctors like Zhu Danxi, among many others, we can admit that they might have used the paradigms of theory of systematic correspondence also as an explanation of their treatments.

81. We cannot discard here the possible influence of other evolutions of non-medical thought and/or cosmovision, like a movement towards reconciling different concepts about the structure of the universe, which could be even ingrained in our most inner brain mechanisms. See details in [14].

82. See, for instance, the anecdote of Hua Shou [滑壽], a famous Ming dynasty physician, were he facilitated a labour prescribing a decoction of wutong leaves, a selection he explained just in terms of qi movement and seasonal analogies [36:37]. Note that wutong –Chinese parasol tree, botanically Firminia simplex (L.) W.F.Wight, or platanifolia– is seldom employed in medical applications, and in any case, the uses of the concoction of its leaves are as a salve in treating carbuncles, sores or hemorroids.

83. In fact, as Le Blanc says, resonance is one of the more important ideas appearing in the Huainanzi: "One topic stands out as pivotal in Huai-nan Tzu, namely the idea of 'stimulus and response', or more simply, 'resonance'" [23:8].

84. In this way of thinking we can then see that the acupuncturist by contrast is especially interested in trying to find the right "ji" [機] or "mechanism" or "dynamic" and getting the dynamic of qi movements timed just right with the use of the needle in order to trigger the desired changes. The "ji", dynamic/mechanism is discussed in chapter one above. Putting these ideas together, and in the words of S. Birch: "yi is fundamental to medicine, it is a property of the mind to welcome the qi (in needling) and to intuit or feel the resonance of the herbs and patient so that they can be properly matched. Qi is fundamental in both cases and basically the two fundamental mechanism associated with qi: ji –in acupuncture and ganying [感應]– in herbs are used." See also [2, 4, 10].

85. Bencao tradition and scholars also used those concepts, but –as shown already- they were many times just alluding to them or using them apparently as only purely functional concepts, i.e., without explicitly exposing its value as structure. This is the reason why I mention only the Shanganhlun in the main text, but the existence of a qi-based structure affects all the herbal traditions, including both, the Shanghanlun and Bencao.

86. Nonetheless, the herbal medicine field is in a game where it cannot dictate the rules. If it wants to be widely accepted, it will have to speak the language of the currently dominant paradigm. It does no good to advocate against research thorough the dominant bio-pharmacological model, on the contrary, it will probably be very useful for the field to embrace this, but in an enlarged and deepened way. This has been part of the reason for writing the current chapter, it will be best to avoid the trap of thinking of the "active principle" as something separate from the biocomplexity of the substances on the one hand but it will also be necessary to embrace the probably still more murky complexity of the physician-plant-patient internal and external relationships.

87. Take, for instance the words of Professor Aiping Lu, Dean of Chinese Medicine School (SCM) and Director of the Institute of Advancing Translational Medicine in Bone & Joint Diseases: "We try to integrate medicines to produce a combination of Chinese and Western medicine" [29].

88. See, as references, the different published reports presented in at the journal "Science" in December 2012: [Vol 338, 21 Dec 2012, pages 1644, 1652, 1653,1654].

89. For more details, see the excellent paper by Marco Bischof on the subject [7].

90. As I finish this chapter I have become aware of new areas of scientific investigation in Chinese medicine that have the potential to open up more inclusive models of action and utilization of herbal medicine. These areas are called "systems biology" and "OMICS" research. They take advantage of the now available computing power coupled with the application of complexity theory [25] formulated through software analysis programs that operate based on complexity theory, and are leading to what is being called 'personalized medicine" [16, 32]. At present these approaches have become fused with the dominant older paradigm of thinking in biology, focusing on complex pharmacological process, and not yet including other aspects that have been described in this and earlier chapters (see in particular chapters one, three, four and five [4, 12, 38]), but systems biology [9, 13, 21] and OMICS [9, 13, 21] have the very possibility of starting to include these non-pharmacological aspects.

CHAPTER SEVEN

# QI [氣] AND STILLNESS [靜]

## Taiji Quan [太極拳] Qigong [氣功] Acupuncture [針灸]

Miguel Angel Cabrer Mir

## Introduction

The evolution of Taiji quan [太極拳], qigong [氣功] and acupuncture [針灸] has been influenced by different schools of thought and social change that have occurred throughout the history of Chinese culture, from the Han and Qing dynasties to the Communist Revolution and up to present times. Influences can be seen not only in the practice of these three disciplines but also in the way of understanding and explaining many of the basic concepts pertinent to all.

One of these basic and omnipresent concepts is qi [氣]. Recent times have seen an abundance of explanations to define the term qi and adapt it to the necessities of Western cultures. The understanding of qi as an intellectual concept has reduced its significance and disconnected it from its practical aspect.

Taiji quan, qigong and acupuncture are disciplines of movement in which action is essential. It is through practice that we can achieve an understanding of abstract concepts such as qi [氣], ji [機], shi [勢]. At the same time we can say that movement cannot exist without stillness, a concept that serves as a constant link in this chapter.

## Stillness-movement

The purpose of this chapter is to show how the practice of stillness enables movement that has greater resonance with our surroundings. Stillness permits a sensitivity-in-action which results in a more harmonic response to the circumstances of the moment. Throughout this text I have deliberately left out the "and" between stillness-movement, as the word "and" may suggest separation. This unity or absence of "and" is reflected in the following text:

> In every movement, there is nothing that does not move, in every stillness, there is nothing that is not still. [8:138].

Many people approach the practice of Taiji quan or qigong in search of this stillness. It is also possible that we seek this stillness from the point of view of our dualistic mentality, and thus we separate stillness from movement. The word "and" is still a barrier. The practice of stillness-movement should be like a meadow covered in snow in the winter: a field without apparent life, without grass or flowers. But this absence of life is not real. The seed, the beginning of movement, is waiting for the opportune moment, the change of season. When spring comes the seeds germinate, flowers begin to blossom and movement fills the meadow which has received the nutrition of stillness.

> Non-action is the real action. One hundred acts are not as good as one moment of silence. One hundred movements are not as good as one moment of standing still. Big movement is not as good as small movement. Small movement is not as good as no movement. [20:58]

## Stillness in Chinese Culture

The following quotations refer to stillness in relation to movement in the disciplines of government, martial arts and medicine. Confucianism and Daoism, traditions that have deeply marked the history of Chinese culture, show an inclination towards stillness as a tool for cultivation from the beginning. Confucius says:

> The master said: one who practices government with virtue can be compared with the Pole star. It resides in this place and all of the stars pay homage to it [25: 46].

While the Daode jing says:

> The myriad living things (wan wu) arise side by side; in this, I see their return. The living things (under the sky/heaven) flourish abundantly and each again returns to its root. This is called "stillness" (jing-靜) Stillness means to return to the natural order (ming-命). To return to the natural order is called constancy [1:141].

This vision of stillness, which arises in both Confucian and Daoist schools of thought, has influenced different arts in Chinese culture. Medical and martial practices were no exception to this cultural pollination. Zhuangzi says:

> The art of sword fighting is to give your opponent the impression of an opening and offer him an opportunity to attack. I move only after he does, but my sword reaches him first [31:4].

While the Sunzi the author of the "Art of War" says:

> I let the enemy initiate the attack, but my blow strikes first [31:14].

And the Wei Liao Tzus says:

> An army gains victory through stillness [31:15].

In the medical tradition we also find this idea, for example Lingshu chapter nine tells us:

> The practitioner must deeply reside in a place of stillness and divine the comings and goings of the spirit with one's (sensory) doors and windows shut. The practitioner's ethereal and corporeal souls must not be scattered, his mind must be focused, and his essence qi undivided, and undistracted by human sounds [6].

## Stillness and qi

Let us explore how we can investigate the practice of stillness in Taiji quan, qigong and acupuncture.

In some of the earliest texts that refer to obtaining qi, the emphasis is on an attitude of non-force.

> therefore this vital energy cannot be halted by force. Neiye –2 [26:48].

> and when the mind controls the qi –this we call using force. Daode Jing [12:72].

Qi is like the fruit from a tree, a result of maturation that requires time. It is like learning a craft or learning to play an instrument. At the beginning, there is no harmony, but through constant practice a day arrives when the music comes with no effort. Qi, like fruit, appears after the cultivation of stillness, relaxation and the unified perception of body movement.

Now days we are living in a world that demands rapid, almost immediate results. This cultivates an impatience that is also reflected in the desire for and the practice to "obtain" qi. But this thirst for obtaining fruit in a few weeks is not an attitude exclusive to our own times. Mencius tells us the story of the man from Song, which illustrates this desire to accelerate processes:

> Pay constant attention to the task. Do not neglect the heart and mind. Do not (make an artificial effort to) help it grow. Do not be like the man of Song. There was a man of Song who pulled at his shoots of grain, because he was anxious for them to grow. Having finished, he went home, not realizing what he had done. He said to his family, "I am worn out today; I have been helping the grain to grow." His son rushed out of the house to look at their plants and found that they all had withered... [13:92].

This acceleration brings with it a change in our physiological rhythms. One of the more sensitive movements, which is easily altered by any exterior changes, is breathing. When we are given unexpected news, when an emotion gets out of control, the rhythm of inhalation and exhalation is modified. For this reason, since ancient times, breathing patterns have been an important element in many corporal practices. One of the first references to the movement of qi in Chinese culture is the following:

> Swallow... it travels; travelling, it extends; extending, it descends; descending it stabilizes, it solidifies; solidifying, it sprouts; sprouting, it grows; growing, it returns; returning, it is heaven. Heaven –its root is above; earth –its root is below. Follow the pattern and live; go against it and die. [11:126].

Some sinologists have interpreted this writing as a set of instructions for a breathing exercise, an important practice through which we can access the dynamism (ji-機) of the two poles of heaven and earth.

In later texts like the Neiye or chapter ten of the Daode Jing, there are some direct references to an internal process for awakening the dao. They also refer to breathing:

> For all (to practice) the Way
> You must coil, you must contract
> ou must uncoil, you must expand
> You must be firm; you must be regular (in this practice)
> Hold fast to this excellent (practice) do not let go of it
> Chase away the excessive; abandon the trivial
> And when you reach its ultimate limit
> You will return to the Way and its inner power. [26:78].
> In concentrating your qi and making pliant, are you able to become
> the new-born babe? (Daode Jing –chapter 10 [2:90]).

Physical relaxation and a calm mind (the image of a new-born baby) permit a more comprehensive deeper breathing that involves the whole body. Calm and stillness are what allow breathing to become integrated without effort throughout our body in a natural way, and so lead to further calming of the mind. A quiet mind and a relaxed body are vital elements for gaining access to the sensitivity of perceiving change. However breathing is a very sensitive tool that cannot be changed from one day to the next. The change is produced as relaxation and stillness become integrated into our person.

## Qi as a dynamic factor

The understanding of qi as a dynamic factor is central to the sensitivity of perception that arises from stillness. The search for order or harmony is one of the oldest characteristics of Chinese thought. All streams of Chinese thought flow towards this point although they differ in the way they put it into practice. I would like to mention the following and their relationship with qi.

### *Correlative Cosmology*

The "correlative cosmology" movement dates from the third century BCE and became firmly established in the Han dynasty. It attempts to find order within the supposed harmony that the cosmos reflects. Yinyang, qi and wuxing (five-phases) make up the language used by texts like the Huainanzi and Lushi chunqiu to relate aspects of society such as the state and the human body to the cosmos.

This connection between the cosmos and aspects of society has a key concept: ganying 感應 (resonance). Qi is an important factor in the concept of ganying.[1]

> The idea of qi is as a conveyor of resonant influence, on the ganying principle of "like responds to like." [19:30].

According to this principal, qi is an element that facilitates communication as well as being a primordial substance. This function allows the quality of qi to have an important role in the continual movement of life, while still maintaining its immaterial characteristics. Its objective is to facilitate harmony with the rhythm of the universe and maintain a balance that influences society in general.

## *Zhuangzi*

In the Daoist movement represented by Zhuangzi there is no concept of resonance (ganying), but there is a reference to a quality of qi that allows us to act according to circumstances.

> Yanqi said "May I ask about the purification of the mind-heart?
> Confucius said "When you unify your will (zhi 志), you do not listen (ie understand) with the ears, but listen with the mind-heart. When you do not listen with the mind-heart but listen with qi, listening will stop at the ear and the mind-heart stop at what tallies with it. As for qi, it is that which being empty, awaits things. Only the way accumulates in emptiness. Emptiness is the purification of the mind-heart" [1:90].

In this text we see that qi is related to the qualities of emptiness and to a sensitivity that allows us "to wait for things to arrive". Normally, our actions are reactions that are dominated by the senses, by desires or by emotions, which prevents us from acting in a way that is complementary to what is around us.

## *Gudang [鼓盪] and Taiji quan*

In the Taiji quan classics we find the following text:

> The qi should be excited (gudang-鼓盪); the spirit (shen-神) should be gathered within. [8:90].

This relationship between qi and gudang has certain similarities with what is described in correlative cosmology and Zhuangzi. Gu [鼓] has several meanings, all of which have a connotations to do with resonance: drum, playing the drum, vibrate, shake... The characteristic of dang [盪] according to Barbara Davis is: "Responsiveness to outside force, such as the way in which a drum-skin vibrates or water stirs" [8:90].

Cheng Man Ching has the following to say on the subject:

> To use the qi to move the body is the root and is internal. Gudang [鼓盪] is the branch and is external. Gathered within is stillness, gudang is movement. They are able to respond to each other and unite as one. However, gudang is not only about one's own qi being gudang, I must also make my qi gudang together with that of the rest of the world. [8:90].

All of these orientations, correlative cosmology, Zhuangzi, the gudang of Taiji quan, help us to understand qi. A qi that allows us to act with sensitivity in resonance with our environment, not something exclusive that circulates along the meridians.

This concept of resonance has implications in the practice of applying qi in tuishou[2] and acupuncture, arts that, in a way, need a strategy of resonance when they are practised. This strategy is not developed through a desire to cure someone or push the other person, but from adapting to the terrain we find before us. It is possible that if these actions are carried out at the right moment, a simple needle, or a simple pressure may cause great changes: relief in the case of therapy, or unbalancing the other person in the case of the martial arts.

In the past, just like Ding the cook below, many practitioners of martial arts and medicine in Daoist and Confucian schools, sought to awaken the sensitivity called qi, shen, jingshen in order to obtain a greater awareness of the present and to act in resonance with their surroundings.

> Butcher Ding put down his cleaver and replied, "What I care about is the Way, which goes beyond mere technique. When I first began cutting up oxen, all I could see was the ox itself. After three years, I no longer saw the ox as a whole. And now... now I meet with my spirit and don't look with my eyes. My sensory knowledge is restrained and my spiritual desires are allowed to move/act... [28:200].

I believe that today, stillness and the quality of "knowing how to wait", or "resonate", are elements that are obscured by an anxiety to obtain qi. It is particularly prevalent in modern times to look for qi right away, talk about qi right away, and perceive qi right away. How can we combine this attitude with the following statements taken from books written at very different times in history, yet despite chronological distance we can see a common idea: "don't focus your attention or your mind on qi".

> And when the mind controls the qi –this we call using force
> (Daode Jing chapter 55 [12:72].

> The whole body's yi is on the spirit (jingshen), it is on the qi, then it is stagnant (zhi). (Exposition of Insights into the Thirteen Postures –Wu Yuxiang [8:140]).

## Stillness-Movement and Taiji Quan

In recent times, the practice of Taiji quan has become very popular. More or less every gymnasium or cultural centre offers classes. This growth is not exclusive to the West. It was in Maoist China that the process began.

When the Chinese Republic was established in 1949 one of the main problems it encountered was in health care. The government urgently needed to create an effective system which would be in keeping with the new ideologies. This urgent need lead them to recuperate certain Chinese medical practices under the guidance of Chinese doctors trained in western medicine.

Amongst the new approaches was the core concept of prevention. In this area, apart from introducing preventive measures typical of the western medical approach, it was decided to recuperate and encourage the practice of physical exercises with a therapeutic objective, from which comes the successful reception of the therapeutic approach to taiji.

The popularity of the therapeutic approach to taiji introduced a new emphasis in the teaching, but at the same time it limited or suppressed other aspects. Taiji quan belongs to the family of internal martial arts. In Taiji quan we find more emphasis on cultivating the qi as opposed to muscular development: "Using external muscular force makes movement clumsy; holding the breath hinders the circulation of the blood. Therefore it is of the utmost importance to sink the qi to the dantian and completely relax the entire body, without exerting the slightest energy" [16:74].

I would like to emphasise the concept of "cultivation" returning to the example of a fruit tree. When we plant a tree, we need to wait for a time before we obtain any fruit. Today, we can accelerate this process, but in the end, there is a great difference between the fruit from a tree that has developed at its natural rhythm and one which has been accelerated by technological means. The technological advances of recent times have helped us to make great leaps forward in many aspects of our lives, but at the same time, they have separated us from others: stillness or the art of waiting.

As is the case in other Chinese martial arts, for example Bagua [八卦] or Yiquan [意拳], in Taiji quan there is an emphasis on performing movements at a slow rhythm. This slowing down is one way to cultivate a stillness that waits for the right moment to initiate a movement. The change, the beginning of the movement, starts with a small action, a small movement. Sensing this beginning can help us to adapt better and to act in greater harmony with our surroundings. Stillness is like a powerful microscope that allows us to perceive the beginning of the smallest sign of change.

Going back to the tree metaphor, the leaves, which move with the lightest touch of wind, serve as an illustration of the kind of perception that is achieved through the practice of stillness. In order to produce leaves, the tree needs time. The practice of stillness also requires time to allow the development of this way of perceiving. Curiously, in the "ji" of the taiji character, [極], we find the figure of a tree (木), an image which in many cultures symbolizes the union between heaven and earth. A translation of taiji would be "the supreme summit", the place where yin-yang are in equilibrium. This equilibrium is not rigid since the balance between yin-yang is constantly changing and hence the symbol for taiji –see figure one. This circular figure illustrates the union of the two aspects of yin-yang as well as evoking movement. If harmony is represented by the yin-yang equilibrium, the practice of stillness also needs to be in equilibrium with movement.

## Taiji quan: a way to balance stillness with movement

### Relax the body

The term most commonly used in Taiji quan texts to refer to a relaxed body is song [鬆] (meaning lax or loose). The question is how to achieve this relaxation. One of the most important indications in the practice of Taiji quan is: "relax the shoulders." Relaxed shoulders not only facilitate the release of the upper part of the torso, the shoulders and cervical spine, but also help arm movement to integrate with the whole body. The arms tend to move independently from the rest of the body. The repetition of movements to integrate the arms with the rest of the body with the objective to achieve complete unification is fundamental. The arms and hands permit tactile contact with the exterior. If arm movement is disconnected from the rest of the body this contact is trapped at the shoulder level limiting our perception.

### Sink the qi in the dantian

Shoulder relaxation not only frees the upper part of the body and facilitates integrated body movement but also influences our ability to work on another important aspect for the unification of stillness with movement: sink the qi to the dantian.[3]

Some taiji masters explain the term "sink" as a state of profound relaxation that includes both mental and physical aspects. The posture of a cat watching a mouse hole is often used as an example of this state of relaxation. The cat is relaxed but attentive to any change that may arise and so is able to act instantly. This physically relaxed state is possible because the body finds a position in which the muscles waste no unnecessary energy in order to maintain balance. Effort invested in finding the alignment of our body enables a relaxation of the muscles, which in turn allows the breathing to descend of its own accord. "Sinking qi to the dantian" refers to preparing the conditions that allow our breathing to find its way down to the lower abdomen.

## Quiet mind/Yi (意) and movement

A relaxed body and low deep breath prepare the ground for keeping the mind still. All these conditions facilitate the state of being in resonance with the moment. A busy mind, jumping from one thing to another is like agitated water, both lose their potential to reflect.

> When water is still, it reflects one's beard and moustache clearly... The mind/heart of the sage is clear! It is the jian mirror of heaven and Earth and the jian–mirror of the myriad living things. [1:53].

Any action we make starts before the movement occurs. The practice of stillness enables us to perceive this initial stage in the process of an action. For example, if we raise an arm, the action begins with minute changes, which grow into the external expression of the arm movement. The first spark of this movement is the action of yi [意].[4] It is easy to lose touch with this initial moment, even to the extent of being unable to maintain contact with it long enough to see through the complete action of the arm.

The distance between the initial moment and its physical expression is full of obstacles: physical tensions in the body or mental activity thoughts, desires, emotions. These obstacles interfere with the resonance of the two moments.

Physical relaxation and a quiet mind enable the unification of these two moments of a movement.

When we throw a tennis ball to the floor the second we hear the sound of the ball hitting the ground it is rising again. The sound and the rising movement are simultaneous. The yi is the moment the ball hits the ground and the bounce back is the qi.

The still mind and relaxed body allow a harmonious union of yi and qi.

The action arises out of the yi of the still mind and the qi circulates thanks to a relaxed body. This yi-qi mix must occur naturally without effort.

Yi shows the way and qi follows it. It is important that the action of yi is to simply show the way to qi, not to try to direct qi or push it

> The whole body's yi is on the spirit (jingshen-精神), not on the qi. If it is on the qi, then it is stagnant (zhi-滞). (Exposition of Insights into the Thirteen Postures –Wu Yuxiang [8:140]).

This affirmation may cause a little confusion because in many current practices, there is an emphasis on putting our intention on qi. Master Cheng Man Ching commented:

> These words are very strange. They imply that the qi is not important, and in fact, it is not. When the qi reaches the highest level and becomes mental energy, it is called spiritual power or "the power without physical force" wherever the eyes concentrate, the spirit reaches and the qi follows. The qi can mobilize the body, but you need not will the qi in order to move it. The spirit can carry the qi with it. This spiritual power is called "divine speed" [8:140].

Qi moved with intention or willpower will become stagnated in every place towards which we direct our intention or will. Like flowing water, qi needs room to move without obstacles to avoid stagnation.

## Stillness-Movement and qigong

Water is a classic metaphoric element in Chinese thought. Some of the first definitions of the term qi make direct reference to water:

> Water is the blood and vapour (qi) of the earth... like what flows through the muscles and vessels. (Guanzi [11:77]).

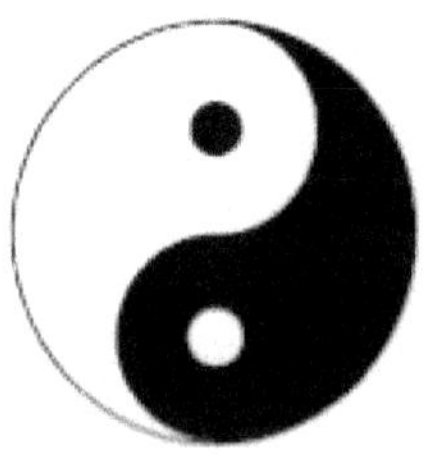

Taiji symbol

> Mountains are the gathering of earth; lowland wastes are where creatures take shelter. Rivers are where energy (qi) is guided... (Guo Yu [15:40]).

One of the characteristic qualities of water is its downward movement. In early texts that refer to health and longevity we find examples that relate qi to a downward action.

> Qi is that which benefits (when) descending and harms (when) rising (it) follows heat and leaves cold, thus the sages cool the head and warm the feet... in order to reap the benefits. (Maifa [7:79]).

Downward movement cannot exist without upward movement (what goes up must come down!). Problems arise when the two actions do not balance each other out. The river descends to the sea. From there, as vapour it rises again. If one of these movements stagnates or is delayed the rhythm gets out of balance and problems arise. Body movement, mostly in terms of the extremities, together with breathing, are the elements that have been used to facilitate this non-stagnated flow.

> Now the reason why flowing water does not become putrid and the doorway pivot is not devoured by bugs is because they move. By moving, you fill the four limbs and empty the five depots. When the five depots are empty, the jade body will benefit. (Maishu [11:144]).[5]

To facilitate this unimpeded flow just any old movement does not suffice, the quality of the movement is paramount. We need to tune our bodies to carry out these movements with an awareness of where the movements originate. If we return to the image of the river, the source is the origin of the movement. It is a movement which appears at the surface but whose origin is connected to the interior in the accumulation of water that surges to the surface. We can relate this interior space to stillness, the exterior to movement. If the channel is free from obstacles the river flows freely. If we use this as a metaphor for the body we can say that movement clears the channel and stillness permits the perception of the origin of that movement.

In recent time the synergy between stillness and movement has been lost and there is a tendency to centre on stillness and forget movement or vice versa. This imbalance between movement and stillness in bodywork in China occurred with the remodelling in the 20th Century.

From the 1950 onwards, changes occurred in the physical exercise known as "qigong" influenced by placing value on movement to the detriment of stillness.[6] Interpretations of the guidelines that appear in this article by Mao Zedong may have influenced this change of emphasis in the practice.

> Human beings are active animals and they love to be active. Human beings are also rational animals and thus they need a reason for their activity. Why is this? Because activity secures survival. Yes, but that is an easy explanation. Because activity secures the fortune of the homeland... Activity is ultimately what nourishes life and satisfies the mind. This and none other is the truth... Sitting in meditation was advised by followers of Zhuxi and Lu Xiangshan over the ages, the most recent example being Master Yinshi´s book. He praises his method as wonderful and highly spiritual and says that activity destroys the body. This is one way of looking at things. However, I do not share these ideas. In my opinion, there is nothing between heaven and earth that is not activity. (Kunio Miura [14:334]).

This emphasis on movement meant that the aspect of stillness began to lose importance. Stillness is not just simply being immobile, nor is it have an exclusively related to religious practice.

Another image that we can use to help us understand the harmony between stillness and movement is the forest. Forests, especially in spring, autumn, or at dusk, have an endless array of colours that combine without any one being dominant. As we pass through the forest our visual experience is of being surrounded by images in constant balance. When we go for a walk, we also alternate between moments of stillness and movement, which, in conjunction with the image of stillness and movement that nature offers us, perform an alchemy within us; our body relaxes and our mind is quietened.

Can we reproduce this state when we perform our corporal practices?

## Stillness-Movement and acupuncture

Acupuncture training starts with the classical theories: yin-yang, five phases, study of the localization of the points, the function of the points and the techniques of needle insertion. The majority of these themes, with the exception of needling techniques, are theoretical and intellectual. The practical application of acupuncture is in studying the localization of the points, needling, and how we enter in contact with the patient. In clinical practice these are physical actions, specifically the use of the hands, as we mainly use the hands for palpation (the pulse, abdomen, meridians, points) and to manipulate the needles.

In the discipline of Taiji quan, especially in the practice of tuishou which we will see further on, the hands serve to give and to receive. In the practice of acupuncture they play a similar role. Through the hands we receive information through palpation and we come into contact with the patient. As in the practice of tuishou this contact is limited if there is tension in the body or an agitated mind. A doctor of the Han, Gou Yu dynasty described the mind hand connection in this way:

> Medicine is yi. The region of the skin is very finely divided. Following the flow of qi requires consummate skill. When inserting needles, an error of a hair's breadth will mean failure. A kind of spirit connects the physician's heart with his hand, and that is something I can know but cannot explain. [27:176-77].

According to this doctor the practice of acupuncture centres on this relationship of the mind (internal state-stillness) and hands (movement-body): "A kind of spirit connects the physician's heart with his hand, and that is something I can know but cannot explain".

The action of the hands in acupuncture has two important phases: first, contact with the patient through palpation (of the pulse the abdomen, the point, the skin...); second the contact with the needles (how we insert the needle, how we carry out the action of tonification or draining).

Placing emphasis in the importance of touch in acupuncture as in tuishou serves mutually to enrich both disciplines.

## Tuishou: the nexus between Taiji quan and acupuncture

Tuishou is the pair-work practiced in Taiji quan. As with acupuncture, contact through touch is an important element to be developed. Listening through touch leads to a greater sensitivity. This sensitivity requires long years of cultivation and a strong base of stillness. In the past, sensitivity was developed within a master/disciple relationship, a direct relationship that allowed for the development of difficult-to-explain concepts in simple words. When the teaching of acupuncture was institutionalized in the 1950s and 1960s, these aspects of apprenticeship were suppressed. In a short period of time the Chinese government needed doctors who could set up and maintain a health system that had just been created [5, 30].

How can we work to develop this lost sensitivity? How can we relate it to the practice of acupuncture and tuishou?

Normally, tuishou [推手] is translated as "push hands", which overshadows any element of sensitivity. Today, some practitioners are starting to translate it as "listening with the hands". Through contact with our hands, we can sense when there is tension or emptiness. Our action is a response which arises according to circumstances. It is not a reaction. The art of tuishou is knowing how to adapt and act in resonance with what is happening at a given moment. In the practice of tuishou there is a phrase that summarises the essential elements that must be awakened, and which can also be applied to the practice of acupuncture.

> Stick, adhere, follow the other, forget yourself, don't resist or separate.

The sensitivity of touch developed through practising tuishou can help us to gather information through touch in acupuncture, in palpation and in the contact we maintain with the needle in insertion and subsequent manipulation. In the past the Taiji quan practitioner did not initiate the practice of tuishou until some years had passed in which they learned the movements of Taiji quan. These movements served to restructure the body, achieve a deeper breathing pattern and a more still mind. All this helped the body to perceive movement in a different way. This way is beneficial to acupuncture and tuishou.

## Palpation of the patient

### *Stick and adhere*

This refers to the way in which we are in contact with the other person. In acupuncture, it could be our contact with the needle, how we touch the other person, pulse, abdominal palpation, palpation of the channels.

When we carry out these actions: do we have the quality of "waiting" referred to previously? –or do we have innumerable theories in our heads? In the story of Ding the cook, this way of carrying out an action is described. An action that is directed by shen.

> Butcher Ding put down his cleaver and replied, " What I care about is the Way, which goes beyond mere technique. When I first began cutting up oxen, all I could see was the ox itself. After three years, I no longer saw the ox as a whole. And now –now I meet it with my spirit and don´t look with my eyes. My sensory knowledge is restrained and my spiritual desires are allowed to move/act" [28:200].

Through touch, we can be more sensitive to the circumstances and movements occurring around us. In acupuncture and tuishou, touch is an important tool. The quality of this touch allows for an attitude of "wait for it to happen" and not a reaction led by theories or emotions.

Adherence or sticking which originates in the hands or arms inhibits neutral contact with the patient. The differences between adhere and stick is subtle. Both are ways to initiate contact but the first is lighter than the second, a little denser. Knowledge of these two different qualities enables us to adapt to the needs of the patient and perceive whether the necessary contact is lighter or denser. As in the practice of tuishou where the signs from the partner tell us if a simple light contact is enough to move them or of we need to use a denser contact. Whether the contact is light or dense we maintain our unity in softness.

### *Follow the other and forget yourself*

Forgetting yourself refers to keeping your mind in stillness. In tuishou, as in acupuncture, the information the other person transmits to us is in constant movement. Our own mind, our emotions and desires are a barrier that impedes resonance with the exterior. A relaxed body and a still mind are essential for resonating with what is around us. The transparency of water serves as a metaphoric image of this quality:

> When water is still, it reflects one's beard and moustache clearly. The mind Heart (xin) of the sage is clear! It is the jian-mirror of heaven and earth and the jian-mirror of the myriad living things. That which, empty and still (xu, jing) insipid and bland, silent and featureless, does nothing (wu wei) is the level (which acts as a Standard for) heaven and earth and it is the culmination of the way (dao) and virtue (de). (Zhuangzi [1:83]).

Gradually, and through constant practice, our responses come from the circumstances of the moment. We are not tied to a theory or a technique. It is important to know the theories or techniques, but it is more important to learn not to be trapped by them. At the beginning, we need to have a base, but later we have to be creative. When referring to constant change, Chinese thought speaks of the alternation between yin and yang, and in Taiji quan of the substantial and insubstantial.

> Yin-yang are not forces or substances, but rather complementary aspects or moments that constitute any orderly, efficient, and "creative" process. [22:35].

The aim of working with tuishou (listening with the hands) is to awaken the sensitivity that allows pair-work to become a "creative" process. When what prevails is force, wanting to impose your action, wanting to win, a destructive process is generated, a process of imposition that cuts off any dialogue with the exterior. Any resonance is lost. The forgetting oneself referred to in this sentence does not mean that we annul ourselves as a person and follow the other without any objection. We simply try to make our ego, with its baggage of emotions and desires, slowly become calmer so that we can act in a creative way with the circumstances.

In acupuncture, something similar may happen when carrying out a diagnosis or treatment. Where does the whole process come from? Does it come out of a creative dialogue between the two, or does one opinion prevail? Are our actions guided by theories or techniques, or by the timing of the moment?

### *Don't resist or separate*

This is the attitude that allows us to develop the above qualities. Acupuncture and tuishou are arts that are developed in action. Resisting or separating cuts us off from the moment, from our surroundings. Not resisting or separating ourselves from the movement of the other person allows us to attain a quality that makes listening for the changes easier. This space or moment is expressed in the Yijing as follows:

> It is by means of the Changes that the sages plumb the utmost profundity and dig into the very incipient (ji-幾) of things. It is profundity alone that thus allows one to penetrate the aspirations of all the people in the world; it is a grasp of incipience alone that thus allows one to accomplish the great affairs of the world. [18:63].

In the taiji classics, there is the following phrase:

> From feet, to the legs, then to the waist, always there must be complete integration into one qi. In advancing forward and retreating back, you will then be able to seize the opportunity and strategic advantage. [10:217].

The unity of a single qi refers to the state of stillness that is achieved within the constant practice of relaxation. A relaxation that includes both our physical and mental aspects. From this stillness we can approach any movement with a different sensitivity. (then be able to seize the opportunity and strategic advantage –deji deshi [得機得勢]).

Stillness and movement. Ji [機] would be the space for stillness that allows us to sense the changes before they are produced, and the shi [勢] would be the propensity for the action that comes out of stillness. This is the action that Chinese thought has defined as wuwei. [無為].

When we carry out an acupuncture treatment, or we practice tuishou, can we maintain this attitude of wuwei?

## Contacting with the needle

In schools of acupuncture various needling techniques are taught, for example tonification and draining, but rarely is attention placed on the way in which we handle the needle during the practice of these techniques. The quality of touch of our fingers and hands allows the needles to become an extension of the body.

### *Stick and adhere*

Previously we spoke of sticking and adhering in the context of our contact with the patient and now we must apply the same concepts to needling. The quality of touch with which we manipulate the needle will permit the classic acupuncture actions in the practice of tonification or draining to reach the very tip of the needle.[7] For this reason it is important to pay attention to how we hold the needle and the sense of touch we have when we carry out the actions of tonification or draining.

The practice of Taiji quan teaches us how to move with a unified body. It is thanks to this quality that, in tuishou, we can put into practice the actions of pushing and receiving with greater sensitivity.

This same tactile perception developed in the actions of pushing and receiving in tuishou can be applied to the way we stick and adhere to the needles in acupuncture. If we are too tense or our contact is too weak the movement will not be unified and will be mechanical, centred on turning the needle or the pressure our hands exert on the needle. If our objective is that the needle become an extensión of our body we need to cultivate the tactile contact we maintain with the needle. The practice of tuishou, with its emphasis on sticking and adhering is one way to to develop this relationship between the body and the needles.

## *Follow the other and forget yourself*

We cannot begin to experience the needle as an extension of our body if we have not first experienced unified movement. In the classical Taiji quan texts there are a number of attempts to describe this unification in movement:

> What is long boxing? It is like the long river or a great ocean flowing smoothly and ceaselessly. (Fu Zhongwen: Mastering Yang Style Taiji quan [10:208]).

Tuishou practice consists of constant movement in unison with the other person, applying the concept "follow the other and forget yourself." This leads to the ability to listen for the smallest movement from the other person until there are no longer two movements but only one.

In the case of acupunture we can ask the question, "can we follow the movements of the needle?" or better still "are the needle and the body moving as one?" The needle should not be a "foreign body." We must forget that we hold an object which is separate from us. The needle must become an extension of our breath and touch.

## *Don't resist or separate*

In tuishou we often come up against problems at the moment of change between receiving or pushing. It is not only important to stick and adhere to the other but also to be able to maintain this tactile quality at the moment of action. We can relate this moment of change or action in acupuncture to the actions of tonification and draining. If we apply these techniques when we manipulate the needles there is a change in the contact with the needles.

In tuishou practice we can monitor the level of harmony existing between stillness and movement. Frequently tensions or separations appear at the moment of receiving or pushing as we feel our personal space "invaded". Both actions result in a loss of contact "stick-adhere" and we go back to making two separate movements. If this separation happens when we are needling we lose contact with the needle and our needle manipulation becomes mechanical.

## The model of Zhuangzi applied to tuishou and acupuncture

### Tuishou and intention

There are many surprises when we begin practicing tuishou after years of practising Taiji quan. In theory prolonged practice of Taiji quan enables us to relax the body and quieten our inner state. The surprise is to discover that in practising tuishou physical and internal tensions resurge causing us to lose the qualities which we thought we had acquired. In the initial stages we learn some physical movements which help us to receive and to push or not be pushed. In acupuncture this would be like learning the mechanical movements involved in tonification or dispersion, using techniques which differ from the teaching model. These techniques rely on experiment and finding the best way through experience. This is a process which requires time and cannot be learned in a book or in a few weekend courses. It is like the process used for learning a craft where the intention is slowly diluted giving way to other forms of learning.

### Tuishou and attention

If we persist in our learning process and have the good luck to find a teacher adept in these arts, then we learn that the attitude at the moment of action, albeit tonification or pushing, comes from our innate nature.

In this phase we begin to listen, not only to the mechanical physicality of our movements but to other more subtle movements, for example our breathing, the relaxation of our shoulders or the breath sinking to the dantian.

In the first phase our attention was on the mechanical physical movement. Now we can place our attention on something more internal which enables us to be more present but can also disconnect us from the external circumstances. The art of Taiji quan is manifest when we break the barriers between the external intention and the internal attention so that they become one and the action we take has both characteristics.

### Tuishou and awareness

This is the phase in which physical movement, technique, has fused with internal perception and a separation no longer exists. The previous phases are important: we need to learn the actions of physical movements and we need to pay attention to our internal state. But even at the beginning it is important to maintain a balance between the internal and external. From the first moment we are working the third phase.

From the start, the opportunity to work with someone who enables you to "taste" the quality of the third phase will help you to feel what you are aiming for. This direct experience will assure that the first two phases do not stagnate in the external or internal. In time and with guidance the actions of Taiji quan or acupuncture will change in a natural way, and our movement expresses unity without intention or attention, simply occurring in the same way that water from a spring accumulates and suddenly starts bubbling to the surface.

## Conclusion

The beginning of change is tiny, silent. That is why the practice of stillness is important. Constant practice enables us to be more sensitive to this beginning.

Stillness does not mean being literally "still". The aim is to be able to apply this stillness to action. In applying stillness to action we are receptive to the signs which invite us to be more aware of, and attentive to, the changes that are produced around us.

## Bibliography

1- Allan S. *The Way of Water and Sprouts of Virtue*. Albany, State University of New York, 1997.

2- Ames RT, Hall DL. *A Philosophical Translation: Dao De Jing –making this life significant*, New York, Ballantine Books, 2003.

3- Birch S, Cabrer Mir MA, Rodriguez M. Chapter one: Qi and the mind –explorations of the links between qi, the mind, mental and emotional states. In this volume.

4- Birch S, Rodriguez M, Cabrer Mir MA. Chapter two: The jingmai –a summary of their development and nature. In this volume.

5- Birch S, Felt R. *Understanding Acupuncture*, Edinburgh, Churchill Livingstone, 1999.

6- Chace C. On greeting a friend, an approach to needle technique. *Lantern*. 2006:3(3):4-7.

7- Daly NP. *Hybridizing the human body: The hydrological development of acupuncture in early Imperial China*. Masters thesis, Department of East Asian Studies, McGill University, 1999.

8- Davis B. *The Tai ji quan Classics*. Berkeley, California. North Atlantic Books, 2004.

9- Fox A. Reflex and reflectivity: Wuwei in the Zhuangzi. In Cook S (ed). *Hiding the World in the World*. Albany, State University of New York, 2003: 207-225.

10- Fu ZW. *Mastering Yang Style Tai jiquan*.Translated by Louis Swaim. Berkeley,California. North Atlantic Books, 1999.
11- Harper D. *Early Chinese Medical Literature: the Mawangdui Medical Manuscripts*. London, Kegan Paul, 1998.
12- Henricks RG. *Lao Tzu's Tao Te Ching*. New York, Columbia University Press, 2000.
13- Ivanhoe PJ. *Ethics in the Confucian Tradition*. Indianapolis. Hackett Publishing Company, 2002.
14- Kohn L. *Chinese Healing Exercises, The Tradition of daoyin*. Honolulu.University of Hawai Press, 2008.
15- Lewis ME. *The flood Myths of Early China*. Albany, State University of New York Press, 2006.
16- Liang TT. *Tai Chi chuan for health and self-defense*. New York, Vintage Books, 1974.
17- Lin ZX, Yu L, Guo ZY, Shen ZY, Zhang HL, Zhang TL. *Qigong: Chinese Medicine or Pseudoscience?* New York, Prometheus Books, 2000.
18- Lynn RJ. *The Classic of Changes*. New York, Columbia University Press, 1994.
19- Major JS. *Heaven and Earth in Early Han Thought*. Albany, State University of New York Press, 1993.
20- Miller D, Cartmell T. *Xing yi nei gong –Xing Yi Health maintenance and Internal Strength*. Burkan,California Unique Publication, 1999.
21- Miura K. "The revival of Qi: Qigong in Contemporay China" in Kohn L. (Ed.) *Taoist Meditation and Longevity Technique*. Anne Arbor, Center for Chinese Studies, The University of Michigan, 1989.
22- Moeller HG. *The Philosophy of the Daodejing*, New York, Columbia University Press, 2006.
23- Olson SA. *The Intrinsic Energies of Tai chi chuan*. Minnesota. Dragon Door Publication, 1994.
24- Palmer DA. *Qigong Fever –Body, Science and Utopia in China*. New York, Columbia University Press, 2007.
25- Puett MJ. *The Ambivalence of Creation Debates Concerning Innovation and Artifice in Early China*. California, Stanford University, 2001
26- Roth HD. *Original Tao –Inward Training (Nei Yeh)*. New York, Columbia University Press, 1999.
27- Scheid V. *Chinese Medicine in Contemporary China*, Durham, Duke University press, 2002.
28- Slingerland E. *Effortless Action*, Oxford, Oxford University Press, 2003.
29- Sommers D. Chapter three: How to become a shang yi or "superior physician," An exploration on the influence of the practitioner in early China. In this volume.
30- Unschuld PU. *Medicine in China: A History of Ideas*, Berkeley, University of California Press, 1985.
31- Wile D. *Lost Tai Chi Classics from the Late Ching Dynasty*. Albany, State University of New York Press, 1996.
32- Wile D. *T'ai Chi's Ancestors: the making of an Internal Martial Art*. New City, New York. Sweet Ch'i Press, 1999.

## Endnotes

1. We saw this in chapter one [3], and again chapter three [29].

2. Tuishou is commonly called "push hands" and refers to the paired practice technique used in for example taiji.

3. The term "dantian" [丹田] refers to a region said to below the navel upon which one concentrates one's breathing in some self-cultivation practices.

4. Yi is discussed extensively in earlier chapters such as chapter one [3].

5. One of the Zhangjiashan texts dating from 186 BCE, see chapters 1-3 [3, 4, 29].

6. "In 'A study of physical culture", published in 1917, Mao attacked the technique of quiet meditation (jingzuo) popular during the Republican period, as instilling passivity... Mao's favouring of active sports may be one reason for the dominance of gymnastic exercises in the qigong of 1950 rather than the still meditation, although the latter certainly did not disappear from qigong" [24:45].

7. Chapter four "The jingmai and qi –acupuncture perspectives" discusses this extensively.

CHAPTER EIGHT

# QI [氣], JINGMAI [經脈]

## Scientific investigation of concepts based in traditional East Asian medicine –challenges to cross-paradigm research[i]

**Stephen Birch[ii], Mark Bovey[iii]**

## Introduction

Traditional medical systems in China developed a core model of the body in health and disease that referred to qi [氣] as a kind of ground substance for all material things especially living things, which was said to concentrate and circulate in the jingmai [經脈], variously translated as "meridians", "channels" and was described in relation to physiology. The diagnosis and treatment of disease was focused on identifying the condition of the qi and jingmai and correcting their disturbances. The principle early therapy was of zhenjiu [鍼灸] or acupuncture and moxibustion. Traditional East Asian medicine (TEAM) is a broad field that refers to multiple systems of practice that have developed out of this core model in many countries over many time periods. Different strategies have been used to investigate the "jingmai" and "qi" scientifically. A number of models have been proposed that aim to bring these concepts within a scientific framework and various efforts have been made to observe or "measure" them. Some studies have attempted to investigate whether qi or the jingmai are "real", meaning whether they can be objectively and reliably measured or observed using acceptable methodologies. Some studies have attempted to show that they are quaint historically based concepts that approximate other well established (real) entities or which act as pointers to those entities. However, attempts to scientifically investigate the "jingmai" and "qi" face a

i. We would like to thank Richard Hammerschlag for comments on an earlier draft of this chapter and give special thanks to Manel Rodriguez for his insightful comments.
ii. Associate Professor, University College of Health Sciences –Campus Kristiania, Oslo, Norway; Chairperson, International Committee for the Study of Traditional East Asian Medicine (ICSTEAM), Amsterdam, Holland.
iii. Research Manager, British Acupuncture Council, London, UK; Coordinator, Acupuncture Research Resource Centre, London, UK; London Southbank University; faculty College Integrated Medicine, Reading, UK; member International Committee for the Study of Traditional East Asian Medicine (ICSTEAM), Amsterdam, Holland.

complex array of problems, few of which have been adequately addressed. This paper will discuss the problems facing any investigation of traditional concepts such as "qi" and the "jingmai". The authors have written on these and related issues before [14, 15, 18, 30, 31, 33, 36, 37, 55, 56, 68, 87].

Although the authors have also written extensively on clinical trials of acupuncture and to a lesser extent on studies exploring the physiological basis of acupuncture [17, 19, 20, 22, 30, 32, 37, 46], this chapter will only touch briefly on those issues at appropriate times. For example some think that clinical trials can be used to test the theories of acupuncture [80], however, it will be proposed below that this is not possible, especially for theories such as those of the qi and the jingmai.

How the terms "jingmai" and "qi" are conceived and then translated affects to a large extent the type of approach researchers have used to investigate them. But as we saw in earlier chapters [29, 34], neither term has an agreed upon Western equivalent and each comes with considerable historical variability. This, in large part, is because the terms were conceived and used in philosophically different contexts than those which frame modern scientific thinking. They were conceived and used under very different socio-cultural pressures and influences than we experience in the modern world. We need to re-examine these differences and influences if we are to perform scientific studies of them.

## Conceptual understanding of the "jingmai" and "qi"

The term "jingmai" has been translated into English using a variety of terms such as "channel", "meridian", "conduit", "sinarteria" [110, 120, 132, 142]. While some of these terms bring with them certain implications such as referring to materially based or non-materially based entities, we leave the term un-translated here since the more important way that the jingmai have been approached in scientific studies appears to lie in their relation to qi. A recent anthropological study revealed a variety of approaches to understanding the concept within an acupuncture school in Norway [115], exposing a variety of ways of using and thinking about jingmai. In general though, the jingmai are said to be pathways for the flow of qi, consequently many approaches to investigating the jingmai appear to have been based on an understanding of the concept of qi. Many terms, in turn, have been used for the translation of qi, such as "pneuma", "vapor", "breath", "influences", "energy", "vital energy", "vital force", "life force".[1] It is not our purpose to reconcile or critique these choices of terms, rather to explore the assumptions involved in how they have influenced scientists investigating qi and the jingmai. A cursory look at this issue reveals that scientists have naturally gravitated towards more familiar scientific sounding terms. The focus of most scientific investigations has been to treat qi as a form of "energy" and the jingmai as an "energy" conduction system.[2] The jingmai were important as a system for imposing or restoring order to the various systems in the body. Chapter two [34] found in the development and early descriptions of jingmai that by nature they are "ordering" in nature, which we can say probably means they were conceived to be part of the body's regulatory systems.[3]

## *Qi as energy*

Is there sufficient justification to see qi as some form of measurable energy? A number of people writing about this issue have been critical of the choice of "energy" as translation for "qi" [30, 53, 132, 133:5].[4] In addition, consider the following. As translation for the term "energy" both the Chinese (qili) and Japanese (kiryoku) use the character for qi in a complex term that means literally "qi power" [气力] [29]. Thus it is natural, both in Asia and the West, that scientists for whom the term "energy" is a known concept in physics, chemistry and the biosciences, should view "qi" and "energy" as related. However, the unsuspecting scientist may not be aware that in Asia the term, "qi power" [气力] was selected at some point as a translation for the Western concept and term "energy". The incorporation of modern scientific thinking into Asia required that terms be translated. Very often words in common use were incorporated into a compound term to translate those new terms from e.g. physics or biophysics.

There is a further argument about the qi = energy assumption that arises out of a study of the historical literatures where the term qi was used. The Maishu of the Zhangjiashan texts (circa 186 BCE), older than the primary medical texts of the Neijing says: "As for vapor (qi)... it follows warmth and departs from coolness." [63:81]. If qi were "energy" it should follow the rules of "energy" as we understand them in science today. One of the principle rules governing the movement of "energy" as expressed in the second law of thermodynamics, is that energy will move from higher concentration to lower so as to create equal distribution.[5] In physics warmth represents a higher concentration of "energy" compared to coolness, yet in this influential [63] Maishu quote, qi moves from cool to warm areas, thus one can reasonably conclude that qi behaves differently from energy (or at least that this kind of conceptualizing of qi as energy does not follow the second law of thermodynamics). This contradicts those authors [48] who believe that qi properties accord with thermodynamic principles. In fact there are indications that it, and related concepts, are "ordering" by nature, which runs contrary to the second law of thermodynamics; Zhuangzi describes: "let your heart/mind wander in a state of lazy contentment, let your qi join with silent stillness. Flow along with the naturalness of things, make no room for selfishness and then the world will be ordered" [122:197]. Such passages are indicative of the role that the concept qi had assumed by the fourth century BCE as different thinkers sought to establish order out of the chaos of the Warring states period and found qi an important concept in these efforts. This theme is discussed and developed in chapter one [29], but is important to bear in mind when we attempt to research qi. Thus we find a commonality for the two concepts, qi and jingmai, they help restore order in the body and can thus be thought to be involved in the body's regulatory systems. These examples from early sources provide enough evidence to raise important questions about whether qi can be considered to be "energy" as traditionally understood in science today. As well as these fundamental problems there is another relatively simple issue: if a scientist assumes that qi is a form of energy and tries to measure it (e.g. electrical or electromagnetic signals) how can what has been measured be assumed to represent "qi"? Is a claim to have measured "qi" justified? And if, for example, no electromagnetic energy is detected, is a claim that qi does not exist justified? Clearly it is not sufficient to say qi is energy. Rather there is an imperative to specify what sort of energy, how could it be measured, in what units and why that particular form of energy should be considered at least, as a surrogate marker of qi. In summary, the assumption that qi can, let alone should, be equated with Western concepts of "energy" appears to confound the design and interpretation of such research[6]. At best, such studies may yield what can be viewed as correlations between Western medicine-defined biomarkers and traditional East Asian medicine-defined phenomena.

## *Qi as vital energy/force*

One way that some scientists have tried to avoid this issue is to envision qi in another of its translated forms as "vital energy", "vital force", or "life force".[7] These terms arise out of the broader concept of "vitalism" which has a long history of use in the West. Although not very precise scientifically, they have equivalent uses among many in the West who propose or support theories of vitalism.[8] However, "vitalism" as a concept was ridiculed over the last century in the West [72]. Despite this, it still has its adherents who use different names to refer to what can be seen as basically the same thing. In homeopathy we find the concept of "life force" [96], various biologists or bio-physicists have proposed concepts such as the "bio-field" [111, 114], "bio-energetic fields" [35], "bio-information fields" [35]. For some, the term qi has fit into the desires of those who believe in "vitalism" as an equivalent concept. This leaves the problem of how to deal with qi in relation not only to "energy" but also discredited vitalistic concepts. A fundamental objection to equating qi with vitalism is that qi is understood to be as much a part of dead and inanimate matter as of living beings [63, 78, 121]. Earth, air, fire and water all have qi but can hardly be said to have a life force.

### *Qi as* "fundamental substance"

In recent decades in China, "qi" along with other related concepts such as "jing" (essence) [精] and "shen" (spirit) [神] have been defined as "fundamental substances", implying a kind of material basis to them [6:36, 71:34]. This reflects modern efforts to make the terms appear more material and thus sound more "scientific", an important interpretation if these concepts were to survive in a communist led country. But questions have been raised about this approach [14:x, 106:122 and following, 121:237].[9] It is not so helpful to assume that modern explanations of the world can substitute for traditional ones. Thus many studies coming out of China on "qi" and the "jingmai" have tended to approach these concepts as materially based entities that must be measurable. In particular, the desire to impress the West with the scientific nature of modern approaches to traditional Chinese ideas and methods [106, 124] has often led to re-definitions of those ideas so that they can be explored and showcased, and then used for promotion in China, as appears to have happened with the "measuring" of "qi" in qigong [42, 106].

## Cross-cultural, philosophical and methodological challenges

A common question that researchers have asked of the traditional qi based models of acupuncture and TEAM is "is qi real?" That is, is qi measurable and can it be objectively demonstrated according to scientific standards? Theoretically, if qi cannot be demonstrated as "real", researchers might feel justified in dismissing virtually all the qi based explanatory models of acupuncture and TEAM. It has been argued elsewhere [30:149] that this is almost a nonsensical question.[10] The emergent models of the body and the cosmos from the late Warring States and Han dynasty periods (400 BCE-200 CE) clearly place qi at their center [29, 136]. In chapter one we saw how the Huainanzi (circa 122 BCE) and the important early medical corpus the Huangdi Neijing (second century BCE) both adopted a model where all things in the cosmos, whether material (animate as well as inanimate) or non-material (mental, emotional) are a construct of qi in one form or another [29]. Thus in the models that laid the foundation for TEAM thinking, everything in the world is seen as a construct of qi. Since every imaginable thing is qi how could it not be measurable? In this model all things measured are "qi" related, all measuring things are "qi" related, all those implementing the experiments are "qi" related. The problems are multi-faceted since providing a precise generalizable "definition" of "qi" does not necessarily lead to what science considers "testable hypotheses".

Ancient concepts like "qi" are, like everything else, forced into the crucible of scientific study. The same questions that are asked of other things in the modern world are asked of qi. However, without proper attention to the subject of study, this tends to introduce questionable assumptions that make apparent the cultural biases of the researcher. Without being aware of it many scientists will tend to investigate only their very limited understanding or model of "qi" and then investigate that understanding or model following conventional scientific procedures.[11] For the remainder of this section we will outline philosophical, cross-cultural problems.

There are a number of core philosophical issues that present conceptual and methodological challenges for any attempts at the scientific investigation and understanding of qi and the jingmai. Four issues basic to TEAM thinking have been discussed elsewhere [29, 33]: a) the virtual lack of "objectivity" in traditional East Asian thinking; b) the virtual lack of the "either-or" concept that is a hallmark of the scientific approach; c) the potential inapplicability of reductionist thinking to the primarily syncretistic approach of traditional East Asian thinking;[12] d) the virtual lack of mind-body dualism.[13]

These four issues have already been outlined as key problems for the biological and medical sciences [54] and pose significant challenges for any scientist attempting to investigate qi or the jingmai. Can we and, if so, how can we use reductionist approaches to investigate qi and the jingmai without losing something of their nature? How can we investigate qi and jingmai within a dualist approach? How can we deal with potentially different answers to our questions that are equally valid and not be faulted for violating the fundamental tenets of "either-or" thinking?[14] Are objective descriptions of qi and the jingmai possible given that they were not conceived in an objective manner?[15]

Foss and Rothenberg [54] argued that it is necessary to develop a model that is capable of embracing and describing the "holistic" dimensions if they are to be investigated and understood. If a medical system such as TEAM has holistic tendencies or holistic components, we must find research strategies and methods that keep intact those holistic dimensions if we are to study it [14, 33, 54, 137]. "Model fit" [69], "model fit validity"[16] [43] or "model validity" [79] is an essential ingredient in any efforts that we might make to investigate the nature and utility of a model of medical practice, but to date it has not been given sufficient attention in research of the field of acupuncture [33:29-30]. Lewith, Walach and Jonas have some discussion of the stages and steps necessary for research to proceed [79] as does the British Medical Research Council [50, 95]. While important and useful in the context of designing valid clinical studies, these recommendations are not sufficient for testing a culturally different therapy like TEAM.

In relation to investigating qi and the jingmai, no one, to date, has solved or addressed these questions. A number of researchers have been developing whole systems based models that partially address the embedded conceptual framework problem [12, 70, 137, 138], but these are more focused around clinical practice, rather than the theoretical claims and underpinnings. One of the authors has been working on an approach that may be able to lay the foundations for investigating the theoretical basis (for a start see [23]), some aspects of which are outlined below.

## *Further challenges*

There are two other important challenges that remain unaddressed. These like the four issues mentioned above relate to our core assumptions about what we are doing and the methodological limitations of our approach. The first involves how the scientific method tests hypotheses [33]: *in all hypothesis testing experiments, one never proves anything, one can only ever disprove competing, alternate or opposite hypotheses*, hence the "null hypothesis" is tested. When the null hypothesis is proven to be wrong, it is assumed that the hypothesis was correct. But a fundamental limitation of this method is that it is entirely dependent on the starting knowledge, assumptions and theories of the researchers. For example, if the researcher does not know theories of qi or the jingmai, chooses to believe only a very limited model of them or chooses not to believe or use the TEAM explanations of how something happens, they will not control for those things and will thus not have eliminated them as competing hypotheses, nor will they have tested them [33:30-31].

The risk is that such studies never actually test the concept or phenomenon that they are investigating, only an acceptable-to-them (often transformed and sometimes irrelevant) model of it. An example of this is seen with the use of electrical stimulation of inserted needles in order to be able to standardize the stimulus input in physiological studies of acupuncture analgesia [30:161]. Much of the early Western physiological investigations of acupuncture [62, 109] utilized this supposedly [83] more standardisable acupuncture stimulus method to map out the neuro-peptide analgesic mechanisms of acupuncture. This literature gradually came by many to be accepted de facto as the explanations of how acupuncture works [38, 62, 109] and even by some as the only defining characteristic of the practice of acupuncture [131].[17] However, most acupuncturists do not use electrical stimulation; it was developed in France in the early 1800s, but was not used much in clinical practice until the twentieth century [30, 82]. Thus this opinion is clearly at odds with the actual practice of acupuncture. Another example is given by Kim [75] in his analysis of Cho et al's [47] fMRI brain imaging studies. Cho and colleagues inadvertently replaced the TEAM explanation by a modern scientific one. Their assumptions about pathways of action led to the selection of measurement approaches that could never test the theory they claim to have investigated.[18]

The null hypothesis approach can also be seen as a particular case of the either-or concept, whereas in TEAM thinking one could accept both (opposing) hypotheses. Stephen Hawking, a proponent of "model-dependent realism" has come to a similar understanding:

> Whenever we develop a model of the world and find it to be successful, we tend to attribute to the model the quality of reality or absolute truth. But... the same physical situation can be modelled in different ways, each employing different fundamental elements and concepts. It might be that to describe the universe we have to employ different theories in different situations. Each theory may have its own version of reality, but according to model-dependent realism, that diversity is acceptable, and none of the versions can be said to be more real than any other [64].

The second issue arises out of the first two philosophical differences above: the lack of objectivity and lack of the "either-or" assumption in traditional East Asian thinking. What role does theory play in such a world view? Historical evidence in the traditional East Asian medical field demonstrates an enormous diversity of ideas, models and methods [16, 26, 30, 116, 117, 118, 132, 133]. Very commonly, competing ideas have existed side by side without problem.[19] This is further evidence that the "either-or" model of thinking and that attempts to formulate "objective" descriptions of the world, both of which are characteristics of modern scientific thinking, did not exist in ancient China and were not influential in how TEAM developed throughout Asia until the modern period [30, 33, 134, 135]. Together this further implies that it is inappropriate to consider traditional East Asian theories about nature or the body and their interactions as describing causally related events. A scientific "explanatory" model or theory is one that describes causal relationships between phenomena or events. Traditional theories and models of the world including the medical theories of TEAM such as the qi and jingmai, play a different role than modern scientific theories. A very reasonable explanation of the role of theory in TEAM and acupuncture is that it refers to functional concepts that are primarily about guiding clinical judgments in order to select what the practitioner considers to be an optimal treatment within the system of practice he uses [30:222, 100, 105, 144].[20] TEAM diagnostic patterns may be correlated with patient characteristics but this does not necessarily imply cause and effect.

The philosophical argument regarding this perspective is that knowledge in ancient Chinese thinking was more "skill-knowledge" (practice-based) rather than "representational knowledge" (descriptions of the world "out there") [122:4] or "how-priority" knowledge rather than "what-priority" knowledge [59:149-150]. Kuriyama shows that in classical Chinese thinking "asking 'what' was inseparable from asking 'how'" [78:96].[21] The Western model of "practice-knowledge" that seems to approximate this and which is commonly referenced is Polyani's "tacit knowing" [122:4]. Slingerland explains it thus: "For the early Chinese thinkers... the culmination of knowledge is understood not in terms of a grasp of abstract principles but rather as an ability to move through the world and human society in a manner that is completely spontaneous and yet still fully in harmony with the normative order of the natural and human worlds –the Dao or 'way'" [122:4].[22]

Given this conclusion, there are immediate implications for scientific investigations. For example, in medical research an "explanatory" (placebo-controlled) clinical trial of a therapy [125, 130] is a trial that tests known mechanisms to establish a cause-effect relationship between the intervention and the measured clinical outcome. Such a trial is, at least at present, impossible in TEAM and its related therapies like traditionally based acupuncture for two reasons. As we have just discussed, the theories of practice cannot claim to be descriptions of mechanisms, thus such a trial could never be a test of the mechanisms of traditionally based acupuncture [24]. This is further reinforced by the arguments of Hammerschlag, Zwickey [61] and colleagues [60] that we don't actually know what the mechanisms of acupuncture are in Western physiological terms even after the many physiological studies that have been performed. We have "correlational" data about the effects of acupuncture, but the actual mechanisms remain unknown [60, 61].[23] RCTs of TEAM therapies can evaluate the performance of actions related to, or that use the TEAM concepts as guiding principles for those actions but cannot evaluate the concepts themselves. Poor performance of the actions (in terms of consistency of application of those actions), and the clinical outcomes of the trial do not allow judgment of the nature or validity of the concepts themselves.

## Ensuring validity

In a study investigating whether the perivascular space might be the anatomical basis of the jingmai [84] the researchers performed experiments on mice and rabbits that required locating the stomach and gallbladder jingmai on the torso of the animals. They include a human based illustration of these two jingmai that is anatomically imprecise and which appears to locate the gallbladder jingmai in a different location than textbooks usually do. This raises questions about how well informed the researchers were about the location of these two jingmai. Additionally with the anatomical differences of different mammals, what are the differences in the location of the jingmai between humans and animals and between different animals? The likelihood of such differences raises questions about projecting findings from different animals onto human theories of the jingmai. The study also does not mention whether any members of the research team were experts in acupuncture and especially veterinary acupuncture with experience on mice and rabbits [84]. These issues raise questions about the knowledge and expertise of the researchers conducting such studies and thus the findings of their studies. This problem exists in clinical research in general and also in acupuncture clinical trials. The solution in medicine was the development of the CONSORT reporting guidelines [98, 119] and for acupuncture the STRICTA guidelines [88] which are now part of the CONSORT guidelines [86]. Given that specific expertise in acupuncture is needed for studies of the anatomical, physiological bases of acupuncture it will be necessary to develop reporting guidelines for these studies to help ensure validity of the findings from those studies and the presence of qualified experts.

## *Validating measurements and findings*

### *Ontological versus practical models*

Since the basis of the medical theories of qi and the jingmai lies in efforts to construct practical approaches to problem solving in clinical situations, using ideas that had evolved or were evolving by the time of the early medical literature of the Huangdi Neijing corpus, we have to incorporate this in any approach to testing them scientifically. Whenever we measure something that we think correlates with either qi or the jingmai, it will also be necessary to test whether the *behavior* of the things measured matches predictions about the *behavior* of the qi or jingmai, based on their traditional theories. It is not enough to simply measure something, for example lowered electro-dermal resistance (EDR), and call it the jingmai. The jingmai are related theoretically to certain functions and responsiveness in the body, not just a topographical location. What is measured at that location should also correlate to behavior predicted by jingmai theory. For example, after evaluating the person on whom the EDR is to be measured it is found that the lung channel is xu (vacuous) and the large intestine shi (replete). Do these observations correlate to differences in EDR of the lung and large intestine channels? And, if treatment is applied and the lung channel xu and large intestine shi conditions judged to be improved, do the EDR measurements show changes that match those observations. This is a highly simplified example, but illustrates the behavior of the lung channel in relation to its yang paired large intestine channel, i.e. acupuncture treatment will tend to restore a more balanced state. Almost all research of the jingmai and qi seem to have missed this necessary step.

What does the literature of TEAM tell us about how to assess the condition of the jingmai in practice? Chapter two [34] sketches the development of and reasons for the development of the jingmai concept and chapter four outlines the uses of the jingmai in acupuncture [26]. The jingmai emerged out of earlier discussions of the "mai"[脈], the vessels, which were seen as a kind of primitive physiological system that could be palpated to grasp something about their condition and then treated to help the patient. The Huangdi Neijing first described the jingmai, ascribing to them an important status for grasping and treating the condition of the patient. Lingshu ten tells us that to grasp their xu-shi state one must palpate the vessels (usually understood as the pulses) [25]. Lingshu nine described a system (not in much use today) that compared the relative strength of the radial and carotid arteries to determine the relative xu-shi state of the jingmai. The Nanjing described a much more sophisticated model of radial pulse palpation to determine the xu-shi state of each of the jingmai, which appears to have been influential in many later developments of pulse diagnosis [133].[24] Later authors have added direct palpation of the jingmai themselves [57, 140]. Thus any scientific jingmai measurement system (e.g. EDR) would have to demonstrate correlated changes to those that a practitioner would pick up by pulse palpation.

We saw above that both qi and jingmai are concepts that at least in part, if not fundamentally, refer to ways that the body regulates itself, and offer a means (via for example needling) for helping restore order to a disordered body. Thus another feature that should be involved in research on qi or the jingmai, is that what is measured should be part of a system that is involved in ordering or regulating the body. Here, the fact that many researchers have approached the jingmai as having a higher electrical conductivity relative to surrounding skin may match this requirement. Non-neurological, low level electrical signals in the body have been demonstrated as being fundamental to growth, repair, development processes and regulation within the body and between the body and its environment [9, 10, 11, 35, 39, 40, 41]. Some researchers involved in EDR measurements of the jingmai have speculated that what they have measured is part of this fundamental regulatory system [9, 10, 11]. Some have made further speculations about the jingmai as being a part of the body's information regulation systems [89, 90]. How well do other findings of the jingmai or qi correlate with bio-physical systems involved in bio-regulation?

*Practical models: subjective judgments and their reliability*

Because acupuncture is rooted in clinical practice and observation, it will be necessary to include correlation of findings with clinical observations made by qualified practitioners. Practitioner pulse reading assessments being subjective will need to be guaranteed to be reliable [102]. This can be achieved either by first conducting reliability studies [103] with as needed remedial studying [145, 146] until reliability between qualified practitioners has been established or to have at least two qualified practitioners make assessments and only take measurements when they agree upon their assessments [104]. Thus for example, two practitioners read the pulses to assess the condition of the jingmai, after they agree, the EDR measurements are made. Next, the treatment is applied according to what was judged from the pulses, then, when the two practitioners agree on the changes in the pulses, the EDR measurements are repeated. This model is more persuasive if a control group is used where either no treatment is given or a "sham" treatment is given and where the two practitioners agree that minimal or no changes have occurred in the pulses [104]. Such a study compares reliable subjective assessments of the condition of the jingmai in two groups where changes have been produced or no changes have been produced and examines whether the EDR measurements show a pattern of changes that matches the subjective assessments. The person making the EDR measurements will need to be blind to group assignment of each patient/subject. There will be a further requirement as well. We know already from studies of the acupoints that issues around reliability of their localizations exist [5, 112]: reliability of localization of the jingmai will face the same challenges. Since the localization of the jingmai for placement of the EDR electrodes is based on subjective judgment, then studies will need two or more experts to locate the jingmai relative to the placement of the EDR electrodes and their agreement must be guaranteed. A few studies have used this method to guarantee agreement in clinical and physiological studies [4, 45, 104, 147].

In the research by Ma and colleagues discussed above [84], there was not only no indication of whether a qualified veterinary acupuncturist performed the topographical localization of the jingmai, but there appears also not to have been other experts present to guarantee reliability of the judgments. Thus we cannot be sure that whatever was found can be said to relate to the jingmai. Also, in this study models of jingmai behavior were not tested so that whatever was observed cannot be assumed to correlate (yet) with the jingmai. The lack of these important steps undermines the ability of the study to draw conclusions about the jingmai.

*Diagnostic validity*

Although there has been some investigation of the reliability of TEAM observational assessment methods such as pulse and tongue diagnosis there is still the larger issue of their validity. For example, how do we know that the left, distal position radial pulse relates to the heart and small intestine jingmai? The possible randomized study described above, investigating whether pulse readings are correlated with giving/not giving a treatment, would provide a starting point to examine this more complex question. This issue is likely a problem to be solved further downstream than the issues discussed in this chapter.

*Technical challenges facing investigations of qi and the jingmai*

Put simply, what is it that we are supposed to measure in any investigation of qi and the jingmai? Today in the fields of physics, chemistry, biology, biophysics etc. we are faced with a bewildering array of different measurement technologies and approaches. In order to make appropriate measurements of something like qi and the jingmai, we first need to have separate hypotheses regarding what kind of physical changes or events we might expect to occur so we can try to match those with appropriate measurement technologies.

If we assume that qi is related to some form of "energy" what is it we are supposed to measure? Electrical resistance of the skin, electrical potential of the skin, bio-photon emissions, bio-magnetic fields, magnetic vector potential, fields visualized under high density charge (Kirlian photography, gas discharge visualization), quantum field changes? The translation of traditional concepts such as qi and jingmai into measurable phenomena will likely develop along several paths simultaneously. Once we have appropriately informed models of qi or the jingmai and derived hypotheses about them, how do we know what we are supposed to measure in order to test those hypotheses? Some methods will be theoretically driven, where instrumentation is chosen or developed to match the theoretical constructions,[25] some will be accidental[26] or by informed guesswork, observations emerging out of exploratory studies, some will miss the point completely by inadvertently using inappropriate technologies.[27] In the absence of acceptable models and reasonable hypothetical physiological/bio-physical translations of the concepts of qi and jingmai, progress will continue haphazardly with often indefensible findings and claims.

A step that will sometimes be necessary is the use of modeling tools and techniques such as non-linear dynamical systems modeling, computer modeling and testing [13, 56, 76]. This step helps refine and make more precise the models to be tested and to help ensure a closer match of theory (of qi, jingmai) with measurement technology.

## Finding solutions: A step-by-step approach

If progress is to be made in the scientific investigation of qi and the jingmai, properly informed models of them need to be constructed that are also able to bypass or solve the various challenges mentioned above. It will be important to deal with the stated or explicit theories of qi and the jingmai, but we will also need to build up implicit theories through deductive and inductive reasoning, observation, qualitative investigations, etc [27]. This necessarily requires the participation of appropriate scholars of the literature and clinicians who practice with those techniques, most likely combined with other research expertise such as qualitative research methods employed, for example, by anthropologists, sociologists, etc. Other experts will be required for developing and using appropriate technologies and for validating clinical observations. In all, a careful step-by-step multidisciplinary approach is needed. Table 1 summarizes this.[28]

Even if the traditional theories of qi and the jingmai do not yield clearly positive results in experiments following the steps outlined in Table 1, it still does not mean that those theories are not useful as guides to practitioners. Clinical utility can be tested in different clinical trial studies. Various pragmatic style comparison studies [85, 125] can be developed to explore the clinical utility of these theories. Questions such as: "do forms of acupuncture that use theories of qi and jingmai yield results that are equal to or better than other forms of acupuncture that do not use these theories?"[29] can be tested. The implicit difficulty in conducting explanatory trials of traditionally based acupuncture was discussed above. Clinical testing of traditional acupuncture concepts can only be achieved in pragmatic trials, where the test is of clinical utility (matching traditional ideas) rather than the validity or reality of hypothetical constructs.

It is also highly likely given the enormous diversity of theories, practice methods and approaches in the field of TEAM that there will be issues around generalizability of results. Take for example the concept of "jingmai". In Keiraku Chiryo, Japanese Meridian Therapy the jingmai are treated as though they are very superficial, in the skin. Disturbances of the jingmai are the principle focus of the diagnosis and treatment [57, 120]. While in TCM acupuncture the jingmai are generally seen in relation to the depth at which deqi sensations are obtained and thus seen in relation to deeper structures. [108, 141]. However the principle focus of diagnosis and treatment in TCM is not the jingmai, disturbances of the jingmai are only focused on in for example pain problems [6, 44, 51].[30] It is unlikely that a general theory of the jingmai can ultimately resolve these different interpretative perspectives. Thus it is probable that studies will develop hypotheses utilizing a particular assumption about depth and will have to test accordingly. When positive evidence for the existence of or correlation to the jingmai is obtained in these studies it will be important to resist temptation to generalize from the results to the overall more diverse concept of the jingmai. It is possible that ongoing studies may reveal something that incorporates evidence from both lines of interpretative investigations so that more insightful theories of the jingmai may evolve, but it is also possible that different lines of evidence develop that support the different interpretations, even though they appear to be contradictory. Not generalizing inappropriately and being open to opposing results will probably be necessary.[31]

**Table 1 –Steps required for hypothesis development and testing within the TEAM explanatory model**

| Tasks | Approaches | Expertise |
|---|---|---|
| 1- literature review and expert surveys to develop "explicit" models/understanding | literature review & analysis; expert surveys & consultation | -access to relevant literatures (multilingual and linguistic skills, medical historians, medical anthropologists, etc)<br>-clinical experts |
| 2- ancillary literature and expert surveys & clinical observation to develop "implicit" models/understanding | Ancillary literature analysis; clinical observation (inductive, deductive reasoning) & additional surveys/questionnaires (qualitative research) | -clinicians<br>-medical sociologists, anthropologists, etc<br>-psychologists<br>-philosophers |
| 3- combining "explicit" and "implicit" theories from 1 & 2 to formulate more complete models | combining of 1 & 2 findings with expert consultation | -clinical experts<br>-theoreticians, philosophers<br>-various scientists (mathematics, physics, etc) |
| 4- testing of the models from 3 to help refine them | mathematical modeling and testing | -clinical experts<br>-mathematicians, physicists |
| 5- repeat 3 & 4 with return to 1 & 2 as needed until a model is developed that matches traditional theories, bypasses philosophical & cross-cultural problems, etc | clinical exploration & testing; theory development & testing; mathematical modeling & testing; | -clinical experts<br>-mathematicians<br>-various research experts (qualitative & quantitative) |
| 6- identify techniques & technologies relevant for measuring the components of the model from 3, 4 & 5,* μ | various biological and physical measurements | -biophysicists, engineers<br>-computer experts<br>-clinical experts<br>-mathematicians |

μ. Step 6 can start earlier while working on other steps.
*Relevant technologies should not include only what is available at the time the experiments were being conducted but may require waiting for or development of appropriate technologies to be developed or become accessible. There has to be a proper match of desired variables to be measured and appropriate technologies for measuring them, not just using what is available now and may be relevant.

| Tasks | Approaches | Expertise |
|---|---|---|
| 7- perform studies to validate use of traditional observations/assessments (necessary for matching of models from 5 with measurements from 6 and full testing of relevant hypotheses) | intra-rater & inter-rater reliability studies with development of methods to improve both and guarantee both, exploration of diagnostic validity | -clinical experts<br>-bio-statisticians<br>-biomedical researchers<br>-clinical instructors |
| 8- perform studies with instrumentation (from 6) to measure phenomena identified in models (from 5) and verified by clinical observations (from 7)** | instrumentation;<br>clinical applications;<br>clinical observations | -engineers, biophysicists<br>-mathematicians<br>-clinical experts<br>-biomedical researchers<br>-sociologists, anthropologists<br>-etc |
| 9- repetition of studies in 8 with revisiting 1-7 as needed & repetition of those studies | same as 8 | same as 8 |

## Summary of primary issues facing the scientific investigations of qi and the jingmai

The primary issues facing any attempts to make scientific observations or measurements of qi and the jingmai can be grouped under three main areas:

1- *Conceptual.* (related to establishing the validity of researcher claims of testing TEAM concepts)
Has an informed and rigorous model of the object of study been developed? Were the hypotheses that were tested accurately reflective of the object of study? Have the researchers drawn properly contextualized conclusions or have they attempted generalizations beyond the scope of what they have done?

**Here it is not only important to make measurements (6) of the phenomena modeled (5) but these must also match predictions from the models (5) verified by clinical observations (7).

2 - *Technical.* (related to establishing the validity of researcher claims to have measured the correct things in scientific terms).[32]
Have relevant measurement instruments or observation methods been used?
Has the evidence for use of that technology been presented and is it sufficient?
Has the instrumentation been shown to be reliable and sufficiently accurate?
Were the measurements free of artifacts or were potential artifacts sufficiently controlled for?

3 - *Methodological.* (related to establishing the validity of researcher claims of having tested qi or the jingmai using scientific methods)
Is there sufficient justification with regards the concepts to be tested for the instrumentation selected to test derivative hypotheses?
Have both correlations between theoretical predictions *and* measured outcomes *and* the *behaviour* of the objects of study (qi, jingmai), been investigated? (Step 8 in table 1 above)
Have the technical measurements been taken in correspondence to clinical decisions and/or observations?
Were those clinical decisions/observations reliable?

Future studies of, for example, qi or the jingmai, can use the steps in Table 1 in their design and implementation phases.[33] Reviews, evaluations of studies investigating qi or the jingmai can use the areas outlined above as criteria for evaluating studies.

## Conclusions

In this paper we have outlined historical, philosophical and cultural issues that make investigations of TEAM concepts such as "qi" and the "jingmai" difficult. We believe that these issues cannot be ignored if valid studies are to be performed. We outlined a series of steps that will allow for valid studies to be conducted. These steps require coordinated multi-disciplinary approaches in order to generate valid testable hypotheses and valid methods of measurement and observation. We have presented a series of arguments based on layers of evidence to support these requirements.

In addition, the steps outlined above can be used as basic guidelines for judging how well studies of, for example, "qi" or the "jingmai" examined the qi or the jingmai. We suspect that in most studies we will see large conceptual and methodological gaps since these critical steps have not previously been followed.

We hope that the arguments above will help researchers involved in investigating TEAM or the traditional concepts of other systems such as Ayurveda and provide a framework for establishing valid scientific investigations.

## Bibliography

1- *Acupuncture*. NIH Consensus Statement 1997 Nov 3-5; 15(5):1-34.
2- Ahn AC, Colbert AP, Anderson BJ, Martinsen OG, Hammerschlag R, Cina S, Wayne PM, Langevin HM. Electrical properties of acupuncture points and meridians: a systematic review. *Bioelectromagnetics*. 2008 May;29(4):245-56.
3- Ahn AC, Martinsen OG. Electrical characterization of acupuncture points: Technical issues and challenges. *J Altern Complement Med* 2007;13:817–824.
4- Ahn AC, Park M, Shaw JR, McManus CA, Kaptchuk TJ, Langevin HM. *Electrical impedance of acupuncture meridians: the relevance of subcutaneous collagenous bands*. PLoS One. 2010; 5(7):e11907
5- Aird M, Coyle ME, Cobbin DM, Zaslawski CJ. A Study of the Comparative Accuracy of Two Methods of Locating Acupuncture points', *Acupuncture in Medicine*, 2000;18(1):15-21.
6- Anon. *Essentials of Chinese Acupuncture*. Beijing, Foreign Languages Press, 1980.
7- Anon, Interview with Ji Sheng Han, *Omni*, February 1988, pages 81 and following.
8- Barnes LL. *Needles, Herbs, Gods and Ghosts*, Cambridge, Harvard University Press, 2005.
9- Becker RO. Electromagnetic controls over biological growth processes. *J Bioelect*. 1984:3(162):105-118.
10- Becker, RO, Marino AA. *Electromagnetism and Life*, Albany: State University of New York Press, 1982.
11- Becker RO, Selden G. *The Body Electric*, New York: William Morrow, 1985.
12- Bell IR, Koithan M. Models for the study of whole systems. *Integr Cancer Ther*. 2006:5(4):293-307.
13- Bell IR, Koithan M, Pincus D. Methodological Implications of Nonlinear Dynamical Systems Models for Whole Systems of Complementary and Alternative Medicine. *Forsch Komplementmed* 2012;19(suppl 1):15–21.
14- Birch S. Introduction. In Manaka Y, Itaya K, Birch S. *Chasing the Dragon's Tail*, Brookline, Paradigm Publications, 1995:ix-xxvii.
15- Birch S. Testing the claims of traditionally based acupuncture. *Complem Ther Med* 1997:5: 147-151.
16- Birch S. Diversity and acupuncture: Acupuncture is not a coherent or historically stable tradition. in AJ. Vickers (ed.) *Examining Complementary Medicine: The Sceptical Holist*. Cheltenham: Stanley Thomas, 1998, pp. 45-63.
17- Birch S. Overview of models used in controlled acupuncture studies and thoughts about questions answerable by each. *Clin Acup Orien Med* 2003a:3, 4:207-217.
18- Birch S. Testing traditionally based systems of acupuncture. *Clin Acup Orient Med*. 2003b:4(2-3):84-87.

19- Birch S. Clinical research of acupuncture: part two –controlled clinical trials an overview of their methods. *J Alt Complem Med.* 2004:10, 3:481-498.
20- Birch S. A review and analysis of placebo treatments, placebo effects and placebo controls in trials of medical procedures when sham is not inert. *J Alt Complem Med*, 2006:12(3):303-310.
21- Birch S. Comment on 'sham device v inert pill: randomised controlled trial of two placebo treatments. February 9, 2006 & Yes let's get real: what placebo isn't. March 10, 2006a. http://www.bmj.com/cgi/letters/332/7538/391#129658
22- Birch S. Reflections on the German acupuncture studies. *J Chin Med.* 2007:83:12-17.
23- Birch S. Filling the whole in acupuncture. Part 1: What are we doing in the supplementation needle technique? *EJOM*, 2009:6(2):25-35 (1st half); 2009:6(3):18-27 (2nd half).
24- Birch S. Sham acupuncture is not a placebo –implications and problems in research. *JAM* 2012;2:5 –9 .
25- Birch S. Traditional needling techniques as practical constructions from reading historical descriptions. *Eur J Oriental Med.* 2013;7(3)26-33.
26- Birch S. Chapter four: The Jingmai and qi –acupuncture perspectives. In this volume
27- Birch S. (In preparation-a). Filling the whole in acupuncture. Part 2: The "treat-ment space" –modeling the treatment process in acupuncture.
28- Birch S, Bovey M. Which are the placebo effects: comments on Kaptchuk et al's IBS placebo study. June 30, 2008. http://www.bmj.com/cgi/letters/336/7651/999.
29- Birch S, Cabrer Mir MA, Rodriguez M. Chapter one: Qi and the mind – explorations of the links between qi, the mind, mental and emotional states. In this volume.
30- Birch S, Felt R. *Understanding Acupuncture*, Edinburgh, Churchill Livingstone, 1999.
31- Birch S., Friedman M. On the development of a mathematical model for the "laws" of the five phases, *Amer J Acup*; 1989:17, 4:361-6.
32- Birch S, Hammerschlag R, Trinh K, Zaslawski C. The non-specific effects of acupuncture treatment: When and how to control for them. *Clin Acup Orien Med*; 2002:3, 1:20-25.
33- Birch S, Lewith G. Acupuncture research, the story so far. In MacPherson H, Hammerschlag. R, Lewith G, Schnyer R (eds). *Acupuncture Research: Strategies for Building an Evidence Base*. London, Elsevier, 2007:15-35.
34- Birch S, Rodriguez M, Cabrer Mir MA. Chapter two: The jingmai –a summary of their development and nature. In this volume.
35- Bischof M. Field concepts and the emergence of a holistic biophysics. Beloussov, L.V., Popp, F.A., Voeikov, V.L., and Van Wijk, R., (eds.): *Biophotonics and Coherent Systems*. Moscow University Press, Moscow, 2000:1-25.
36- Bovey M. Deqi. *J Chin Med* 2006; (81): 18-29
37- Bovey M. *Researching practice: the good, the bad and the masterful.* Eur J Orient Med 2010; 6(4): 6-15

38- Bowsher D. Mechanisms of acupuncture. In Filshie J, White A. (eds). *Medical Acupuncture*. Edinburgh, Churchill Livingstone, 1998 pp 69-83.
39- Burr HS. *Blueprint for immortality: The electric patterns of life*, Daniel, Essex, 1972.
40- Burr HS, Lane CT. Electrical characteristics of living systems, *Yale J. of Biology and Medicine*, 1935;8(1):31-35.
41- Burr HS, Northrop FS. Evidence for the Existence of an Electro-Dynamic Field in Living Organisms. *Proc Natl Acad Sci U S A*. 1939 Jun;25(6):284-8.
42- Cabrer Mir MA. Chapter seven: Qi and stillness –Taijiquan, qigong and acupuncture. In this volume.
43- Cassidy CM. *Methodological Issues in Investigations of Massage/Bodywork Therapy*. Evanston, American Massage Therapy Association Foundation, 2002.
44- Cheng XN. *Chinese Acupuncture and Moxibustion*. Beijing, Foreign Languages Press, 1987.
45- Cheng SC, Lin CH, Chang YJ, Lee TH, Ryu SJ, Chen CH, Chang HK, Chang CJ, Hu WL, Hung YC. Fire-Heat and Qi Deficiency Syndromes as Predictors of Short-term Prognosis of Acute Ischemic Stroke. *J Altern Complem Med*. 2013:19(8)721-728.
46- Chmelik S, Bovey M. *Acupuncture and Traditional Chinese Medicine for treating migraine*. In: Fernández-de-las-Peñas C, Chaitow L, Schoenen J (eds) Multidisciplinary management of migraine: pharmacological, manual and other therapies. Jones & Bartlett Learning, Sudbury, MA. 2011.
47- Cho ZH, Chung SC, Jones JP, Park JB, Park HJ, Lee HJ, Wong EK, Min BI. New findings of the correlation between acupoints and corresponding brain cortices using functional MRI. *Proc Nat Acad Sci USA*, 1998:95:2670-2673.
48- Cohen M. Energy Medicine from an Ancient and Modern Perspective. In Cohen M. (Ed) *Prescriptions for Holistic Health*, Monash Institute of Health Services Research. Clayton, May 2002 ISBN 0 9580841 06. pp 97-108.
49- Comunetti A, Laage S, Schiessl N, Kistler A. *Characteristics of human skin conductance at acupuncture points*. Experientia; 1995;51:328-331.
50- Craig P, Dieppe P, Macintyre S, Mitchie S, Nazareth I, Petticrew M: Developing and evaluating complex interventions: the new Medical Research Council guidance. *BMJ* 2008;337:979–983.
51- Ellis A, Wiseman N, Boss K. *Fundamentals of Chinese Acupuncture*; Brookline, Paradigm Publications, 1988.
52- Falk CX, Birch S, Avants SK, Tsau Y, Margolin A. Preliminary results of a new method for locating auricular acupuncture points. *Acup Electrother Int Res J*. 2000:25:165-177.
53- Felt RO. Is qi energy? *Thieme Almanac 2008: Acupuncture and Chinese Medicine*. Stuttgart, George Thieme Verlag, 2008:303-308.
54- Foss L, Rothenberg K. *The Second Medical Revolution*, Boston, Shambhala Publications, 1987.
55- Friedman M, Birch S, Tiller WA. Towards the development of a mathematical model for acupuncture meridians, *Acup Electrother Res Int J*; 1989:14:217-26.

56- Friedman M, Birch S, Tiller WA. Mathematical modeling as a tool in basic research in acupuncture. *J Alt Complem Med.* 3, Suppl 1: 1997:S89-S99.
57- Fukushima K. *Meridian Therapy*, Tokyo, Toyo Hari Medical Association, 1991.
58- Gleick J. *Chaos: Making a New Science*, New York, Viking, 1987.
59- Hall DL, Ames RT. *Thinking from the Han*, Albany, State University of New York, 1998.
60- Hammerschlag R, Langevin HE, Lao LX, Lewith G. Physiological dynamics of acupuncture: correlations and mechanisms. In MacPherson H, Hammerschlag.R, Lewith G, Schnyer R (eds). *Acupuncture Research: Strategies for Building an Evidence Base.* London, Elsevier, 2007:181-197.
61- Hammerschlag R, Zwickey H. Evidence based complementary and alternative medicine: back to basics. *J Alt Complem Med.* 2006;12(4):349-350.
62- Han JS. Physiology of acupuncture: A review of thirty years of research. *J Alt Complem Med.* 1997:3, Suppl.1, 101-108.
63- Harper D. *Early Chinese Medical Literature: the Mawangdui Medical Manuscripts.* London, Kegan Paul, 1998.
64- Hawking S, Mlodinow L. The (elusive) theory of everything. *Scientific American*, October 2010, pages 51-53.
65- Hsu E. Pulse diagnostics in the Western Han: how mai and qi determine bing. In Hsu E, (ed). *Innovation in Chinese Medicine*, Cambridge, Cambridge University Press, 2001:51-91.
66- Hsu TL, Bau JG, Wang WK, Li SP, Wang YYL. Similarity between coffee effects and qi-stimulating events. *J Altern Complem Med.* 2008;14(9):1145–1150.
67- Jahn RG, Dunne BJ. Sensors, filters and the source of reality. *J Scientific Exploration*, 2004:18;4:547–570.
68- Jia J, Yu Y, Deng JH, Robinson N, Bovey M, Cui YH, Liu HR, Ding W, Wu HG, Wang XM. A review of Omics research in acupuncture: The relevance and future prospects for understanding the nature of meridians and acupoints. *Journal of Ethnopharmacology* 2012;140:594–603.
69- Jonas WB. Balancing quality research in acupuncture: Matching methodology with goals and materials; *Proceedings of the Second Symposium of the Society for Acupuncture Research.* Society for Acupuncture Research, 1995:212-229.
70- Jonas WB, Beckner W, Coulter I. Proposal for an integrated evaluation model for the study of whole systems health care in cancer. *Integr Cancer Ther*, 2006:5(4):315-319.
71- Kaptchuk TJ. *The Web That Has No Weaver*, New York, Congdon and Weed, 1983.
72- Kaptchuk TJ. Historical context of the concept of vitalism in complementary and alternative medicine. In: Micozzi MS. (Ed). *Fundamentals of Complementary and Alternative Medicine,* New York, Churchill Livingstone, 1996:39-45.
73- Kaptchuk TJ, Kelley JM, Conboy LA, Davis RB, Kerr CE, Jacobson EE, Kirsch I, Schnyer RN, Nam BH, Nguyen LT, Park M, Rivers AL, McManus C, Kokkotou E, Drossman DA, Goldman P, Lembo AJ. Components of placebo effect: randomized controlled trial in patients with irritable bowel syndrome. *BMJ*, 2008:336(7651):999-1003.

74- Kaptchuk TJ, Stason WB, Davis RB, Legedza ART, Schnyer RN, Kerr CE, Stone DA, Nam BH, Kirsch I, Goldman RH. Sham device v inert pill: randomized controlled trial of two placebo treatments. *BMJ* 2006; 332:391- 397.
75- Kim JY. Beyond paradigm: Making transcultural connections in a scientific translation of acupuncture. *Soc Sci Med.* 2006:62(12):2960-72.
76- Koithan M, Bell IR, Niemeyer K, Pincus D. A Complex Systems Science Perspective for Whole Systems of Complementary and Alternative Medicine Research. *Forsch Komplementmed* 2012;19(suppl 1):7–14
77- Kumar M. *Quantum –Einstein, Bohr and the great debate about the nature of reality*, London, Icon books, 2009.
78- Kuriyama S. *The Expressiveness of the Body and the Divergence of Greek and Chinese Medicine*, New York, Zone Books 1999.
79- Lewith G, Wallach H, Jonas WB. Balanced research strategies for complementary and alternative medicine. In Lewith G, Jonas WB, Walach H. (eds) *Clinical Research in Complementary Therapies*, Edinburgh, Churchill Livingstone 2002:3-27.
80- Li Y, Liang FR, Yu SG, Liu XG, Tang Y, Yang XG, Tian XP, Yan J, Sun GJ, Chang XR, Zhang H, Zhang HX, Ma TT. Randomized controlled trial to treat migraine with acupuncture: design and protocol. *Trials*, 2008, 9:57. http://www.trialsjournal.com/content/9/1/57
81- Lin ZX, Yu L, Guo ZY, Shen ZY, Zhang HL, Zhang TL. *Qigong: Chinese Medicine or Pseudoscience?* New York, Prometheus Books, 2000.
82- Lu GD, Needham J. *Celestial Lancets*; Cambridge, Cambridge University Press, 1980.
83- Lytle CD, Thomas BM, Gordon EA, Krauthamer V. Electrostimulators for acupuncture: safety issues. *J Alt Complem Med.* 2000:6(1):37-44.
84- Ma WT, Tong H, Xu WY, Hu JM, Liu N, Li HY, Cao LX. Perivascular Space: Possible Anatomical Substrate for the Meridian. *J Altern Complem Med.* 2003; 9(6):851–859.
85- MacPherson H. Acupuncture research: time to shift from theoretical to practical questions. *J Alt Compl Med.* 2006:12(9), 837–839.
86- MacPherson H, Altman DG, Hammerschlag R, Li YP, Wu TX, White A, Moher D; on behalf of the STRICTA Revision Group. Revised STandards for Reporting Interventions in Clinical Trials of Acupuncture (STRICTA): extending the CONSORT statement. *Acupunct Med* 2010 28: 83-93, originally published online June 3, 2010, doi: 0.1136/aim.2009.001370
87- MacPherson H, Sherman K, Hammerschlag R, Birch S, Lao L, Zaslawski C. The clinical evaluation of East Asian systems of medicine. *Clin Acup Orient Med* 2002:3, 1:16-19.
88- MacPherson H, White A, Cummings M, Jobst K, Rose K, Niemtzow R. for the STRICTA Group. Standards for Reporting Interventions in Controlled Trials of Acupuncture: The STRICTA recommendations. *J Altern Complement Med* 2002;8:85–90.
89- Manaka Y, Itaya K. Acupuncture as intervention in the biological information system. (Meridian treatment and the X-signal system), Address given at the annual assembly of the Japan Meridian Treatment Association, Tokyo, March 29-30, 1986. Published in English in the *J Acup Soc New York* 1994:1(3-4):9-18.

90- Manaka Y, Itaya K, Birch S. *Chasing the Dragon's Tail*, Brookline, Paradigm Publications, 1995.
91- Manheimer E. Selecting a control for in vivo fertilization and acupuncture randomized controlled trials (RCTs): how sham controls may unnecessarily complicate the RCT evidence base. *Fertil Steril*, 2011: doi:10.1016/j.fertnstert.2011.04.040.
92- McCarroll G, Rowley BA. An investigation of electrically located acupuncture points. *IEEE Transactions on Biomedical Engineering*. 1979;26:177-181.
93- McFadden JJ. *Quantum Evolution: life in the multiverse*. London, Flamingo Publishers, 2002.
94- McTaggart L. *The Field*, London, Element Publishers, 2001.
95- Medical Research Council. A framework for development and evaluation of RCTs for complex interventions to improve health, 2000. Accessed October 5, 2005 via internet: http://www.mrc.ac.uk/pru/pdf-mrc_cpr.pdf.
96- Milgrom LR. Toward a unified theory of homeopathy and conventional medicine. *J Alt Complem Med*, 2007:13, 7:759-769.
97- Miller FG, Colloca L, Kaptchuk TJ. The Placebo effect: illness and interpersonal healing. *Perspect Biol Med*. 2009 ; 52(4): 518.
98- Moher D, Hopewell S, Schulz KF, Montori V, Gøtzsche PC, Devereaux PJ, Elbourne D, Egger M, Altman DG. CONSORT 2010 explanation and elaboration: updated guidelines for reporting parallel group randomised trials. *BMJ* 2010;340:c869. doi: 10.1136/bmj.c869.
99- Motoyama H. A biophysical elucidation of the meridian and ki energy. What is ki energy and how does it flow? *Research Relig. & Parapsych*. 1981:7:1.
100- Murakami M. Lecture given in Newton, Massachusetts, October 1998.
101- Nordergraaf A, Silage D. Electroacupuncture. *IEEE Transactions on Biomedical Engineering*. 1973;20:364-367.
102- O'Brien KA, Birch S. A review of the reliability of Traditional East Asian Medicine diagnoses. *J Altern Complement Med*. 2009;15(4):353-366.
103- O'Brien KA, Abbas E, Movsessian P, Hook M, Komesaroff PA, Birch S. Investigating the reliability of Japanese Toyohari Meridian Therapy diagnosis. *J Altern Complem Med* 2009;15(10):1099–1105.
104- O'Brien KA, Birch S, Abbas E, Movsessian P, Hook M, Komesaroff PA. Traditional East Asian Medical pulse diagnosis –a preliminary physiological investigation. *J Altern Comp Med*. 2013;19(10):793-798. DOI: 10.1089/acm.2012.0141.
105- Ogawa T. Workshop given at the New England School of Acupuncture, Watertown, MA., April, 1996.
106- Palmer DA. *Qigong Fever –Body, Science and Utopia in China*. New York, Columbia University Press, 2007.
107- Paterson C, Dieppe P. Characteristic and incidental (placebo) effects in complex interventions such as acupuncture. *BMJ* 2005;330:1202–1205.
108- Pomeranz B. Scientific bases of acupuncture. In Stux G, Pomeranz B. *Basics of Acupuncture*, Berlin, Springer Verlag 1990, pages 4-55.
109- Pomeranz B, Berman B. Scientific basis of acupuncture. In: G Stux, B Berman, B Pomeranz. *Basics of Acupuncture*. Berlin, Springer-Verlag, fifth edition, 2003, pp 1-86.

110- Porkert M. Theoretical Foundations of Chinese Medicine. Cambridge, MIT Press, 1972.
111- Rein G. Bioinformation in the biofield. *J Alt Complem Med.* 2004:10(1):59-68.
112- Rivers WE, Zollman F. Reliability of surface acupuncture point location. *Medical Acup.* 2013;25(2)134-140.
113- Rodriguez M. Chapter six: Qi, jingmai, yaoyi –a study of their relationships. In this volume.
114- Rubik B. The biofield hypothesis: its biophysical basis and role in medicine. *J Alt Complem Med*, 2002:8,6:703-717.
115- Sagli G. The establishing of Chinese medical concepts in Norwegian acupuncture schools: the cultural translation of jingluo ("circulation tracts"). *Anthropology and Medicine*, 2010;17(3):315-326.
116- Scheid V. *Chinese Medicine in Contemporary China*, Durham, Duke University press, 2002.
117- Scheid V. Not very traditional, nor exactly Chinese, so what kind of medicine is it? TCM's discourse on menopause and its implications for practice, teaching and research. *J Chin Med.* 2006;82:5-20.
118- Schnyer R, Birch S, MacPherson H. Acupuncture practice as the foundation for clinical evaluation. In MacPherson H, Hammerschlag.R, Lewith G, Schnyer R (eds). *Acupuncture Research: Strategies for Building an Evidence Base.* London, Elsevier, 2007:153-179.
119- Schulz KF, Altman DG, Moher D, for the CONSORT Group. CONSORT 2010 statement: updated guidelines for reporting parallel-group randomized trials. *BMJ* 2010;340:c332.
120- Shudo D. *Introduction to Meridian Therapy*, Seattle, Eastland Press, 1990.
121- Sivin N. *Traditional Medicine in Contemporary China*, Ann Arbor, Center for Chinese Studies, University of Michigan, 1987.
122- Slingerland E. *Effortless Action*, Oxford, Oxford University Press, 2003.
123- So EW, Ng EH, Wong YY, Lau EY, Yeung WS, Ho PC. *A randomized double blind comparison of real and placebo acupuncture in IVF treatment.* Hum Reprod. 2009 Feb;24(2):341-8.
124- Taylor K. *Divergent interests and cultivated misunderstandings: the influence of the West on modern Chinese medicine.* Soc Hist Med. 2004:17, 1:93-111.
125- Thomas K, Fitter M. Possible research strategies for evaluating CAM interventions. In Lewith G, Jonas WB, Walach H. (eds) *Clinical Research in Complementary Therapies*, Edinburgh, Churchill Livingstone 2002:59-91.
126- Thomas KJ, MacPherson H, Thorpe L, Brazier J, Fitter M, Campbell MJ, Roman M, Walters SJ, Nicholl J. Randomised controlled trial of a short course of traditional acupuncture compared with usual care for persistent non-specific low back pain. *BMJ*, 2006;333:623-626.
127- Tiller WA. On the evolution of electrodermal diagnostic instruments. *J Advancement in Med.* 1988:1(1):41-72.
128- Tiller WA. On the evolution and future development of electrodermal diagnostic instruments. In *Energy Fields in Medicine*, Kalamazoo, Michigan, John E. Fetzer Foundation, 1989:257-328.

129- Toulmin S. *The Philosophy of Science*, London, Hutchinson University Library, 1953.
130- Treweek S, Zwarenstein M. Making trials matter: pragmatic and explanatory trials and the problem of applicability. *Trials* 2009, 10:37 doi:10.1186/1745-6215-10-37.
131- Ulett G. *Beyond Yin and Yang*; St. Louis, Missouri, Warren H. Green Inc, 1992.
132- Unschuld PU. *Medicine in China: A History of Ideas*, Berkeley, University of California Press, 1985.
133- Unschuld PU. *Medicine in China: The Classic of Difficult Issues*, Berkeley, University of California Press, 1986.
134- Unschuld PU. Traditional Chinese medicine; some historical and epistemological reflections. *Soc Sci Med*; 1987:24, 12:1023-1029.
135- Unschuld PU. Epistemological issues and changing legitimation: Traditional Chinese medicine in the twentieth century. In Leslie C, Young A, (eds) *Paths to Asian Medical Knowledge*; Berkeley, University of California Press, 1992:44-61.
136- Unschuld PU. *Huang Di Nei Jing Su Wen –nature, knowledge, imagery in an ancient Chinese medical text*. Berkeley, University of California Press, 2003.
137- Verhoef MJ, Lewith G, Rittenbaugh C, Thomas K, Boon H, Fonnebo V. Whole systems research: moving forward. *Focus on Alt Compl Ther*, 2004:9(2):87-90.
138- Verhoef MJ, Vanderheyden LC, Fonnebo V. A whole systems research approach to cancer care: why we need it and how to get started? *Integr Cancer Ther*, 2006:5(4): 287-292.
139- Volkov MV, Oganesyan OV. *External fixation: joint deformities and bone fractures*, Madison CT, International Universities Press, 1987.
140- Wang JY. *Applied Channel Theory in Chinese Medicine*. Seattle, Eastland Press, 2008.
141- Wang KM, Yao SM, Xian YL, Hou ZL. A study on the receptive field of acupoints and the relationship between characteristics of needling sensation and groups of afferent fibres. *Sci Sin*[B] 1985;28:963–9.
142- Wiseman N, Ellis A. *Fundamentals of Chinese Medicine*; Brookline, Massachusetts, Paradigm Publications, 1985.
143- Yan X, Lu F, Jiang HJ, Wu XC, Cao W, Xia ZQ, Shen H, Wang J, Dao M, Lin H, Zhu RS. (2002). Certain physical manifestation and effects of external Qi of yan xin life science technology. *J Scientific Exploration* 2002:16
144- Yanagishita T. Lecture given in Tokyo, July, 1997.
145- Zhang GG, Lee WL, Bausell B, Lao LX, Handwerger B, Berman B. Variability in the Traditional Chinese Medicine (TCM) Diagnoses and Herbal Prescriptions Provided by Three TCM Practitioners for 40 Patients with Rheumatoid Arthritis. *J Alt Complem Med*. 2005;11(3):415–421.
146- Zhang GG, Singh B, Lee WL, Handwerger B, Lao LX, Berman L. Improvement of Agreement in TCM Diagnosis Among TCM Practitioners for Persons with the Conventional Diagnosis of Rheumatoid Arthritis: Effect of Training. *J Alt Complem Med*. 2008;14(4):381–386.
147- Zhong MC, Tang NY, Liu CH, Huang WH, Hsu YT, Liu YL, Li TC, Hsieh CL. Relationship Between Chinese Medicine Pattern Types, Clinical Severity, and

Prognosis in Patients With Acute Cerebral Infarct. *Explore: The Journal of Science and Healing*, 2013;9(4):226-231.
148- Zhu ZX. Research advances in the electrical specificity of channels and acupuncture points. *Amer J Acup*. 1981:9,3:203-216.

## Endnotes

1. Barnes has a very useful discussion with examples of how early translations of concepts such as qi, jingmai etc were so colored by the concepts of vitalism that were current at the time of their attempts as to distort the meanings of the original [8:87-92]. These examples are instructive of how problems of understanding can arise.

2. This is most obvious with the assumption that the jingmai should be measurable electrically as lines of lower electrical resistance, and thus as conductors of electrical energy.

3. Recall also from chapter two how the term "jing" [經] is often translated by scholars using terms that invoke an understanding of the jing as something that orders or brings regularity to things [34].

4. There is of course a much more fundamental problem as well. The term "energy" is a general term that has been used in distinction with "matter" as a kind of duality. But since the time of Einstein (early 1900s) with his theories of relativity and the famous "$e=mc^2$" it has been shown that matter and energy are interchangeable. The term "energy" is thus loaded with a conception based on a duality known in physics and related disciplines to be less meaningful and thus outdated. The fields of biology and medicine have been very slow to catch up with this and other twentieth century developments in physics [Foss, Rothenberg 1987]. Scientifically speaking to ask, as many have done, whether qi might be some form of measurable "energy" is thus problematic. The same problem holds for the notion of qi as a "substance", some kind of "matter," see discussions below. Possibly of more relevance is the notion of "force". In physics there are the four "fundamental forces: "gravitational", "electromagnetic", "strong nuclear" and "weak nuclear". The notion of "force" might be more fruitful, but needs to be more carefully conceptualised –see also endnote 7 below.

5. Kumar has a good discussion of this issue [77:10-11]. It represents a fundamental property of energy as related to heat/cold, which is important in our discussion because one of the bases for understanding qi that was used historically was experiential. For example one of the qi properties of herbal medicines was their thermal nature, i.e. in terms of heat and cold (see chapter six for discussions of this [113]). Although as we have described above to talk of "energy" can be scientifically unclear or vague, the notions of qi as "energy" and that one of the characteristic properties of the "qi" of an herb is its thermal quality, suggests a problem for the equation of qi as "energy" given the second law of thermo-dynamics. For energy to move from cool to warm considerable energy is needed,

which is the principle of the refrigerator, it is not what "naturally occurs". Developments in mathematics and physics notably in the areas of complexity theory and chaos theory have also demonstrated that the second law of thermodynamics is not in fact a universal law [58].

6. For further discussions of this issue see: Birch, Felt [30:148-150] and Unschuld [132:72].

7. In endnote 4 above, we highlighted the problem of conceiving of qi as "energy". Here the notion of qi as some kind of "force" could hold more value, but "vital force" and "life force" are not recognizable in the fields of physics, at least not in terms of testable and potentially measurable concepts.

8. For a good review and overview of this area see Bischof [35].

9. Sivin states the problem of considering qi as a "substance" thus: "This account, although typical of recent writing, differs considerably from the classical understanding" [121:237]. Palmer has more extensive discussions in relation to the making of qigong scientific "By adopting the ideology of scientism, whether by conviction or by opportunism, the qigong sector engaged in a new dynamic in its internal and external relations. A new discourse on scientific orthodoxy could be felt, giving materialist interpretations to practices and concepts inherited from Chinese popular traditions... superstitions had been mixed into qigong owing to past feudal and religious influences, deforming the true nature of qigong. The renaissance of qigong thus required the elimination of such impurities and the eradication of the superstitions in order to create a scientific qigong." [106:122].

10. The notion that if something cannot be measured it is not "real" is a common mistake among scientists pursuing an agenda of their own devising. Many things established and later measured in science have over time, not been measurable because of the lack of the right tools for making the appropriate measurements, this is found repeatedly in the history of science. The fact that in an experiment using technology "X", the object of investigation "A" could not be measured is often a limitation of the technology and/or the knowledge base and conceptualising of the scientists, not the lack of existence of "A." All the more so when the object of investigation "A" is "qi" or the "jingmai", which we have seen above and in earlier chapters, to be conceptually complex (see chapters one, two, four and six [26, 29, 34, 113]). Conversely, scientists have often made the opposite mistake. While using technology "X" to investigate "A" something is measured that fell within the acceptable limits of their model or conceptualising about "A", then those scientists often declare that they have measured "A" and that its nature is related to the thing that they have measured. In examples and discussions below we examine studies that have made these mistakes.

11. See the following studies as examples: Hsu and colleagues assumed that measurement of something related to "qi stimulation" (as they define it) is sufficient to make generalizations about the nature of qi [66]; Motoyama assumed that the electrical signal he could measure with his AMI device was qi [99] based upon his models of the meridians and qi;

Yan et al. assumed that alteration of a number of physical systems at the level of atomic emissions (half-life of radioactive isotopes), molecular structures (aqueous solution structure) during external qi-gong informs us about the nature of qi [143]. On what basis were those technologies selected as indicative of qi effects or the nature of qi? This last area of research has been severely criticized already [81].

12. It is tempting to use the word "holistic" here. But, as we will see, this term seems to be unclear in how it is used and unclear in its applicability to TEAM and investigations of qi and the jingmai. For this reason, while we use the term "holistic" here and there to contextualise the discussion for some readers, help them see familiar territories, we inherently recognize the limitations and problems in the use of this term (see also next endnote).

13. In chapter one the case was made for seeing qi as something related to all bodily things and all emotional-mental things, and that outside the more speculative cosmological models for the concept of qi, it is commonly used in ways that associate it with how one experiences the world, and is thus fundamentally involved in mind-body conceptions [34]. This has immediate implications for research on qi, however it is conceived for the purposes of research, it should also be seen in relation to the mind-body and not only mental or bodily things.

14. The issues are more complex. In either-or thinking it would seem quite acceptable to ask a question like "is qi real or not?" But, given that the term qi is used to refer to all phenomenal things, not in either-or terms, we can raise questions regarding the underlying assumptions inherent in the question. The scientific method and its assumptions require a focus and narrowing down of the question tested, but with a concept like qi, this automatically starts violating the concept investigated so that it is no longer accurate. The typical approach of researchers has been to focus on one kind of statement about qi and ask the "is qi real?" question. Then naturally the either-or influenced scientist will likely not even imagine that there could be completely different ideas about qi so that the next step is to treat answers to the question as indicators of the reality of the broad concept rather than the more limited subset that the researcher was actually trying to investigate. Both skeptics and supporters have been guilty of this mistake. The either-or assumption tends to encourage treatment of something like the concept of qi inaccurately. An additional important methodological problem is one of making generalizations from studies where they cannot be made.

15. This is not to say that "science" is exclusively dualistic and reductionistic (non-"holistic"), clearly "science" is not. Within the whole field of "science" there is a polarity of approaches. On the one hand there are disciplines, approaches and scientists that have tended to take advantage of methods and assumptions based in dualistic, reductionistic thinking such as chemistry, many areas of physics, biology, medicine etc. There are also other disciplines, approaches and scientists that have tended to non-reductionist, non-dualist thinking seen in quantum mechanics, anthropology, sociology, psychology etc. Typically scientific disciplines or scientists tend to adopt one approach or the other. They tend not to read much about the other and make little effort to fit the findings and theories of both

together or showing how they relate to each other. These two tendencies have naturally been in opposition and many have had difficulty reconciling them, just as bio-medicine and biology have had difficulty reconciling them [54]. Since it is usually through the disciplines of the biological and medical sciences that a treatment system such as acupuncture is investigated, then it too has been subjected to the same difficulties. What is clear is that neither perspective is right or wrong, they each lead to limitations in how one asks questions and seeks answers to those questions. The two approaches are complementary, but that is not the tendency of how they have been used in medical research. While the modern physicist often has less difficulty seeing both sides of this due to developments in physics over the last hundred or so years [35, 54, 93, 94] often the biological and medical sciences continue to struggle with this [35, 54]. Thus for the most part, the more reductionistic-dualistic type thinking and its approaches and methods have tended to be used in investigations of something like acupuncture and TEAM. Clearly this creates difficult practical and conceptual challenges for investigations of TEAM and especially its concepts like qi and the jingmai.

16. Lewith, Walach and Jonas describe model validity as "the likelihood that the research has adequately addressed the unique theory and therapeutic context" of the system being investigated [79:12].

17. Hammerschlag and Zwickey highlighted an additional issue that emerges out of this work [61]. Since the methods of stimulation (electro-acupuncture) are not usual methods of practice, the mechanisms they exposed (various neuro-peptide pathways) cannot be considered as actual mechanisms by which acupuncture works. They also argue that the kinds of studies that have been done examining the "physiological mechanisms" of acupuncture yield correlational data. With the application of particular stimuli we see a correlated change, but the mechanisms in the body remain unexplored or untested (like a "black box" model) [61]. At the very least we must acknowledge that the mechanisms by which acupuncture have been found to work "lie considerably 'downstream' from where the needles are inserted" [60:182]. To date the link between demonstrated mechanisms of action of acupuncture and acupuncture practice are correlational at best as they lack plausible links or actual mechanisms between the practical application of the therapy and the measured physiological changes [60]. We come back to this again below.

18. The problems with physiological studies and even some clinical trials of acupuncture are more complex. Sometimes despite appearances and funding sources, acupuncture was not even the object or focus of the study rather it was a convenient tool for investigating other things. Early physiological studies of acupuncture focused especially on pain mechanisms, but some researchers openly admit that they chose this line of inquiry not because of an interest in acupuncture or seeing how acupuncture works but because they saw acupuncture as a good tool for exploring the body's pain control systems [7, 30]. Recent clinical studies tried using acupuncture as a tool to study placebo [73, 74], despite being listed with their funding sources as acupuncture studies [http://nccam.nih.gov/clinicaltrials/alltrials.htm –search "acupuncture", see numbers 25, 47 (searched 06/01/2009)]. Arguably these trials failed completely to achieve their goals due to confusion of placebo and non-placebo effects [21, 28], but many still consider them as trials that show acu-

puncture triggers little more than placebo effects [97]. Obviously when acupuncture was not the focus of study, these different studies were designed in such ways as to not investigate acupuncture per se.

19. Unschuld stated it thus: "The unique feature of the Chinese situation-and this should receive more attention from historians and philosophers of science-is the continuous tendency towards a syncretism of all ideas that exist (within accepted limits). Somehow a way was always found in China to reconcile opposing views and to build bridges." [132:57]. Recently Scheid presented evidence for some exclusional-type thinking in Chinese medicine [Scheid, lecture May 18, 2012] so that we must question the exclusive validity of Unschuld's statement, so, like many other things in TEAM, there seem to be exceptions to every attempted rule or generalizations we might try to make, due largely to such a diverse and extended history.

20. The NIH consensus development conference on acupuncture in 1997 drew similar conclusions about traditional ideas when they concluded that concepts such as qi "are difficult to reconcile with contemporary biomedical information but continue to play an important role in the evaluation of patients and the formulation of treatment in acupuncture" [1].

21. An example of this is seen with the description of qi by Chunyuyi of circa 150 BCE: "As for the so-called qi, one ought to harmonise drink and food, and choose clear days for coach rides and walks to broaden the mind in order to adjust the tendons, bones, flesh, blood and vessel-pulses for bringing qi into flow" [65:76], the what of qi is the how of its development.

22. Hall and Ames state it clearly in different ways: "'Knowing," then in classical China is not a knowing *what* that provides some understanding of the environment conditions of the natural world, but is rather a knowing *how* to be adept in relationships, and *how* in optimizing the possibilities that these relations provide, to develop trust in their viability" [59:150] and again quoting Chang Tung-sun: "The Chinese are only interested in knowing the will of Heaven in order to seek good fortune and to avoid misfortune. As to the nature of Heaven, they are indifferent. This fact shows that the Chinese have not applied the category of substance to the idea of Heaven and have not taken Heaven as the ultimate stuff of the universe" [59:149].

23. Putting aside the complex issues involved in the concept of "placebo" and "placebo controls" in trials of acupuncture [20, 107], "sham" acupuncture studies cannot be valid "explanatory" trials that test the mechanisms of acupuncture. "Sham acupuncture" trials are instead a form of comparative trial where attempts are made to control for variables thought to be involved in how acupuncture might work (such as needle location, needle technique) so that two forms of acupuncture are compared to each other rather than testing the mechanism of one. For example, in an adjunctive IVF trial [123] "verum" acupuncture was compared to "sham" acupuncture delivered at identical points but using "stage dagger" needles that only pricked the surface of the skin. Hence this was a comparison of penetrative and skin-pricking varieties of acupuncture, not a placebo-controlled trial [24] and of questionable value as a sham-controlled trial [91].

24. Chunyu Yi was described as palpating the "mai" in his case histories in the Shiji [65], sometimes this appears to be palpation of the mai (not jingmai –see chapters two and four [26, 34]) directly and sometimes the pulses. It is not clear the extent to which the jingmai were palpated in the Neijing or Nanjing for the purposes of diagnosis. Certainly pulse diagnosis appears to provide the information needed to assess the state of the jingmai.

25. The investments of time and resources necessary to do investigations of lower electro-dermal resistance has fostered a climate where commercially available products have dominated the field of electro-dermal research of the jingmai. While not unusual in medical technology, the scientific claims of most devices such as the Dermatron, Royodoraku, AMI, are not scientifically defensible. Clinical utility has come to replace scientific rigour leaving the area open to question –see reviews below and for example the review of Ahn et al. [2].

26. Russian doctors accidentally discovered that when metal pins are left at the site of acupuncture points on surgically repaired limbs this can trigger unwanted side effects, but when the acupoints are carefully avoided, these side effects are eliminated [30:164, 139].

27. The fMRI studies have already been discussed [47, 75], another example is the association of endorphins with acupuncture, where some researchers attempted to claim that this provides evidence for the existence of the acupoints [108].

28. In a sense this is similar to the process that Toulmin describes [129:40-43]. First one must do a "natural history" of the subject to be investigated (descriptive science) to make the object clear. Once it is clear, then studies can begin to examine how it works, to establish how it functions, behaves etc. (explanatory science). This brings together a natural blend of what are also called "qualitative" approaches and "quantitative" approaches.

29. Gradually we see more studies emerging that have employed pragmatic type approaches involving traditionally based forms of acupuncture. An interesting study by MacPherson and colleagues [126] demonstrated evolving long term changes following the use of traditional Chinese (TCM) acupuncture for low back pain. This may well be the first study that captures the long term effects of the "root treatment" of a traditionally based system of acupuncture, which is aimed at improving the body's ability to heal itself [30]. This study potentially illustrates the clinical utility of treatment based on traditional theories. Hopefully we will see more studies of this type.

30. See also chapter four in this volume for a contrast of styles of practice, especially appendix one [26].

31. Jahn and Dunne discuss the mental attitudes of the researcher if they want to approach something like consciousness research, including being open to opposing positions [67].

32. If we take for example the measurement of the electrical properties of the skin (possibly related to the jingmai and their acupoints), there are a lot of technical issues that need to

be addressed that have not, to date, been adequately addressed. A number of authors have written about this [2, 3, 49, 52, 56, 90, 92, 101, 127, 128, 148].

33. Although not directly the theme of the workshop, the authors organized a workshop along with Terje Alraek (Norway) at the University College of Health Sciences –Campus Kristiania, Oslo. The workshop was titled "Back to Basics –exploring teaching and practice of TEAM-acupuncture in order to develop appropriate research methods" –A Research Workshop". Drs Claudia Witt (Berlin), Hugh MacPherson (York), Peter Wayne (Boston), Lixing Lao (Baltimore), Chris Zaslawski (Sydney), Sarah Price (Edinburgh) were the other participants in the workshop. Four papers will be published by the nine participants from this workshop addressing general theoretical and conceptual issues, diagnosis related issues, treatment related issues and outcome assessment related issues. This landmark workshop overlapped to some extent with the theme of the current chapter.

CHAPTER NINE

# SUMMARY OF CORE PRACTICAL CONCEPTS

Manuel Rodríguez Cuadras, Miguel Angel Cabrer Mir, Stephen Birch

This chapter has been combined from contributions by each of the authors. Miguel Angel Cabrer Mir has a long standing Taiji quan, Qigong and Yiquan practice and has been teaching for many years. He is also an experienced acupuncturist and has been engaged in teaching over the last few years. Manuel Rodriguez had long standing practices in Judo, Taekwan do, Qigong, Aikido and the Japanese sword form Iaido, teaching Judo, Aikido, Iaido and Qigong. He is also an experienced acupuncturist and herbalist with a lot of teaching experience. Stephen Birch is a long standing practitioner of acupuncture who has trained with many very experienced practitioners and has extensive teaching experience. His additional work of scholarship and research in acupuncture also helped form his contributions in this chapter. As the chapter unfolds it is mostly written as though from the perspective of the three authors, but, at times, it is necessary to let the individual author express himself. We hope you do not find this confusing. Although we have prepared a reasonably lengthy introduction we have tried to remove the heavy scholarship that is found in each of the earlier chapters. There is a short bibliography at the end of the chapter, but we do not use our normal system of referencing in this chapter, we do not want to distract you from the practical issues. You can find most of what we refer to in earlier chapters and the other sources we have listed in the bibliography.

We have also broken the chapter down into a series of sections, these are:

1. Why this chapter (introduction)
2. Bodily and mental aspects
    - 2.1. Acupuncture and Taiji quan
    - 2.2. The vessel: working with the body
    - 2.3. Skills and abilities to be cultivated by the acupuncturist
        - 2.3.1. Alertness, concentration
        - 2.3.2. Calmness (dynamic calmness)
        - 2.3.3. Sensitivity
        - 2.3.4. Alignment
        - 2.3.5. Grounding

## 1. Why this chapter?

In the chapters above we have seen that something like the practice of acupuncture requires the development of certain skills and abilities if the traditional techniques are to be reproduced and we are to maximise the way that we can influence the qi of a patient with a tool like a needle. Chapter four described a number of different ways that needling was discussed in the historical literature, the role of the practitioner and different aspects of practitioner involvement. Appendix two of the same chapter described a needling technique and showed that it was probably constructed through practice based on practical interpretations of a number of historical descriptions of needling.[1]

In summary of the contents of that chapter and its appendix, we can say that the well applied needle technique requires:

1. A developed sensitivity to subtle influences, changes and the ability to respond precisely.
2. The development of a certain inner state.
3. Application of certain mechanical processes.
4. The procedure that comes through repeated practice.

In the same chapter on acupuncture various passages from the Suwen, Lingshu and Nanjing were cited to explain how the authors thought qi could be engaged with a needle and then influenced to produce optimal changes. In Nanjing seventy-eight and eighty it is clearly described how one must first palpate the acupoint to be treated and get the qi to arrive. After the qi has arrived, the needle is then inserted applying a number of different technical skills to influence the qi and to produce the desired effects of bu [補], supplementation/tonification or xie [寫], draining. Rather than repeat these descriptions or repeat the needling techniques described in the chapter, we would like to break down the whole process into a kind of action oriented process. Following this we will describe some practical exercises that lay the groundwork for the whole needling technique. The initial processes described will form the foundation for the needling, regardless of what kind of acupuncture system one practices and regardless of the specific technique within that system that one intends to apply.

The more common forms of needling today do not attempt to reproduce these needling methods, usually the needle is inserted and then manipulated until the patient describes certain sensations which are taken as a sign of the obtaining of qi (deqi [得氣]). What we will attempt to describe are exercises and actions to help train your ability to sense and feel the arrival of qi and engage the qi during treatment to maximize treatment effects. These are quite subtle phenomena and require a lot of careful study and practice to be developed. As cited above, Shudo states that it took him many years on his own to be able to do this, so we can see that it is not something one can simply do without training and experience. The same is true for the person studying the piano. It takes time and a lot of practice before the person's fingers start to find the right notes with the right sequencing, touch and timing. It takes considerably more practice and time before the performance might rise to the level of a concert performance. If we want to improve our abilities to influence the qi of a patient with a needle, using historically based ideas, we need to be patient, diligent and be willing to learn from our mistakes. While some people have natural talents that allow them to perform at a higher level than others more quickly, there is still no short cut: **practice, practice, practice**. How can we best prepare ourselves in order to try to shorten the time it takes to achieve the desired goals?

## Needling: an action oriented description[2]

In order to highlight the aspects of practice that we will be focusing on and to help describe a more rounded picture of the act of needling, we break down the act of needling into four stages, which are each sketched out below:

1. Decisions
2. Engagement
3. Enactment
4. Completion

Each system of practice has its own theories, reasons, methods and techniques that inform what is done at each of these four stages; it is part of the nature of "acupuncture" that there is such tremendous diversity in these four stages are enacted.

### 1- Decisions

Before the treatment begins a series of decisions need to be made:

Decision about the pattern of diagnosis.
Decision about treatment side(s).
Decisions about treatment points and their variations.
Decisions about treatment techniques and their variations.
Assessment of the overall condition of the patient, judgments about dose and prognosis and decisions about modifications of the treatment according to those judgments.

### 2- Engagement

Following these decisions one needs to position oneself and get ready to engage the qi of the patient in preparation for needling.

*The preparation for needling:*
Bodily work:
- One's body position relative to the patient and acupoint to be needled.
- One's body posture.
- Scan one-self to identify and release tension.

Mental work:
- Calming oneself.
- Alert and focused.

*Begin engagement*
Touching to achieve engagement:
- The manner of touching and placement of finger-tip to find the acupoint.
- Locating the channel with the finger tip.

Increasing one's engagement:
- Maintaining one's touch/contact.
- Moving the finger-tip along the channel as one looks for the acupoint.
- Finding the acupoint with one's finger-tip.

Maintaining one's engagement:
Placing the finger and thumb at the acupoint in preparation for needling.

In this process, one touches so as to begin engagement with the qi of the patient; naturally as one does this one feels something with respect to this. How one touches, with what you touch and the procedure that comes through repetitive practice help maximize that initial engagement. The starting point behind this lies in how one positions and holds oneself and how one prepares one's body and mental focus before starting to touch. Then as one starts to move the finger to find the acupoint, the patient's qi responds, you keep attention to the initial feeling and observe how it changes with your finger movement. Finding and then moving your finger along the channel should increase those feelings, then as you find the acupoint, the feelings increase again as you more directly contact the place where "qi enters and exits". These are very subtle phenomena and require that the mind not be distracted, require a certain kind of focus, and that the body is in a relaxed and observant/receptive state. Modern practitioners Shudo and Wang both describe in their own ways, based on their own experiences, how to touch and find the acupoint and how this process of finding the acupoint can get the qi to arrive, and that this is the qi arrival that Nanjing seventy-eight and eighty refer to. Throughout this process, you keep your attention quietly focused on the subtle feelings that began with the initial touch and which (with repetitive practice and training) increase as you move the finger to find the acupoint. Never let your finger leave the skin, maintain a smooth constant contact with all that you do and stay relaxed. This sounds easy, but, it is far from easy as we all tend to hold tension without realizing it and these very subtle slow actions take time to master and become second nature.

### *3- Enactment*

Following the above actions you are now ready to start needling. The qi has already been contacted (the first "qi arrival"). Then there are a series of other actions you perform as the needling technique.

*Starting to needle:*
Placing and advancing/inserting the needle to correct depth.
Seeking a secondary engagement as the qi starts to be influenced by the needle.
Increase that engagement as the needle starts to influence the qi again.

Adjustment of your posture, left hand, right hand so that you can maintain your focus and awareness.

"Gathering the qi":
Allow the needle to increase the engagement.
Pay attention to adjust your posture, release tension as needed –bodywork.
Pay attention to maintain a quiet focus.
With the right and left hands perform the various actions needed for the needle technique.

Here the initial feelings you had as you started touching and which you increased with your movements and locating of the acupoint, now start to increase again as the needle starts to influence the qi further and as this influence builds up (the second "qi arrival"). Following this build-up of these qi reactions/feelings, you begin the specific needling technique according to what change you decided was needed through this acupoint (bu-supplementation or xie-draining). When the actions have been sufficiently performed and the intended changes produced, the needle needs to be removed all following precise timing and responsiveness.

*Getting ready for and removal of the needle:*
Maintaining a maximal engagement.
Adjustment of your body in preparation for removal.
Actions of the left and right hands in preparation for removal.
Having good timing for the removal and actions of the left and right hands.

Removal of the needle and closure (or not) of the acupoint:
Optimising one's timing and body actions.

Maintaining the engagement at removal:
Finger/cotton pressing the acupoint/"hole".

### *4. Completion*

Removal of the finger from the acupoint:
Separation from the engagement.
But with preparation for re-engagement as one readies to needle the next acupoint.

Maintaining all bodily/mental states.
Readying to needle the next acupoint.

Continuing re-enactments.

Once one has made one's decisions of what to do and where to do it, one readies oneself in preparation for first finding the next acupoint and then needling it. These actions all require an initial contact or engagement with the patient's qi, which one maintains throughout as one seeks to increase it and then utilize it through mechanical manipulations of the needle. In a very important sense these initial feelings of engagement and their increase are the foundation for all the actions involved in needling. It is this first contact that will be described below with a series of practical exercises to help you develop your skills.

## 2. Bodily and mental aspects

### 2.1 Acupuncture and Taiji quan

"Needling regulates the qi (tiao qi)" (Lingshu 75)

The above sentence relates needle insertion to the regulation of qi. This regulation is implied in the character tiao [調], which expresses the action of regulating, of tuning a musical instrument, or mixing in precise proportions. This regulation or balance is not achieved simply by inserting needles. There is a whole process involved: palpation of the channels, the pulse, looking for the point, the arrival of qi; all of this is culminated by the moment of insertion. All of these actions can be influenced by the physical and mental state of the acupuncturist.

The objective of the exercises that follow is to obtain a better connection between body and mind. A connection that can be achieved by relaxing the body and calming the mind. In this way, we seek to open the way to a more finely tuned state, to a more sensitive perception; qualities that can be useful when inserting needles or practicing Taiji quan.

## 2.2 The Vessel: working with the body

In Chinese writing, we find three different ways of writing the word body, one of which is ti [體]. We would like to emphasise the similarities that exist between "ritual" (li [禮]) and "body" ti [體]). These two characters have one part in common, whose meaning refers to a vessel.

In ancient times, vessels were of great importance in rituals. Their function was to serve as a vehicle for feeding and communicating with spirits or ancestors. A vessel has an external part, which gives it physical shape, and an internal part, which is the recipient. The food was placed in the interior of the vessel and consumed by the spirits in the form of the vapour rising from its cooking. This nutrition of the spirits was called yangshen (nourish the spirits [養神]). This communication was a way to solve problems that affected the maintaining of order or harmony. These could range from individual health problems to more social matters impeding the smooth running of government.

But from the third century BCE, new ideas arise which break the monopoly held by the rituals of the previous era, which could only be performed by the shaman or the king.

One of the most important changes was to consider that any individual, not just the king or the shaman, could participate more actively in the construction of order or harmony. A change which led to a new way of looking at the body. The body as an individual being becomes an important element; it is transformed into an active tool for the conservation of health and at the same time, it can enter terrain that had previously been the exclusive domain of the spirits. The body becomes the vessel that can contain the subtle, or a mind in calmness. A clear example of this process is found in the Neiye, where we are given direct references on the importance of maintaining the body in a good position, in order to create a space where the mind can become calm and settled.

Neiye: XI
When your body is not aligned
The inner power will not come
When you are not tranquil within
Your mind will not be well ordered
Align your body, assist the inner power
Then it will gradually come on its own

## *The mind: yi* [意] *and zhi* [志]

If we consider a metaphoric image that relates the mind to water, we could say that turbulent water, the elements that prevent us from seeing the riverbed, are the movements of yi or zhi. Calming the yi-zhi allows the dirt to settle to the riverbed, and enables the water to reflect like a mirror again. The origin of this turbulence (yi-zhi) comes from our desires or emotions, which use our senses as a gateway to the exterior.

The problem is that we need our senses, our emotions and our desires in order to live, to feel. It is not a question of proposing austerity, simply not allowing the mud or dirt to dominate, but rather allowing the crystalline part of the water to reappear. Our emotions or desires are still there, but within the river, not on the surface. Calmness of mind produces not only a better harmony with the body, but also helps to calm the yi - zhi. A phrase which illustrates the importance of calming yi or zhi, and its relationship with the mind and body, is found in chapter three of the Daode Jing.

> they empty the hearts-mind of the people and fill their stomachs
> They weaken their (zhi) aspiration and strengthen their bones…

These examples from the Neiye and Daode Jing, speak of the mind and body working in unison. Throughout history, things have always begun with the physical aspect, the most palpable, our body structure, our tensions. Once we relax the physical part, we can become more sensitive to the movements of our mind. We can find examples in a variety of texts.

> refined essence to transform into vital energy, refined vital energy to transform into spirit, refined spirit to return to emptiness

This sentence comes from the literature of internal alchemy, which began in China in the twelfth century, but there are texts from previous eras which already refer to a similar process. The Wenzi tells us:

> The highest learning listens with the spirit, the middle learning listens with the mind, and the lowest learning listens with the ears

We can compare this development with the three levels referred to in Zhuangzi:

listen with your ears, no don't listen with your ears, listen with your mind, no don't listen with your mind listen with your vital energy (qi [氣])

The Liezi also has a similar theme:

my body merges with my mind, my mind merges with my vital energy, my vital energy merges with my spirit and my spirit merges with nothingness (wu [無])

They all speak of beginning with the body followed by the involvement of the mind. This combination of body and mind causes the body to become more aware, knowledge from perception loses ground and the mind abandons its exclusively rational aspect. This combination awakens what Zhuangzi calls listening with qi, which allows us to wait for things to happen, not to react.

The form of consciousness, yi [意], is discussed in many martial arts and medical texts, is the result of unification between the body and mind. Relaxing the body and calming the mind produces a different type of yi from that produced by a tense body or an agitated mind. A practical example, which has already been mentioned in this book, is the story of Ding the Butcher. His mastery does not come from his ability with his body, in this case his hands, nor does it come from his mind. Ding says that he is guided by shen [神]. The problem is that in the west, whenever we see the word shen or qi, we immediately forget about the two initial stages.

The creation of the vessel and its interior space allows us to work with our body, our mind and at the same time to create a space where the two can be combined.

## 2. 3 Skills and abilities to be cultivated by the acupuncturist

What can we do in order to listen with qi, so that we are capable of perceiving and participating in the dynamics, benefit from propensity, perform naturally and effortlessly in that empty space where things originate and around which things happen? We must first cultivate a series of skills and attitudes that favour the event. Following tradition, and allowing for the fact that they can be called by different names in different texts and periods, we can say that these basic skills are:

Alertness, concentration
Calmness (dynamic calmness)

Sensitivity
Alignment
Grounding
Presence
Awareness

In reality, the last two are a consequence of the preceding ones. All of them involve physical, mental and psycho-emotional aspects, although we may find some that are more related to mind-spirit (alertness, concentration, calmness) and others that have a clear structural or corporal component (alignment, grounding), leaving sensitivity as a common factor that participates in both indivisible aspects.

### 2.3.1 Alertness, concentration

It is clear that in order to detect, understand and more importantly to participate in the dynamics of the acupunctural event, an intentional act of concentration is required. The following texts come from the classics and can be found in various sources already cited in the book [1, 2, 3, 4, 5, 6, 7, 8].

Let the classics speak:

We must not forget that, according to the Suwen 25:

Applying acupuncture is like approaching a precipice; your hands must be firm and strong, as if you were holding down a tiger, and your mind must be free of any interferences

Lingshu 9 tells us:

Practitioners are deeply immersed in a place of stillness and are aware of the comings and goings of the spirit 神 with their own (sensorial) doors and windows shut... Their minds must be focused

Lingshu 1 says:

Those who are going to examine the illness must calm their minds when observing the patient, without looking to the left or the right

Suwen 54 and Lingshu 9 both inform us:

The practitioner's internal state must be calm and focused, without being distracted by sensorial information or emotions and *The intentions (yi)* must remain stable –Suwen 62

We need correct focus and attention –Lingshu 1 *Given that what is observed is very subtle* Suwen 25 and one has to remain very alert and focused –Suwen 27

Lingshu 1 tells us that

The subtlety of needle insertion resides in its speed... in order to understand its comings and goings, emphasise its frequency

### 2.3.2 Calmness (dynamic calmness)

It is not possible to maintain attention on an event if we cannot remain calm. Calmness is necessary in order to listen, so that the mind, or better, the hands themselves, are able to form a faithful reflection of the reality of which it is part. Like still waters... but alive. The calmness that an acupuncturist requires is more like that of a warrior than that of a meditator, and its expression is closer to dance and harmony than to stillness.

Suwen 25 tells us:

> A doctor must be like a crossbowman pulling the trigger at exactly the right moment, neither a moment before nor a moment too late

And how is this achieved? The Nei Ye tells us[3]:

> Relaxed and loose, but caring,
> In solitude you delight in your own person.
> This is called "revolving qi":
> Your attention and your actions seem celestial
> When the four limbs are aligned,
> and blood and qi are calm,
> One may unify one's attention and, concentrating one's mind.
> Ones eyes and ears will not be sullied.

### 2.3.3 Sensitivity

An acupuncturist's work is not about strength; we already know that qi is not achieved through strength. Awareness, presence, participation in an act that cannot happen in any other way, given that its propensity and its dynamics require sensitivity, refined perception and bringing it to a state of cohesion with the action. Once again, the classics are quite clear:

> Calmly and attentively contemplating the patient in order to observe any minute change when qi arrives. These changes are so obscure that they can hardly be seen. Suwen 25

Within these changes, it is essential to perceive the arrival of qi:

Perceive the arrival of qi before inserting the needle. Nanjing 78, 80

> As soon as one [perceives] with one's left hand that the influences (氣) have appeared, one inserts the needle. Nanjing 80

and

> As soon as the arrival of the influences [氣] [perceived by the left hand] give form [to pulsation in the usual locations] where the movement [in the] vessels [can be perceived under the skin], one inserts the needle. Nanjing 78

### 2.3.4 Alignment

In classical Chinese thought, the idea of alignment is very important; it is only through correct alignment that Heaven and Earth can communicate through a person, impregnating him or her with their virtue (de [德]). The idea that if you are aligned with Heaven, you can create a bigger and better order in yourself and in your surroundings is a fundamental one. This can be seen in many ancient texts. For example:

> Heaven in one is de, earth in one is qi, de flows downwards and qi rises, and then there is life. Lingshu 8

Remember the instruction in Neiye:

> When the four limbs are aligned,
> and blood and qi are calm,
> One may unify ones attention and, concentrating ones mind.
> Ones eyes and ears will not be sullied.

Alignment simultaneously implies a composition of body structure, a disposition which will favour the propensity of the event; this is particularly visible in the study of martial arts.[4]

### 2.3.5 Grounding

The taller a tree grows, the deeper it sinks its roots. Alignment, calmness, attention must be built on a solid base. But for an acupuncturist, solid does not mean immobile; once again there is a similitude with martial arts, where it is essential to be rooted, but at the same time extraordinarily mobile. If not, how would you be able to adapt yourself to constantly changing circumstances? Yes, grounding means lowering your centre of gravity. But it also means "sinking" the mind at the same time, the shen within oneself. For the grounding to be real, its physical, mental and psycho-emotional aspects must go hand in hand, and that comes with a progressive feeling of confidence and security. Grounding also allows you to receive, and to have the perception of a contact "channel" with and between Heaven and Earth, reminding us about and facilitating alignment and calmness.

### 2.3.6 Presence

While this is a difficult quality to define, it is very easy to appreciate. It is often expressed in the well-known phrase "here and now", which is simultaneously the objective and the path, and refers to both the volatility and importance of the present moment and also the need for the subjective sensation of "I am".

Largely a consequence of good grounding, correct alignment and a calm mind-spirit, presence is that quality which not only causes another human being who is nearby to sense that we are there, it also spreads out and fills the environment. The quality of presence not only says "I am here now", it also shows "I am", and if it is positive, it extends to "we are". We have all experienced the sensation produced by being close, or even seeing a true master, the things he does that make him loved and respected, the things that make us feel better and feel like better people. That is presence.

As practitioners, presence is useful to us in various ways:

As confirmation that the qualities of alertness, calmness, alignment and grounding are present, active and integrated.

To transmit our vocation to our patients: I am here, I am here to help, we are together in this.

And as a result of all of that, to improve the results of the therapeutic intervention.

In a very normal way, so that our work is not so tiring.

### 2.3.7 Awareness (yi)

If presence is difficult to define, how do we approach awareness? Or, what do we mean when we say "awareness"? As we will see below, in a way we are talking about "yi", a concept so important in Chinese medicine as to be the subject of a separate section.

## 2.4 Yi

When introducing yi, we have chosen to write "awareness" and not "consciousness", to stress that this is not just a reflexive quality. Awareness includes, but is not limited to, consciousness of oneself, the perception of your own self. It expands further and further, and in its higher state, it blends with the rest of the universe, and eventually even the idea of "I am aware" disappears. This state is the objective of many traditions of mysticism, and this is not the place to study the matter in greater depth. However, we can affirm that a perfect clinical action, which produces results that go beyond technique, are often linked to this sensation of disappearing separation; we can say that intention and consciousness have given way to natural action and awareness.

Awareness is empty, which is the same thing that Zhuangzi says about qi. It is thanks to this emptiness that one can perceive the whole and move effortlessly within it.

It is possible that, in spite of their similarities, the awareness of a mystic, a warrior and a doctor will not be exactly the same. And, of course, they are not expressed in the same way. A doctor's awareness should be revealed in his or her clinical work. We can venture to suggest that this need is a great help for the doctor's personal growth, a true, clear mirror which gives them a more objective way to evaluate their progress at any given time.[5]

In clinical work, awareness, the expression of all the previous qualities, can be useful in:

–Confirming the degree of development and application of the other qualities (presence, grounding, etc.)
–Clearly perceiving the notions that we have found in the classical texts: ji, shi, qi, shen. And as we have seen, this is because these categories do not easily fit into any intellectual definition. They are only accessible via direct perception, i.e. the quality of inclusive, integrated awareness that we have to develop, practice and maintain.[6]

The quality of awareness is inseparable from its more basic expressions, i.e. alertness, consciousness, grounding, alignment, presence. Awareness participates in all of them and integrates them into a state that is able to find different, specific manifestations depending on the type of reality concerned.

Actually, although we have separated them to make them easier to explain, these basic qualities, these skills you need to work on, are inseparable. You cannot be aligned if you are not calm, and you cannot be calm if you are not rooted, etc. It is not possible to reach a determined state of presence and awareness if no attention is paid to more physical or purely mental aspects. It is necessary to practice the different components, as we do. But we must be aware that we cannot even speak about one of them without all the others being present. In the end, we are trying to improve our clinical work, and as a by-product improve ourselves as people. And to achieve this, we have the guidance of classical thought and the tools of, for example, acupuncture.

> "...When inserting the needle, don't look, don't listen, don't talk and don't move. Just pay careful attention to focusing on the point of the needle, in order to feel the comings and goings of qi." Denmei Shudo, commenting on Lingshu 9[7]

Yi may be partly considered as an internal state that arises with calmness, alert attention and awareness, which may be expressed as good position (body alignment), a calm mind and emotions and a kind of unfocused alertness. Yi is, or can be, the conceptual summary of the presence and activity of the skills needed for subtle acupuncture, (alertness, sensitivity, presence, consciousness) and we have seen that, in one context or another, all of them have been defined using that term. Working with yi means bringing all of these capacities and skills into play, by using the most visible aspects: alignment, grounding and calmness. But yi itself does not act, it needs to manifest itself through something else,[8] especially for its action to have a specific result:

> Medicine is awareness (yi), prescription is methods (fa). The divine makes its meaning clear within the methods. Ye Tianshi[9]

We have to bring yi into play, we have to express it through technique and we have to see how things develop using the tangible world as a basis. But this can be a pitfall. We have seen the principle that Lingshu speaks of:

> The crude attend to the form, the superior attend to the spirit.

This can be confusing or even frustrating. We clearly need to pay attention to subtle, and even spiritual, aspects of acupuncture actions. But doesn't the action take place in the material world? In the end, aren't we going to interact with another human being of flesh and blood like ourselves? Does the fact that the acupoint is not always an anatomical reality, place it automatically beyond tangible reality? We don't think so. After years of frustration and defiance,[10] I have reached a different interpretation: The Lingshu is not condemning or contrasting; it is just suggesting a path. We all begin as "crude", with the objective of becoming "superior", slowly working day by day in order to progress from a state where we are placing all of our attention on material structures and technical details, to an eventual state where we are aware and able to take part in a healing activity that is performed without effort or opposition, as if it was happening by itself. According to this interpretation, the phrase proposes a path of technical and personal growth.

This vision of a "path" also allows you to sort out some aspects of yi that may be difficult to reconcile, such as: Should we concentrate, or is it better to be "open"? While intention, attention and awareness are all yi, is it possible for us to do everything at the same time? Is one aspect superior to the others? It helps to consider these aspects as phases or facets of a single reality. They are all present all of the time, but they are visible to a greater or lesser degree according to the moment and circumstances, and this includes the practitioner's specific state of development. Allowing for the inaccuracy of numbers in this area, we could say that in the different phases of the treatment act, they work in different proportions, finally reuniting the different aspects of yi into a visible result: that characteristic of "presence", the state they are all part of; the "distribution" could be something like the following table:

| | **Focus-Intention** | **Intention-Attention** | **Attention-Awareness** |
|---|---|---|---|
| **The mind in the state of** | Organised intelligence | Consciousness of alertness | Integrating awareness |
| **Diagnosis (initial)** | 33 | 33 | 33 |
| **Acupuncture treatment (initial)** | 20 | 45 | 35 |
| **Needle insertion** | 10 | 35 | 55 |
| **Feedback** | 10 | 45 | 45 |

This idea resolves, or may help to resolve, some of the apparent inconsistencies about the concept of yi; it is not about it being intelligence, or intention, or attention, or concentration, or consciousness or awareness. It is rather that every one of these aspects is more visible in different phases of the process of interacting with things. It also constitutes a path (in Chinese, [道], dao) for development as a person and as a therapist. Once again using the stratagem of the three aspects of yi, we can relate it to qualitatively different ways of performing acupuncture.

**2.4.1 The three phases or aspects of yi and their influence on acupuncture treatment**
Treatment can be carried out in three phases, each one producing observable changes in the patient.[11]

The first state or phase helps to create changes in the therapeutic objectives of the diagnosis (the objectives and actions are guided by the intellect and intention), in the tissues and areas treated and in the system of channels. In this first level, actions are limited to the use of techniques to stimulate and manipulate the patient's physiological qi. A certain level of regulation can be reached, due to the self-regulatory effects of the channels where the treatment is applied, similar to the relationships shown through the theories of yin-yang and five-phases. The effects of needle insertion on a channel can therefore cause a certain degree of change in other channels. Acupuncture theories used to diagnose and define treatments are mainly related to these effects.

The second state adds the effects of the resonance between the practitioner and the patient.[12] In this way, the action of non-physiological qi is introduced (interactions at the level of "global vitality", shengqi or zhengqi), which helps to create additional, higher-level regulatory effects in the patient. With practice and improving skills, focusing intention becomes a more routine experience and starts turning into attention (yi) and manipulation helps to obtain better regulation of the patient's channel and physiological systems (physical and functional). The specific theories used in acupuncture for diagnosis and selecting treatments (yin-yang, five-phases, zangfu, jingluo functions, etc.) do not explicitly describe the actions and/or the influences of qi at this level. These qi influences are clearly visible through the practice and analysis of insertion techniques, and are therefore implicit in the treatment.

The third state adds the dynamic effects of acting naturally through calmness and non-action (wuwei). This provides access to a third level of qi: (what we might simply call) cosmological qi. This qi (yuanqi or tianqi) is the matrix that contains all the systems with their specific movements and actions. Harmonising with this by means of the correct dynamics (ji) and a more passive/reflective focus (yi as awareness), the natural state (ziran) of the systems contained in this cosmic qi matrix emerges or becomes apparent again. This makes it possible for a higher level of ordering and regulation and the infusion of this background, non-physiological qi in the patient. As with the second stage, these influences and sources of qi are not explicitly described in the acu-

| | Phase | Influence on insertion | Possible actions and mechanisms |
|---|---|---|---|
| 1 | **INTENTION [Organised intelligence-focus]**<br><br>**Listen with your ears** | Stimulation of the patient's qi | Insertion directly affects physical systems and their physiological components, and also acts on the jingluo system, increasing or reducing the flow of qi, triggering yin-yang and 5-phase type regulatory and restabilising actions. This helps to regulate and improve the functioning of the internal systems (zangfu, qi-blood, etc.). Tonification is present as changes in the movement of qi and an increase in physiological functions |
| 2 | **INTENTION - ATTENTION**<br><br>**Listen with the mind/ heart (shen)** | The patient-therapist interaction gives rise to a set of reciprocal influences between physiological qi (specific) and non-physiological qi (overall vitality) | The role of touch. The role of acupuncture as an entry point and exit point for qi. The role of the xieqi and zhengqi interactions. The role of shen and its interactions. The probable role of simple resonance (xiangying/ying). Tonification is the result of better regulation and an increase in physiological functions |
| 3 | **CONSCIOUSNESS -ATTENTION**<br><br>**Listen with qi** | The opening of the cosmological and environmental cycles of qi produce non-physiological interactions that increase and regulate physiological qi | Pure awareness spontaneously harmonising with natural movements and rhythms, without intention, through non-action. The probable role of total or cosmic resonance (ganying) the dynamic (ji) and propensity (shi). Tonification is due to regulation and improvement in physiological functions at the highest level, and to realignment or harmonisation with the matrix of yuanqi allowing this qi to permeate the body |

puncture theories used to guide and select treatments. They are simply implied. However, they become visible through the practice of more highly developed practitioners, and they are mentioned in the basic theories of acupuncture. They become clear through the detailed analysis of the requirements needed to reach "proper" insertion techniques, the techniques of a superior practitioner.

During a treatment at least one, and even all three, phases can become active to varying degrees. A beginner will only activate phase 1, so the qi at this level will be the prime mediator of the effects of the treatment. It is only when the person relaxes and begins to enter the rhythm of treatment that phase 2 will start to become active, and phase 2 qi will begin to act more, gradually increasing the effects of the treatment applied by the therapist. With more training, and the repeated experience of long years of practice, phase 3 will naturally start to play a bigger role, as a function of the individual only needing to bring consciousness to the process. At level 3, qi now has an increasing influence on the treatment effects.

It is possible that some people, because of their background or prior experiences, may be able to use level 1 and 2 qi from the beginning and sometimes have access to level 3 qi early on in their careers. There will be a huge variety in the manifestation of these treatment phases, mainly depending on the practitioner's state of development. The degree to which the qi of each of the three levels participates in the treatment depends on many factors. An advanced practitioner with a lot of experience may be able to bring the three phases of qi into play routinely and on demand. An intermediate practitioner may be able to bring levels 1 and 2 into play routinely and occasionally, and probably with ever increasing frequency, attain level 3. A beginner will have access to level 1 qi from the start of the treatment, and occasionally (but with ever increasing frequency) bring level 2 qi into play. On very rare occasions, a beginner will be able to bring third level qi to the treatment.

It is quite possible that there will be many, complex factors influencing this grading for any given practitioner during each of his or her treatments. One of them will be the condition of the patient. It is likely that part of the learning and development process that a practitioner experiences will involve coming across different patients, some of whom may have an influence on the process. The practitioner may not understand this influence at first, but over time, understanding will develop along with experience.

Many patients come for treatment in very poor condition, so that their manifestations are mostly limited to level 1. With these patients, it is unlikely that a beginner will be able to bring influences of level 2 and 3 qi to bear. Many patients are very "sensitive", showing level 2 manifestations. With these patients, a beginner may be able to experience influences of level 2 qi, but it is unlikely that he or she will be able to easily reproduce them with other patients. Occasionally there is a patient in a more elevated state who shows level 3 manifestations. Beginners and intermediate practitioners may be able to experience level 3 qi with this patient, although it will not be easy for them to reproduce this with other patients. The interaction between patient and practitioner will probably increase or reduce these superior effects of qi. Due to the internal state of some patients, the practitioner will be able to access qi from higher sources "accidentally or unintentionally", but will then be incapable of doing the same thing with other patients. Only more highly developed practitioners will be able to overcome these nullifying effects in order to have constant access to the superior effects of qi, whatever type of patient is being treated. It is very likely that time will be needed for lesser-developed practitioners to develop a sense of what is happening with those more developed patients and learn to reproduce the effects with other patients.

Although the patient's state is not taken into account in this model, we can see that his or her specific situation and circumstances can also have an influence on how, and to what degree, the effects of qi manifest themselves during treatment, depending on how the different stages of his or her own physical and interior development are manifested.

### 2.4.2 Cultivating yi

#### *2.4.2.1 Through its expressions: grounding, alignment, presence, consciousness, sensitizing*

Yi is a multifaceted quality and ability that is difficult to pin down. Its discovery and development, which in classical terms would be called its cultivation, must be undertaken using its manifestations, beginning with its more material manifestations. Although structure and function are really two sides of the same thing, structure is normally more accessible to us, the gateway that allows us to enter the whole. Working on yi involves working with and on qi. This therefore offers various possibilities. Of these, we have chosen the ones that have proven more real, simple and related to clinical practice, according to our experience.

Above all, we have to practice the qualities of presence and awareness, and we know that they are rooted in the more structural qualities of alignment and grounding. But even these resist capture in the beginning. We need a method, a path which helps us to progress from "crude" to "superior". Based on both classical indications and personal experience in acupuncture and Aikido, I (MR) call this the "Three-Level Method."

### *2.4.2.2 Levels of practice: a pathway from the crude to the superior*

Remember the words of Zhuangzi:

> Make your will one! Don't listen with your ears, listen with your mind. No, don't listen with your mind, listen with your qi. Listening stops in the ears and the mind stops with recognition, but qi is empty and waits on all things...The way is gathered in emptiness alone. Emptiness is the fasting of the mind.

In other words, the mind, or at least the conscious mind, should get away from the path, to allow a correct perception of reality. This is what Krishnamurti tells us, using other words, about the art of listening.

This means, in order to bring yi and qi into play, we have to reach a state of consciousness that seems to be reserved for a fortunate few. But this state can be understood not as a static reality, but as an objective. And everyone can find their place on the path to this goal. In terms of acupuncture, we have seen that Lingshu one can be seen to refer to a progression. One starts off as a beginner ("crude") and one must pay attention to form and its details. With time, work and luck, one can gradually evolve and find and incorporate more and more subtle forms of qi, such as dynamic qi, shen or propensity. This means that the more physical aspects of the process progressively cease to be the centre of attention and become the place where things happen, where qi and its dynamics can be observed and where they can be influenced from a natural state. The point to which technique becomes "spiritual" is of no importance. As practitioners we always have a relationship with substance, with form.

It was on reaching this point, that I (MR) recalled my experiences with Aikido. From the start, my teachers insisted that I should not use force, but only Ki.[13] Anybody who has practiced an internal martial art knows how frustrating this instruction is. But, although it is sometimes forgotten, in Aikido there is a path, an idea that can serve as a guide for the difficult task of combining structure and spirit into a model that integrates and harmonises them. A way of bringing together the abstract idea of evolution with the very solid idea of clinical work.

There is no need to enumerate or repeat the numerous examples of how East Asian culture tends to conceptualise reality as three states or phases. Of course, reality is in itself a continuum, and these phases only show the milestones, successive landscapes that appear along the same path. However, both tradition and pedagogical experience confirm the practical aspect of this order when defining the path. For this reason, I present this progression which is based on the denominations used in Aikido, an art which has a very structured way to think and practise around this "stages" model, showing, interestingly enough, a close parallelism with Zhuangzi's admonitions and stories. Also, in Aikido these three stages are clearly presented as an evolution, the lucky, perseverant and enlightened practitioner going thorough each of these periods without ever really forgetting the initial ones. This staging will help to organise and guide our passage from crude to superior without forgetting that we work in the real world, where form and spirit are one and the same thing.

Aikido tradition presents a four stage development: Kotai, Jutai, Ekitai and Kitai. Because one can see Ekitai[14] as a refinement of Jutai, an evolution from physical flexibility to a mental fluidity, these two stages are combined in one, characterised for fluidity, and thus allowing what can be a more useful model in the context of therapeutic practice, and better matching the particular fields of Neidan when integrated in therapeutic activity. Ekitai, in fact, will be in the schema a bridge between Jutai, the start of more fluid qualities, and Kitai, the supreme art of not being personally (meaning the "I") involved in the action.

*The crude attends to the form, the superior attends to the dynamics. Lingshu...*

Then, the stages of going from the crude to the superior, can be structured in three phases: one, the initial, characterised by the more physical aspects of the art and the learning of its techniques, two, the intermediate, when the techniques are no longer an obstacle and the practitioner slowly starts flowing with the circumstance, and a third one, the master's stage, where the distinctions between patient, acupuncturist, etc. progressively blur merging into a kind of global reality. Following this model, and using Aikido nomenclature, the stages are:

–Kotai. This is the first and absolutely necessary stage, like constructing the foundations of a building. The focus is in learning and improving all the aspects of the art, with emphasis in its more tangible aspects: theory, point location, techniques, posture, timing, etc. From the mental standpoint, this phase is directed by intention (focus, concentration, posture, repetition) and organised thought, and there is duality between acupuncturist and patient. If we follow Zhuangzi's admonitions, will be like "hearing with your ears".

–Jutai and Ekitai. Once technique is acquired and secure, the physical (jutai) and mental (ekitai) fluidity work starts. In Aikido both stages are, at least on the theoretical level, differentiated, but they can both be characterized by:

- Softness and fluidity, both physical and mental.

- Perception of the tendency of the other ("aite", or the patient) and progressive perception of the situation's propensity (shi).
- Progressive evolution (from jutai to ekitai) from flexibility and softness to natural fluidity.

This is a stage directed by the fluidity, attention and stillness (physical and mental softness, mobile center and axis) with little or no participation of the intention or the organized thought. Distinction between acupuncturist and patient start dissolving into the larger reality, the dynamic (ji) appears and acts, one starts grasping more subtle aspects of the situation, like the propensity (shi) and incipience (ji). It somewhat matches Zhuangzi's "hearing with your mind-heart".

–Ekitai. Once one has reached the fluidity grounded in the knowledge, the work becomes something natural (ziran) that happens by itself. In this stage appear:

- "Ki awase" (get together with ki).
- Action as natural and hazy in the situation, in accordance with its tendency and dynamics.
- Techniques, posture or intention are no longer mentioned.

This stage is one of integration and awareness without the involvement of intention or organized thought. In Zhuangzi's words, it would be like "hearing with your qi", a stage when the practitioner is in a different state ("kimusubi"), and the healing act is something unavoidable, which happens naturally (ziran) and without effort (wuwei).

We can see how this model also shows the different aspects of Yi engaged in the stages of learning process. I want to emphasize that, although maybe useful for understanding and explaining the progression, the division in three stages is only an artifact, an artificial construct where the different aspects of the reality separated by the columns are always present, although mixed in different proportions. We can put together into a table the different stages of practice, the correspondent aspects of yi, and also several related aspects of the total action:

Although somewhat artificial, this three stage model brings us some conceptual and practical advantages, mainly:

1) There is a clear track from the physical and the intention to the ethereal and the awareness; there is no longer a contrast between "the crude" and

| Work Stages/ Feature | Kotai | Jutai-Ekitai | Kitai |
|---|---|---|---|
| Definition | -First level of work<br>-Work solid and precise<br>-Physical aspects developed<br>-Learn to harmonize the own physical structure<br>-Attention to oneself | **Jutai**<br>-Act swiftly, without contraction, in any circumstance<br>-Intention directed to the partner (Aite, patient)<br>**Ekitai**<br>-Action before the event<br>-Acting according to circumstances<br>-Action: guiding the partner towards the desired most natural direction (using the partner-actor propensity) | -Envelope the partner like a mist<br>-Move with the partner in the natural direction (following Universe's propensity) |
| Image | Making the foundations of a building | Flowing like water | "I don't have to do anything but to stand in my feet and be silent"' |
| State | Solid | Liquid | Gaseous |
| Virtue | -Clarity<br>-Precision<br>-Structure | Flexibility | Fluidity |
| Yi acting as | -Intention<br>-Concentration, focus | -Attention<br>-Consciousness | -Awareness<br>-Disappearance of awareness |
| Centre of attention (qi manifestation most observed) | Form | Dynamic | Shen |
| What to look for and evaluate in the situation | Propensity | Dynamics | Emptiness |
| Learning | -Techniques<br>-Mechanics | Fluid use of techniques | Unity (techniques melt) |

"the superior", but a clear pathway from the initial stages of learning to better ways of practicing. This pathway, clearly resonating with self-cultivation, but also with both martial and healing arts, can be characterized according different conceptualizations:

–From doing to not doing.

–From duality to integration.
–From tangible to intangible.

2) Each stage is based and rooted in the preceding one. In all the stages, the preceding ones are present, as are, to a lesser extent, the subsequent ones. In practice, no matter the level achieved by the practitioner, one always continues working and refining all the levels, including the more physical, basic ones. There is a life-time commitment for the practitioner wishing to develop their skills. The concert pianist continues practicing their "scales", the master martial artist still practices the basic as well as advanced forms and movements, so too the very experienced acupuncturist still practices their basic skills.

## 2.5 Timing, the right moment, Ji and Shi (機 勢)

So far, we have spoken about the elements we are going to work with (body-mind), but there is one more important point: its practical application, the moment for performing the action, whether it be a movement of Taiji quan or inserting a needle. A relaxed body and a calm mind produce an action at the right moment. This is a vital concept in the practice of acupuncture or martial arts. A second too late can be a decisive factor in martial practice, too many needles or too large a dosage can negatively affect a treatment.

Some of the key concepts which help to understand the importance of timing are ji [機] and shi [勢], concepts which appear in the literature of acupuncture and Taiji quan, as has been stated in previous chapters. Now we look at their practical aspect and apply them to an action that involves the use of our body-mind. One of the necessary components that allow our body to perform movements are its joints. Open joints will allow us to perform an action in resonance, without impediments. A Taiji quan master said "articulations should always be free of stagnation, without tension, since a closed joint leads to collapse and blockage, which prevents us from responding to the situations that arise around us."

Flexible, open joints allow our body to adapt to the changes that are produced around us. The concept of propensity (shi) refers to the potential for movement that arises according to circumstances. We do not know how or where we are going to move, but we have the potential for initiating the movement readily available. In its physical aspect, this potential needs our joints to be open and relaxed. Any movement or change needs a space for transformation. Being able to perceive this space, where the beginning of the change develops, requires a very finely tuned sensitivity. This first indication of movement is implicit in the concept dynamic (ji) which is related to the mind. More specifically with calmness of mind, because it is thanks to this calmness that we can be more sensitive to the slightest sign.

A calm mind that can perceive the slightest sign and a relaxed body with open joints, which can adapt to any potential movement, are the essence of the exercises presented below. But like the examples we have seen, we will begin with the physical part; our body. An aligned body is the first step towards creating a vessel that can contain a calm mind.

## Bibliography

1- Birch S. Traditional needling techniques as practical constructions from reading historical descriptions. *Eur J Oriental Med.* 2013;7(3)26-33.
2- Birch S. Chapter four: The Jingmai and qi –acupuncture perspectives. In this volume.
3- Birch S, Cabrer Mir MA, Rodriguez M. Chapter one: Qi and the mind –explorations of the links between qi, the mind, mental and emotional states. In this volume.
4- Cabrer Mir MA. Chapter seven: Qi and stillness –Taijiquan, qigong and acupuncture. In this volume.
5- Chace C. On greeting a friend, an approach to needle technique. *Lantern.* 2006:3(3):4-7.
6- Chace C, Bensky D. Chapter five: An axis of efficacy. The range of meaning in chapter one of the Lingshu. In this volume.
7- Matsumoto K, Birch S. *Hara Diagnosis Reflections on the Sea*; Brookline, Paradigm Publications, 1988.
8- Roth HD. *Original Tao –Inward Training (Nei Yeh)*. New York, Columbia University Press, 1999.

## Endnotes

1. The appendix outlined the historical passages from the Suwen, Lingshu and Nanjing, cited with translations and shows how they were combined practically to form the needling technique [1].

2. What we say here arises from having studied and practiced acupuncture for over thirty years and having studied with many teachers with considerably more experience than that. However, while the focus here is on acupuncture it is also relevant for anyone performing

a hands-on therapy that uses qi based models and their reasoning and methods. Thus, what is described here can be of use for massage therapists (tuina, shiatsu etc) as well.

3. In these verses from the Neiye, we can find nearly all of the key factors concerning an acupuncturist's attitude that we are describing in this section. To avoid being repetitive, it is better to refer to a specific line in every section. See [6, 8].

4. There are numerous, fruitful analogies between the martial arts and acupuncture. Most of the requirements a practitioner needs (such as structure, calmness, focus, etc.) are the same. It is no accident that the Suwen compares the work of an acupuncturist to that of a crossbowman. Nor that the language used in classical medicine is influenced so greatly by martial terminology.

5. This is an important difference in types of awareness. When one is oriented towards personal growth, depending on one's state and who one works with, it is relatively easy to fantasise about progress. The warrior or doctor both live far away from the land of fantasy. The reality they move in constantly gives them information on how real their evolution is, at least in terms of their fields of action. It is possible that, in spite of the ultimate unity of all things, awareness shows different nuances, or at least different expressions. This is the advantage of moving in the real world: one can have an elevated awareness in the plane of personal growth, but if one does not also have it in one's chosen field, this will become completely obvious –the warrior loses the fight, the doctor is unable to act effectively. It seems possible, at least in theory, for one to develop great awareness of oneself, while his or her awareness as a warrior or as a doctor is at a lower level; this is what material results show. It seems that the levels of awareness that one reaches are different in different areas of his or her specific life and field.

6. It is very good to experience almost mystical moments of awareness and presence, but how can we maintain that state when, on leaving the treatment room, we are bombarded by telephone calls, emails, bills... This is an authentic challenge. One possible solution may be to gradually train ourselves to use an "awareness switch", for example taking a simple deep breath just before "changing state" can be useful when trained as a trigger.

7. For information on the role of ones psycho-emotional state in the practice of acupuncture and its relation to physical structure, see [5].

8. It would be more appropriate to say that its action is easier and more obvious through a more material medium. A number of reliable modern experiments have proven the existence of mind-material interactions, while physics has spent the last hundred years or so disproving the idea of the separation of mind and body (see [2]).

9. Linzheng Zhinan Yian (Medical Records as a guide to Clinical Work), 1766.

10. My (MR) first serious contact with this phrase was in 2007. From the beginning, I defined myself as belonging in the "crude" group. I considered that the sentence, apart from its arrogance, only emphasised an elitism that to some extent pertained to the culture of that

time. My attitude was: "all right, that may be so, but as I'm not good enough to be 'shang' (superior), I'll try to be the best 'cu' (crude) I possibly can." It has taken me nearly four years to find another interpretation of that sentence. While, emphasising this evolving aspect might not be very original, I feel it is necessary since in all the years I was struggling nobody stated this, which means that maybe it is not such a common interpretation after all.

11. The following explanations are elaborations of what can be found in this book, beginning in chapter one and in more detail in chapter four and is a repetition of what is found in these.

12. This can be seen as part of what is called in clinical practice and research "patient-practitioner interactions".

13. Ki is the Romanisation and Japanese pronunciation of the Chinese word qi, 氣.

14. The stages of working with Ki in Aikido are:

- Kotai: solid, precise, physical work
- Jutai: Smooth work, without contractions
- Ekitai: Fluid, liquid work
- Kitai: Integrative, vaporous work

CHAPTER TEN

# PRACTICAL EXERCISES

Miguel Angel Cabrer Mir, Manuel Rodriguez Cuadras, Stephen Birch

The primary aim of the exercises in this chapter is to help keep the body relaxed and alert during clinical practice.

In this chapter you will find exercises to:

Relax and align the body.

Maintain this state of relaxation and alignment during needling.

Fine tune the sense of touch (pulse, abdominal palpation, the way of holding the needles).

# 1. Exercises

## 1.1. Creating the vessel

In order for the body to act as a vessel, all its parts must become unified, the structure must be consistent both internally and externally. We can organize this process into two main aspects: establishing a solid but movable base (or root), and building upon it an aligned, coherent posture

### 1.1.1. The base: a movable root

#### *1.1.1.1. Grounding qi*

Structure provides coherence, mobilisation and activation awaken alertness, and both of them contribute to a self-perception of integration and openness that are favourable for contact with the patient. We have the trunk and branches, grounding will give us roots.

By grounding qi, we understand the sensation of descent and continuation of the base, the perception that structure and alertness are firmly based and grounded to the centre of the earth. A powerful tree has deep, extensive roots, and those roots are what we seek with grounding.[1]

Apart from bringing consciousness to that quality when we practice it, we can also perform a simple, specific procedure that will prove very useful in day-to-day clinical work.

#### *1.1.1.2. Perceiving your base*

This can be done in a sitting or standing position. If you stand, start with the basic working posture.

We first describe the "sitting" procedure, because if we start with the basic standing posture (our working posture) our attention will tend to go directly to the soles of our feet, with greater attention needed on alignment of the spinal column.

The interesting thing about this exercise is that it promotes a sensation of grounding and as this grounding is combined with an awareness of structure and alertness we also acquire these related qualities on the way.

If you have the colour of soles in your mind, then in any given situation, if you want to be grounded, all you have to do is invoke the colour. In this way, you will start a cascade of events, your attention will automatically be directed

**Sitting procedure**

1. Sit comfortably. The ideal position is to sit on the edge of the seat with a straight vertebral column with proper muscle tone (as if we were standing), not touching the backrest. But the most important thing is to be comfortable.
2. Close your eyes, relax your arms, your hands, your legs, your face. It is a good idea to smile slightly.
3. Direct your attention to your buttocks, to the area in contact with the seat. Ask yourself:
   - Can I feel the contact pressure?
   - Do I feel the same pressure in both buttocks?
   - What sensation does the seat transmit to me? Cold, hot, rough, polished, hard, soft, pleasant, unpleasant? The idea is to perceive, not judge.
4. When you have a clear perception of the sensation in your buttocks, direct your attention to the soles of your feet. Ask yourself the same questions as before:
   - Can I feel the contact pressure?
   - Do I feel the same pressure in both feet?
   - What sensation does the floor (or the soles of my feet) transmit to me? Cold, hot, rough, polished, hard, soft, pleasant, unpleasant? The idea is to perceive, not judge
5. Once you have the sensation of touch in the soles of your feet, see if a colour appears in them (it can be the same colour or a different one. They are frequently different shades of the same colour). It may appear, it may not.

If the soles of your feet have a colour, add it to the other sensations and remember it all again.
   - If no colour appears, see if you want to mentally paint or dye the soles of your feet in a particular colour. If you don't feel like doing so, don't worry. Continue with tactile sensations.
   - If you do want to paint the soles of your feet, mentally choose the colour and imagine yourself painting them in that colour. Depending on the person, these may be everyday images, like picking up a paintbrush, dipping it in the chosen can of paint or ink and painting your feet with it. Other people may just visualise the chosen colour applied to the soles of their feet. It is better to think of a gloss (transparent colour) rather than a paint (opaque colour).
   - Clearly remember the colour, add it to the other sensations and remember it all again.
6. Stay with this perception of the soles of your feet for a few minutes.
7. Breathe deeply three times and on exhaling for the third time, open your eyes. The exercise has finished.

to the soles of your feet, and all the mechanisms you have created will enter into action: attention directed to your soles will ground your qi, and this will help produce structure and alertness.

## 1.1.2. The structure: alignment (standing posture), fluidity, mental attitude

Always keeping the idea –and fact– of a movable root or base, the next step is how to build upon this base.

We have already seen that structure is very important, and that the acupuncturist must work on his or her own structure assiduously and constantly in order to evolve in the more subtle aspects of needle insertion. This involves the alignment, calming and relaxing we saw before in the Neiye. Depending on the individual, this can be seen in many different ways, but in any event, it has to result in a comfortable and relaxed attitude. The way in which alignment promotes calmness is the physical basis that allows us to root within ourselves. The alignment described in the Neiye and the mental attitude suggested by the Neiye and Lingshu can be studied and worked on through posture, suppleness and attitude.

### *1.1.2.1. Standing posture (Shishei)*

This is translated as position, attitude, posture. It comes from *sugata* (shi), which expresses form, and from *ikioi* (sei), which expresses strength, vitality, vivacity. Two masters have this to say about it:

Tamura Nobuyoshi:

> Above all, order the body, which is the container of ki. To do this, extend your spinal column and keep it straight. If you feel you are pushing the sky with your head, your spinal column extends in a natural way. Do not puff out your chest like a soldier standing to attention. Your shoulders are relaxed, and drop slightly, the anus is closed, your kidneys are not curved (no lordosis), ki is comfortably positioned in the seika tanden, your whole body is calm and relaxed.

Miramoto Musashi:

> Your face is calm, neither looking up nor down nor in any direction, your eyes slightly closed, your eyeballs unmoving, your brow unwrinkled, the bridge of your nose straight, without pushing your chin too far forward, the nape of your neck is also straight, your cervical vertebrae full of strength. Below your dropped shoulders,

your body is perfectly relaxed, your spinal column is in the correct position, your buttocks drawn in; from knees to toes, your legs are firmly set on the ground, your hips are not blocked, your belly is firmly rounded.

In Aikido, this supple, balanced posture allows you to move freely, like a tetrahedron, which on turning is like a cone. Acupuncture postures tend to favour parallel feet, although it is useful to remember that the acupuncturist's relation to the couch means that not all balanced postures can be included in the typical parallel feet posture.

In order for the body to act as a vessel, all its different parts must first become unified. There are two areas which make this unity difficult to achieve: the shoulders and the lumbar region, places where our musculature easily accumulates tensions.

**Shoulders:**

One of the important points in the practice of Taiji quan is relaxing the shoulders. The objective is not simply the relaxation of the region, it is to become aware of moving our arms as one with the whole body. In every-day life, we perform many actions using our arms. In general, these movements do not involve the rest of our body; they are performed from our shoulders. This is why it is normal for tensions to slowly accumulate in this region. Becoming aware of how we use our arms is the first step towards slowly integrating them into a unified movement:

**Awareness of our shoulders:** ***pair-work***

If you can find someone to pair up with then you can perform the following simple exercise.

One person performs movements with their arms, trying to observe and perceive when they begin to use their shoulders to carry out these movements. The other person puts one hand on the first person's shoulder and helps him or her to perceive when the movement is being performed from the shoulders. We do the same on both sides and then change roles.

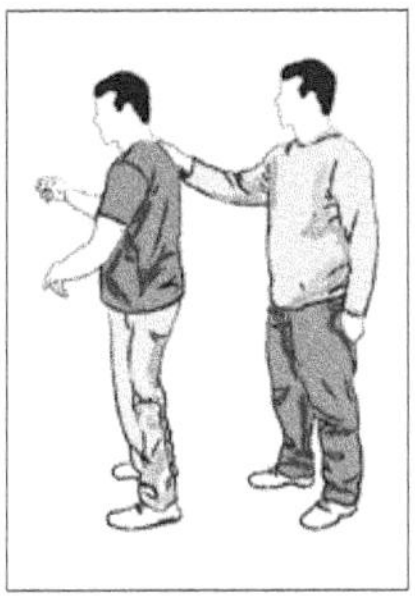
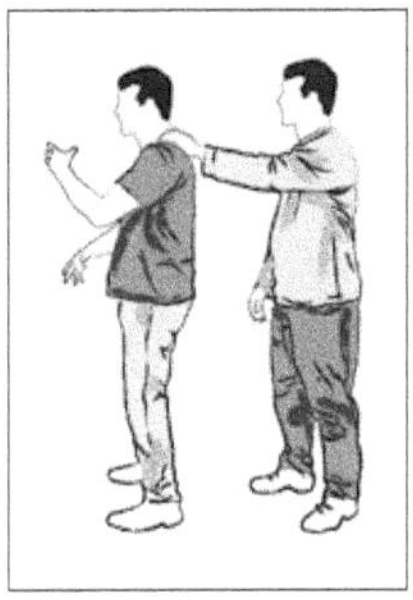

**Awareness of the position of the knees and its effect on the lumbar region:**

The other region referred to above is the lumbar region. When we stand with our knees tense, with no space, our posture causes the lumbar vertebrae to become blocked and tense.

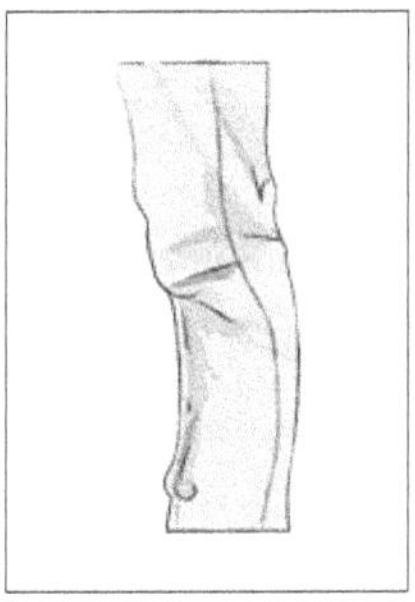
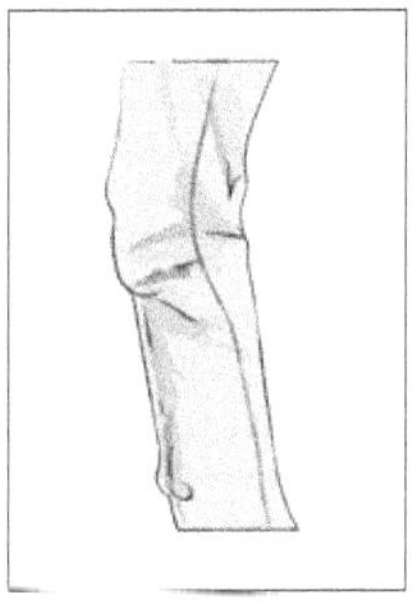

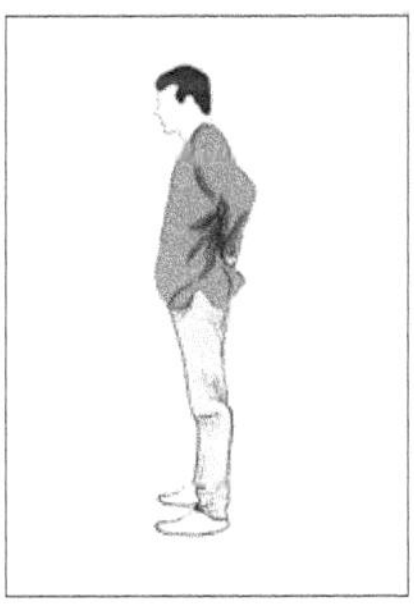
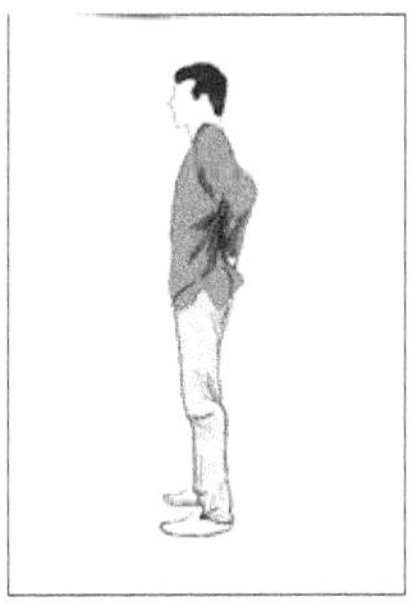

We stand in a comfortable position and place one hand on our lumbar region. We relax our knees a little and observe, with the aid of our hand, if there has been any movement in the lumbar region. Just by relaxing our knees, without performing any other movement, our lumbar region relaxes a little.

With these simple exercises we have opened, or become aware of, two basic regions for connecting our extremities to our torso. All the different parts have been unified. Now it is important for the structure of the vessel to be well aligned.

A vessel needs to be well aligned so that its structure can relax without any of its parts having to do extra work. Having our body well aligned will enable our musculature to perform only the work it needs to do. An excess in some areas makes our musculature do extra work which, over time, leads to the formation of areas of tension.

**Observing and perceiving an aligned structure: pair-work**

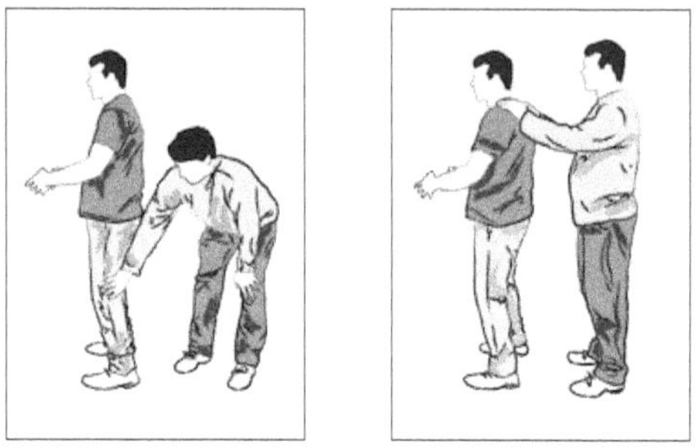

One person stands with his or her feet in parallel. The other person observes and helps their partner by touch, not with words, to adjust their body structure to a position that is aligned with gravity. Once we have made the necessary changes, we give the person time to feel how he or she perceives the new position. It is important to be aware of the physical sensations that arise when we change our posture. There are sometimes differences between our perception of being aligned and the reality that our partner perceives.

### *1.1.2.2 Basic working posture*

This is a posture useful for practice. The details are:

- Hold the feet parallel, meaning the lateral borders of the feet should be parallel, (Fig. 1) separated at approximately the width of the shoulders. With the weight on the center of the soles.
- The knees are slightly bent, without going further than the tip of the feet.
- Try to get them aligned with the feet.
- The pelvis in slightly tilted forward (balanced to the front, like initiating a sitting action), with relaxed gluteus. (Fig. 2).

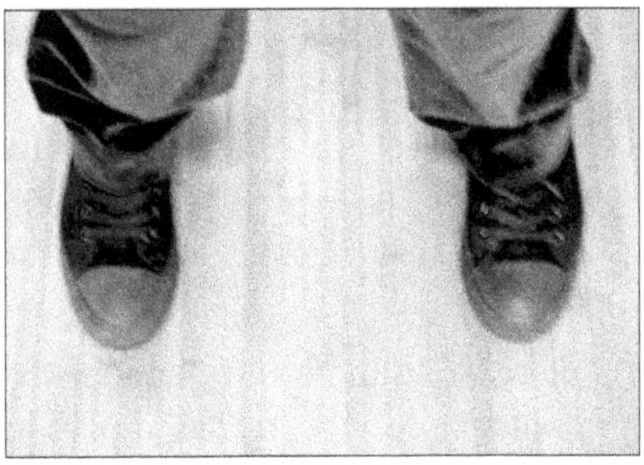
1.

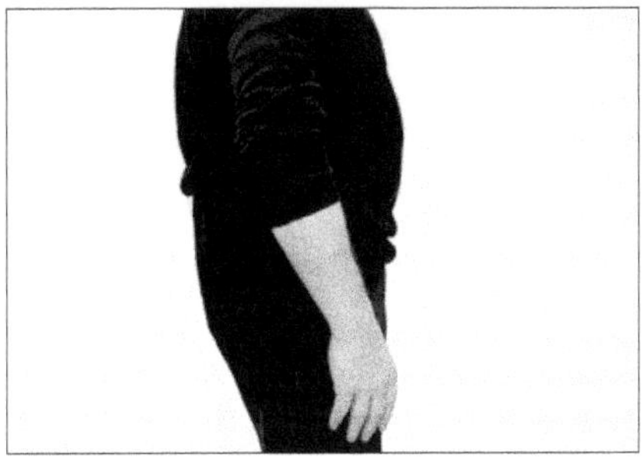
2.

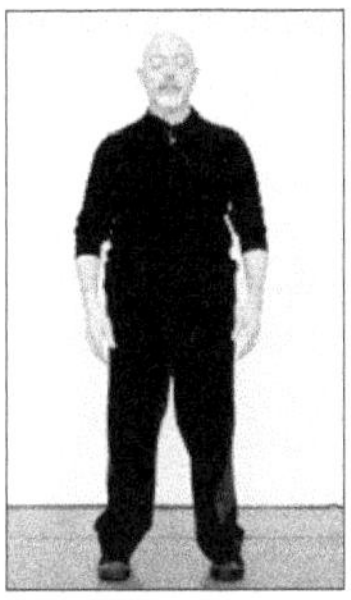
3.

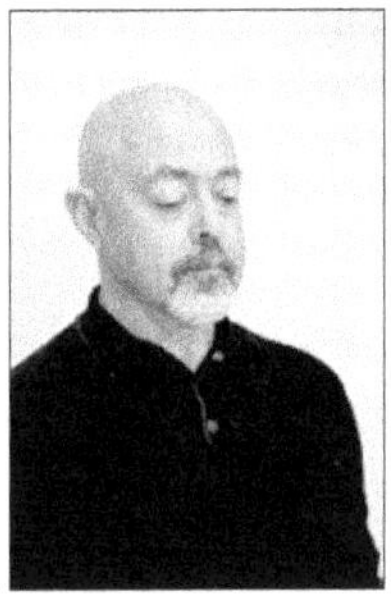
4.

• The spine is straight, avoiding its collapse, in a correct tension, like the string of an instrument.
• The nape of the neck is held firm.
• The shoulders are relaxed, slightly down, with the back slightly rounded (Fig. 3).
• Hold the head as thought it is light, with the intention of slightly pushing up. In this way the head induces some mild tension in the spine, which helps to avoid its collapse and promote its correct tension.
• The top of the head (around the acupoint GV-20 [Baihui]) should be poin-ting upwards, making the jaw slightly drawn.
• In terms of distribution of weight/density, it should be increased from the waist to the feet, and decreased from the waist to the head.
• The mouth is held closed, lips in contact without pressure (there could appear a slight smile), molars in contact, without pressure, tongue touching the roof of the mouth.
• Keep the eyes half closed, looking towards oneself, pupils without movement, avoid being distracted. It is possible to close the eyes at the beginning (Fig. 4).
• Breathing. At the beginning avoid putting too much attention on this. Gently try to go towards a regular, subtle, soft and continuous breathing, uni-ting inhalation and exhalation. Later it is possible to lend more attention to these aspects, starting with regulation of the exhalation.

### *1.1.2.3 Mental attitude*

We repeateadly saw the insistence of texts like the Lingshu, Suwen and Neiye of keeping an appropriate mental attitude, which we defined as states of yi. For instance, Lingshu Chapter 9 says:

> [The practitioner must] deeply reside in a place of stillness and divine the comings and goings of the spirit with one's [sensory] doors and windows shut. [The practitioner's] ethereal and corporeal souls must not be scattered, his mind must be focused, and his essence qi undivided, and undistracted by human sounds. By concentrating his essence, he must unify his mind and direct his will entirely toward needling.

Chace comments how this can be interpreted as the need for inserting from a place of stillness and how doing it in this way we can "welcome the qi" acting without imposing our intention.

### *1.1.2.4 Stillness*

The standing meditation we are going to work with has two positions.

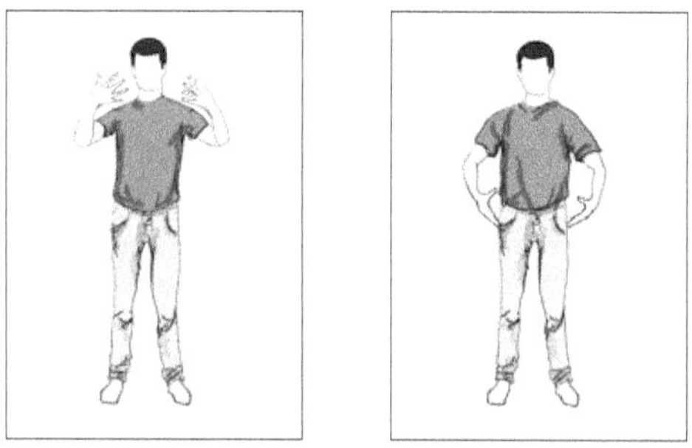

Firstly, we want to assume a position where our body structure is well aligned. To this end, we need to perceive that the weight of our body is on the centre of the soles of our feet. It helps if another person checks that our posture is well aligned. This is important, as it will help our musculature to relax.

We slowly raise our hands with the backs of the hands touching. In this way, we open up the area of the shoulder blades and relax the chest area, which in Taiji is known as "rounding the back and relaxing the chest." When the arms are raised, we try to relax our shoulders. Every so often we do a running check downwards and try to relax any areas that are tensing up. Our fingers are slightly extended, but without being tense. This will help all the tendons in our arms to become active.

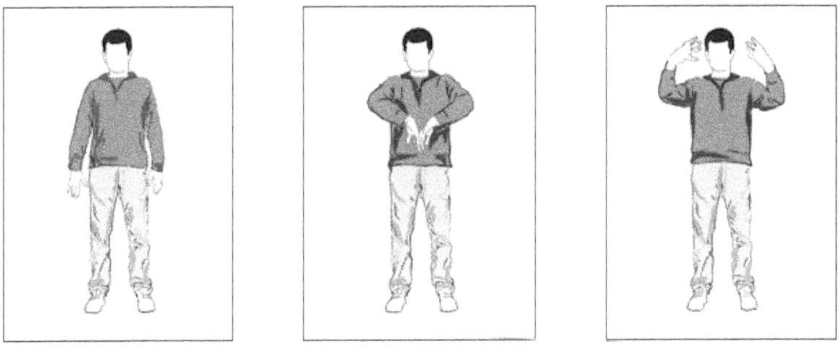

Stand quietly and calmly in the first posture with the arms raised for up to ten minutes, checking periodically about tensions, rhythm of breathing etc. From this posture we then slowly lower the arms to the second posture. Here it is important to observe how we lower our arms. First, we lower our arms from the elbows, then we relax our shoulders and form a circle with our arms in front of our torso. It is as if we are holding a drum; the strap holding the drum is tied at the base of the neck (acupoint GV-14). In this way, we can maintain the unity of our whole body; we are not bearing the weight of the drum with our shoulders. Stand quietly and calmly in this second posture for up to ten minutes, checking periodically about tensions, rhythm of breathing etc.

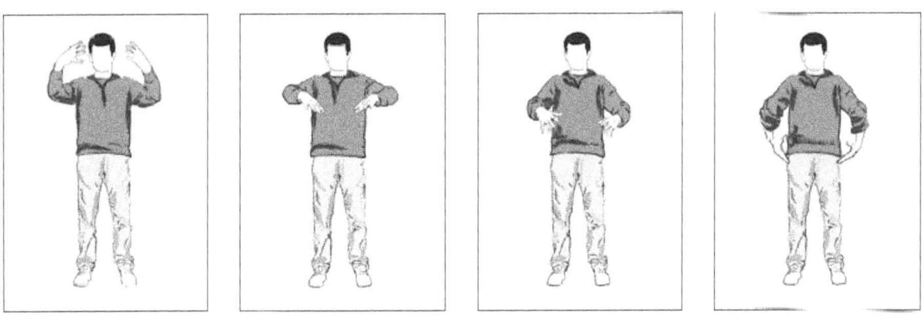

The transition sequence from posture 1 to posture 2

This second posture is important in acupuncture as it similar to the posture we assume when we are performing needle insertions. Practicing this posture can help us to keep our shoulders more relaxed and integrated within our body structure and to be more sensitive to small changes. We always perform a running check downwards to relax any tense areas and at the same time to try to ensure that our body is well aligned.

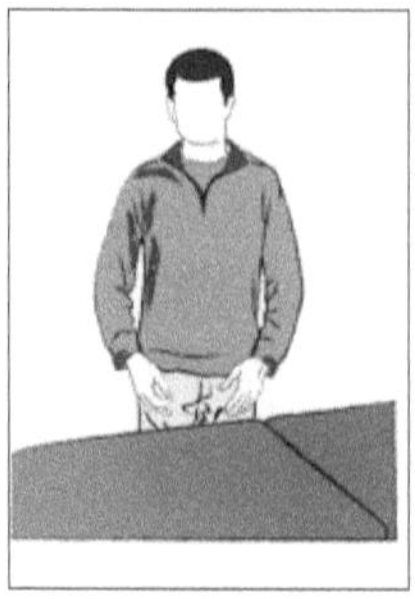

Continual practice of these postures will slowly provide us with a more unified perception of our body and the integration of our arms into our body structure. This last point is important, as we generally use our arms in everyday life to give or take, but these movements usually involve only the arms, not a global movement of the whole body. The practice of standing meditation opens the way to perceiving this body unity and then integrating it into our movements. For this reason, we now propose two simple movements from Taiji quan for integrating the practice of stillness within movement. We should not forget that both disciplines, Taiji quan and acupuncture, are performed through movement.

After unifying our structure, it is important to start working on the other component of the vessel; the inner part. We start by opening up our joints. The circular movement of our joints allow the tendons and ligaments attached to them to enjoy a little more space, which in turn allows our muscles to become a little more relaxed.

## 1.2 Flexibility, fluidity

Placing stress on trying to keep the alignment and stability can risk us getting stuck, either loosing the mobility or needing a conscious effort to go from stillness to movement. The situation is always changing, and our mental and physical attitudes are just the same thing, so, in our job, like in combat, it is essential to get a mobility grounded in balance. Sun Simiao says:

The way of cultivating life requires one to stay as fluid and flexible as possible. Not to spend too much time on, and avoid the exhaustion of trying to achieve impossible goals. It is necessary to learn how to exercise by contemplating nature, observing that the flowing water never becomes putrid, and that an often used door, with active joints never rusts. Why? Because they are always exercising, and almost always moving.

### *1.2.1 Opening our joints*

First we perform the movement with one arm. We imagine that our hand is a paintbrush that is painting a circle, and within the circle a figure of eight. Stand as shown in the photo. Holding one arm at the side, raise the other arm and quietly, gently and slowly move the arm so that the hand moves through the figure of eight movement followed by a circle, repeated by the figure of eight movement, etc.

Repeat this to a total of three or five times. When finished, bring the arm back to the side and perceive how your arm feels and compare it to the other one. Then perform the same movements with the other arm.

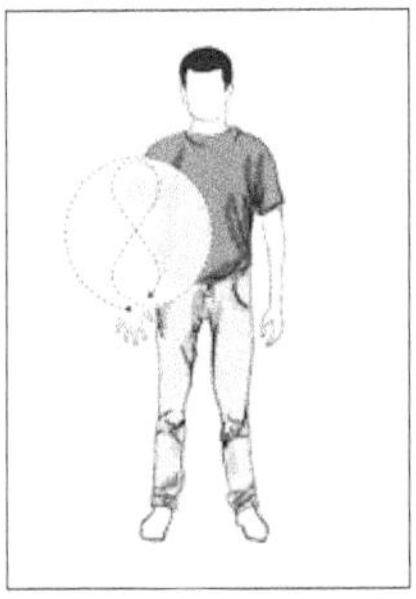

The same movements are performed using the feet to draw figures of eight and circles. Stand on one leg. With the other leg raised slightly in front of you, move the foot slowly and quietly so that it describes a figure of eight, followed by a circle and then the figure of eight again, etc. The circle and the figure of eight are drawn three or five times with the ankle. When you have finished quietly bring the foot back to the ground and stand on both legs to observe how they feel. The same movements are then performed with the other leg.

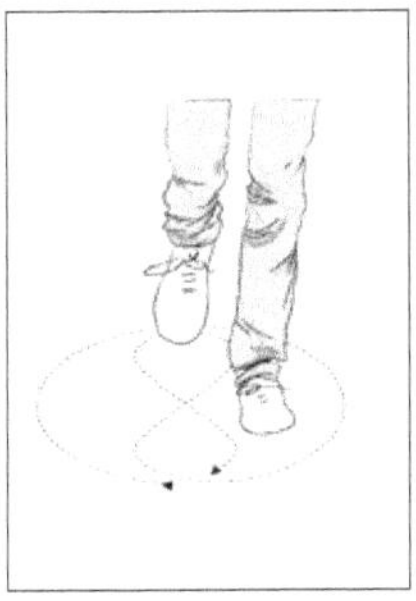

Using these simple exercises, we start to open up all the joints in our extremities.

### *1.2.2 Opening the spine*

In order to open the spine and create more space in its articulations there are a number of simple exercises we can use. The first is extremely simple and is done standing. The others require more explanation and introduction of some simple concepts.

The following exercise will help us to become more aware of the articulations that make up our spinal column. Without forcing the shoulders, that is, without using them to move the spinal column, we try to perform a wave motion rising from the sacrum to the cervical vertebrae. It may be that at first this movement can only be perceived up to the thoracic vertebrae. As the body becomes more relaxed, the movement will go higher. Make sure to not use your shoulders as you perform this simple exercise.

Creating an aligned, unified structure and at the same time opening our articulations in order to create space within. We have begun to construct our vessel. We will now look at other proposals which will help to further the construction of the vessel.

### *1.2.2 Vitalizing the spine and joints: San Guan (three passes)*

The term "guan" means a place where there is a wall, a border crossing or a gorge. It simultaneously represents a pass and a barrier, something which separates and unifies at the same time.

In some schools of Qigong (Luohan gong, for example) guan is compared to articulations (guanjie) and the term is defined as "door" or "pass". Working on the steps or passes can be very helpful as you try to achieve completely relaxed muscles and a skeleton adjusted to the Heaven-Earth alignment, which is a basic condition for unblocking internal channels.

Adjustment of the skeleton is based on aligning the bone structure in a natural way and readjusting its different parts, creating openings that allow the free circulation of qi. This process of modifying qi distribution, which brings with it minute adjustments that are often imperceptible to the naked eye, implies opening the three internal passes (san nei guan, or simply san guan) and the six external ones (liu wai guan).

**San nei guan:** lumbar, dorsal and cervical regions (C1-C2, T2-T3, L2-L3 spaces) [SKLT 1].

**Liu wai guan:** shoulder-elbow-wrist and hip-knee-ankle articulations [SKLT 2].

*Internal passes*

Upper pass: located in the space between C1 and C2. Regulates the movement of qi and blood from the trunk to the head and from the head to the trunk.

Middle pass: between T2 and T3. Regulates the movement of qi and blood from the trunk to the arms and from the arms to the trunk.

Lower pass: between L2 and L3. Regulates the movement of qi and blood from the back to the legs and from the legs to the back.

*External passes*

They are related to the large articulations of the extremities:

Superior: shoulder, elbow and wrist.

Inferior: hips, knees and ankles.

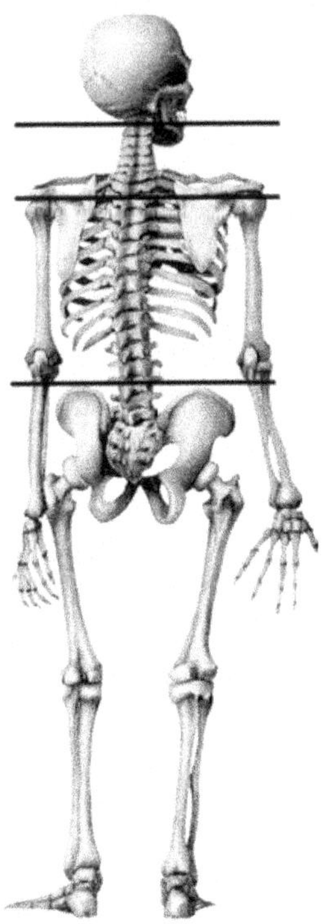

SKLT 1

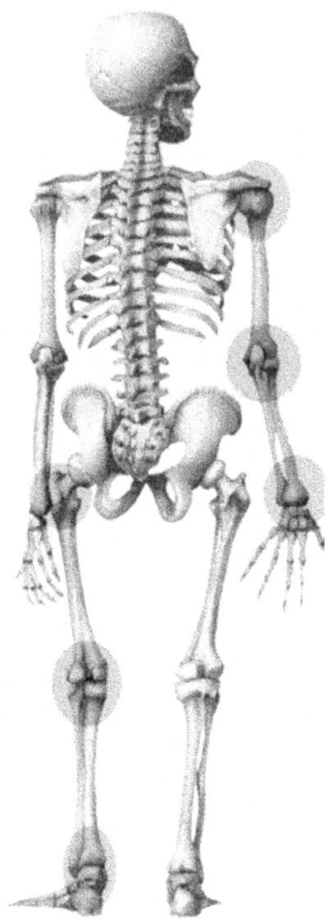

SKLT 2

## San Guan. Exercise: Working on the passes

The basic function of the passes is to regulate and condition the internal structure, creating and stimulating the spaces that allow the free circulation of qi. This is achieved using simple exercises. It is better to start with working only on the internal passes, and then gradually to move on to complete activation.

Activation of the internal passes should be done in the following order:

- Activation: Lumbar-dorsal-cervical.
- Deactivation: Lumbar-dorsal-cervical.

*Activation of internal and external passes:*

In this model, the internal and external passes also coordinate or correspond with each other and efforts should be made to activate corresponding passes at the same time:

- Lumbar: coordinates with shoulders and hips.
- Thoracic: coordinates with elbows and knees.
- Cervical: coordinates with wrists and ankles.

To be able to gradually progress, it is better to start by focusing in the internal passes; the work on the external ones will come mostly by itself as an extension of the practice.

*Working on each pass separately*

Adopt the basic working standing posture (see 1.1.2.2 above): feet parallel and separated to shoulder's width, knees slightly flexed, pelvis slightly pointed to the front, straight spine, strong nape of the neck, chin slightly drawn, vertex (baihui) pointed to the heavens, tongue touching the superior palate, looking at a space about one meter in front of your feet, or closed eyes. Natural and smooth breathing. From this starting point we can activate one, two or the three passes.

**Activating the lumbar pass** (first pass): coordinating the breathe with movements, certain movements are done on the inhalation and others on the exhalation, everything is performed as slowly as you can manage.

As you breathe in slowly, draw, tilt the coccyx backwards (Fig. 5) while relaxing the abdomen (this helps mobilise and open the lumbar pass). At the same time, bring the relaxed arms up from the shoulders, palms facing each other, until the hands reach up to the level of dantian (just below the navel). While you are doing this also let the eyes progressively open so that when the abdomen is full, the eyes are wide open, the hands at the level of dantian, the coccyx tilted as far backwards and upwards as possible (like a dog lifting its tail). Then begin to exhale through the mouth letting the abdomen empty by itself. As you do this exert a slight pressure from your abdominal muscles while the coccyx gradually tilts forwards, ending up a bit more forward than its natural position (like a dog setting its tail between its legs). At the same time allow your knees to bend slightly more. Once you have finished the exhalation, you can repeat the exercise: breath in, arms go up from the shoulders, etc.

When you mobilise the internal lumbar pass, you are also mobilising two of the external passes, the hips and shoulders. When starting this practise, you don't need to pay attention to these, but with repeated practice they can gradually become more involved in the exercise.

After the repetitions you have decided to do in your session, straighten your body adopt the basic standing working posture, put your hands over your navel and take about three smooth and calm breaths, feeling how the qi moves and how the qi of your hands communicate with the qi inside your abdomen. (Fig. 6).

After these three calm breaths, make a deep inhalation opening your eyes widely while presenting your palms to the front (adopting a Yang attitude) (Fig. 7 + Fig. 8). When you feel full of air, let it smoothly escape from your mouth while relaxing the whole body, the hands and the eyes (adopting a Yin attitude) (Fig. 9 + Fig. 10).

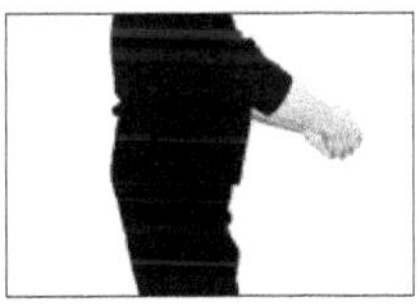
5.

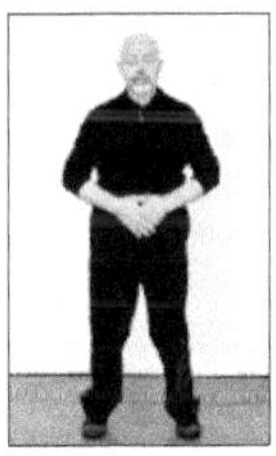
6.

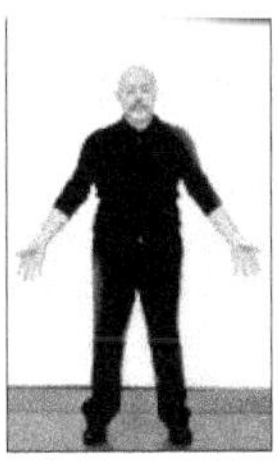
7.

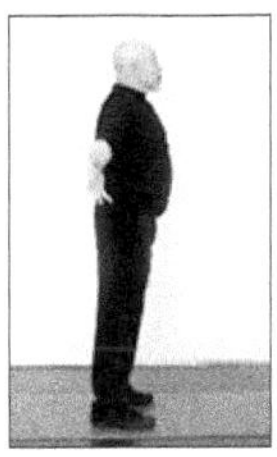
8.

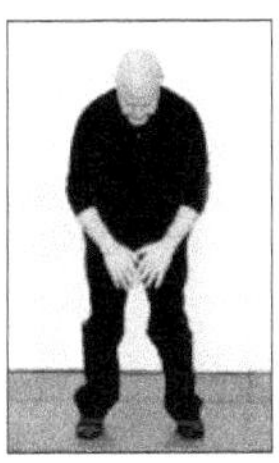
9.

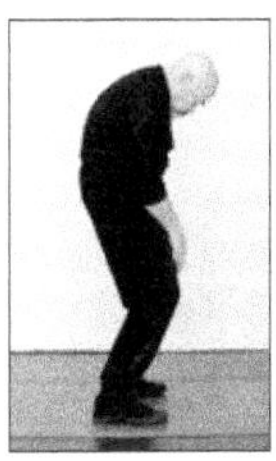
10.

**Activating the thoracic pass** (second pass). Like the previous exercise, movements and breathing are done slowly with coordination between specific movements during inhalation and exhalation.

Inhale slowly, lifting the arms in a relaxed manner from the shoulders up to when the hands reach about the level of Ren17 (middle of the chest) (Fig. 11). Continue breathing in and extend the arms to the sides with the palms facing forwards (Fig. 12). Continue taking air in and stretch the arms with the palms facing out to the sides (Fig. 13), as though you were pushing two far away walls (Fig. 14), thus opening your interscapular area. Pay attention to avoid tension in your shoulders when stretching the arms. When you reach the maximum extension and you are full of breath, start letting the breath smoothly escape via the mouth, and at the same time relax your elbows and knees as you let the arms slowly go down by the sides, while your sight is slowly looking into yourself, kind of looking inwards. The eyesight goes with the muscular movement, becoming more open and outward when inhaling and progressively going inward as you exhale. When finishing the exercise, bend your knees a bit more.

With the internal thoracic pass, the external passes of the elbows and knees can also be activated. When starting this practise, you don't need to pay attention to these, but with repeated practice they can gradually become more involved in the exercise.

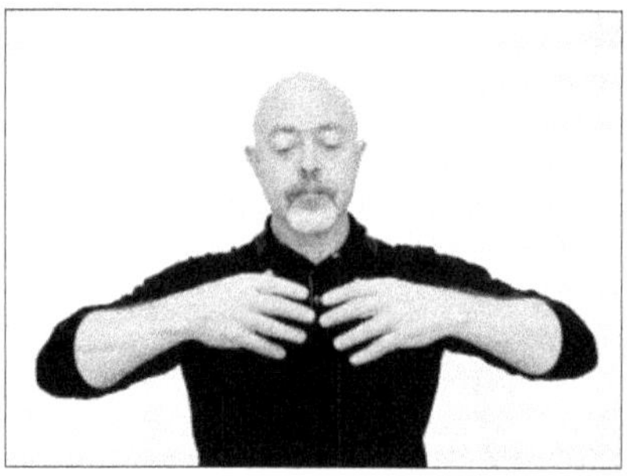

11.

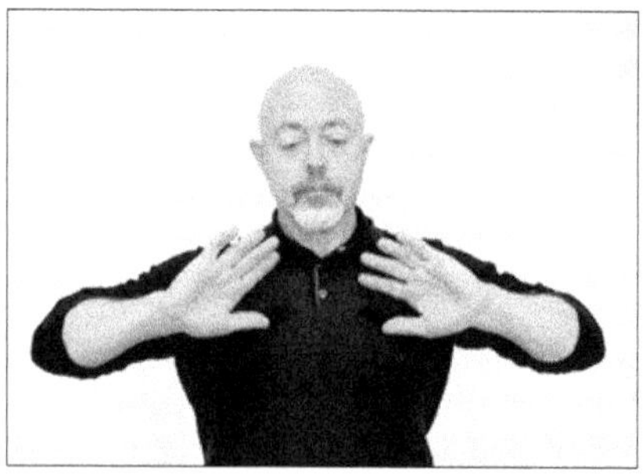

12.

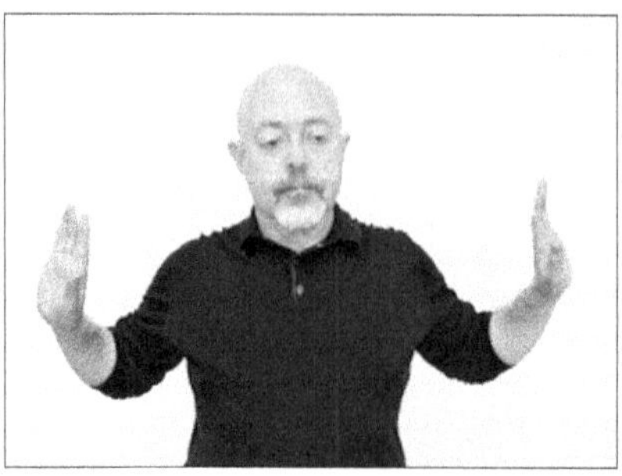

13.

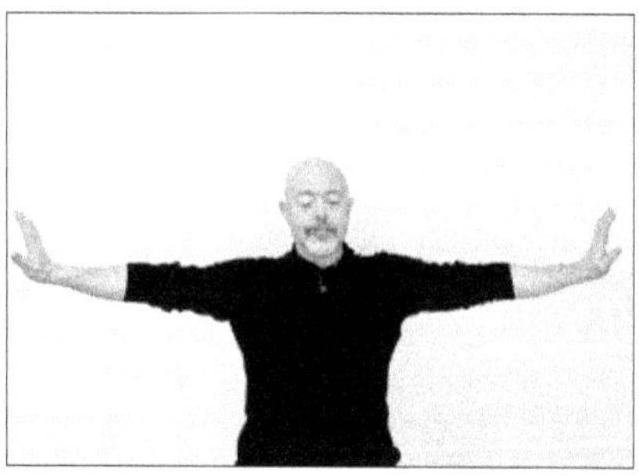

14.

After the repetitions you have decided to do in your session, straighten your body, adopt the basic standing working posture, put your hands over your navel and make about three smooth and calm breaths, feeling how the qi moves and how the qi of your hands communicate with the qi inside your abdomen.

Make a deep inhalation opening wide your eyes and presenting your palms to the front (a Yang attitude). When you feel full of air, let your breath out smoothly from your mouth while relaxing the whole body, the hands and the eyes (a Yin attitude).

**Activating the cervical pass** (third pass). As above, the breath and movements are slow and coordinated.

Starting with the basic standing working posture, breath smoothly in while lifting the arms in front of you with the palms facing each other. When the hands reach the level of the throat (Fig. 15), turn the palms upward and continue breathing in and lifting the arms (Fig. 16), tilting the head backwards and following the hands with your sight up to when you are fully vertically extended, with the palms looking to the heavens and the points of your fingers touching (Fig. 17), feeling at the same time fully extended upward and deeply rooted from your feet. Stay here a second and start breathing out, breathing smoothly from the mouth while relaxing the arms from the shoulders (Fig. 18), elbows (Fig. 19) and wrists when descending along the body, at the same

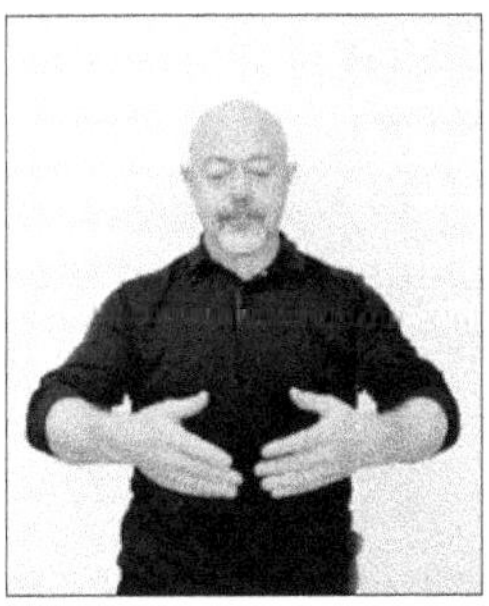

15.

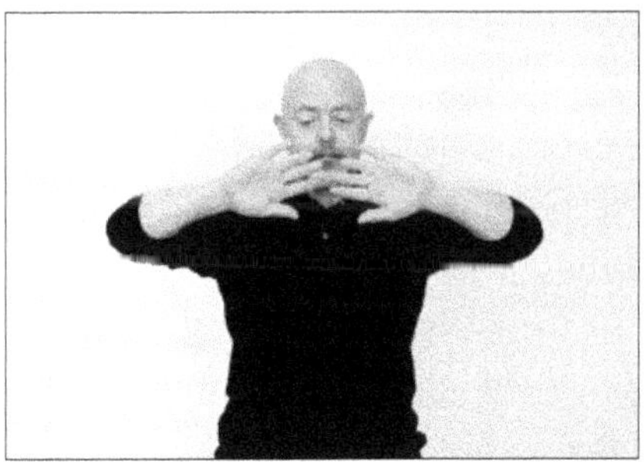

16.

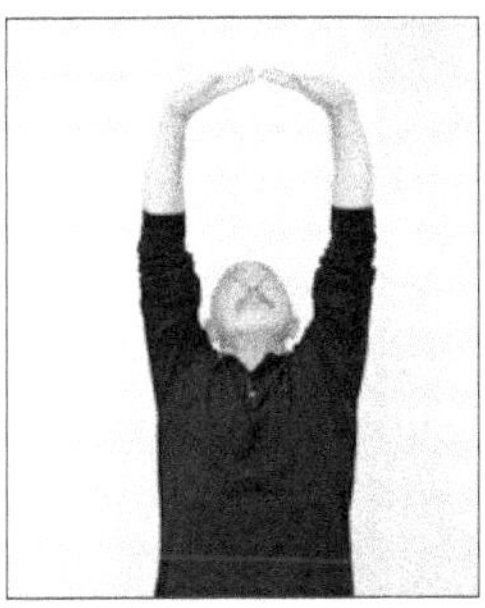

17.

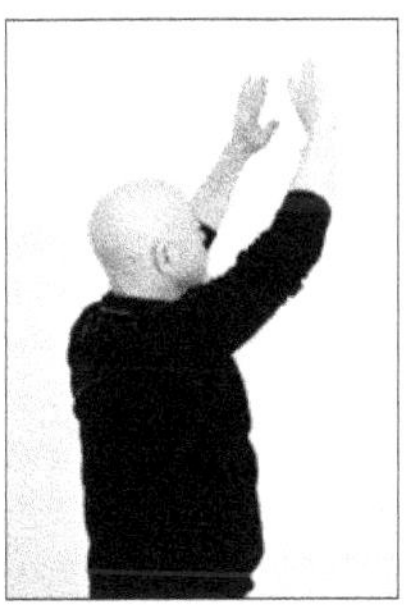

18.

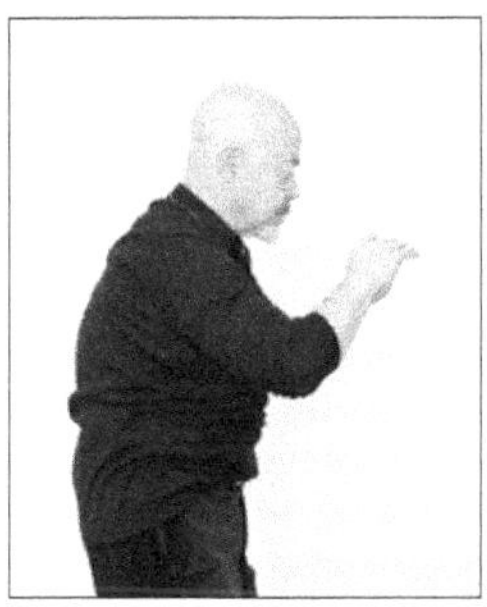

19.

time bring the head back to its natural position and let the knees recover usual to the standing working posture slightly bent. The eyesight goes with the muscular movement, getting more and more alive with the inhalation and progressively going inwards with the exhalation.

With the internal cervical pass, the external passes of wrists and ankles can also be activated. When starting this practise, you don't need to pay attention to these, but with repeated practice they can gradually become more involved in the exercise.

After the repetitions you have decided to do in your session, straighten your body, adopt the basic standing working posture, put your hands over your navel and make about three smooth and calm breaths, feeling how the qi moves and how the qi of your hands communicate with the qi inside your abdomen.

Make a deep inhalation opening wide your eyes and presenting your palms to the front (a Yang attitude). When you feel full of air, let your breath out smoothly from your mouth while relaxing the whole body, the hands and the eyes (a Yin attitude).

*Working with the three passes in a continuous mode*

If there is nothing specifically contraindicated, like a sprained disk at some section of the spinal column you don't want to move excessively, continuitity should be the usual way of doing this exercise. When we say "the exercise of the three passes", we are usually talking of performing these three exercises as a complete set. They are done sequentially and one after the other as a single exercise in three parts.This can be difficult if you have not developed the ability to do a very slow and long inhalation, broken into three parts, with the corresponding movements to open them performed during each of the three inhalation sections and a long exhalation with the three movements to deactivate the passes in succession during three exhalation sections.

When you are activating the internal passes, you will also be activating the corresponding external passes, but when you are starting to do this exercise, you don't need to pay too much attention to these. What is important is to work with the internal passes as well as posible, the external ones will come in time, mostly by themselves.

Adopt the basic working standing posture (see 1.1.2.2 above): feet separated to shoulder's width, knees slightly flexed, pelvis slightly pointed to the front, straight spine, strong nape of the neck, chin slightly drawn, vertex (baihui) pointed to the heavens, tongue touching the superior palate, looking at a space about one meter in front of your feet, or closed eyes. Natural and smooth breathing. Now, from this starting point we will successively activate the three passes.

**Activating the lumbar pass** (first pass): coordinating the breathe with movements, certain movements are done on the inhalation and others on the exhalation, everything is performed as slowly as you can manage.

As you breathe in slowly, draw, tilt the coccyx backwards while relaxing the abdomen (this helps mobilise and open the lumbar pass). At the same time, bring the relaxed arms up from the shoulders, palms facing each other, until the hands reach up to the level of dantian (just below the navel) (Fig. 20). While you are doing this also let the eyes progressively open so that when the abdomen is full, the eyes are slightly open, the hands at the level of dantian, the coccyx tilted as far backwards and upwards as possible (like a dog lifting its tail). Now, with the abdomen half full, the eyes slightly open and the coccyx tilted up and back (lifting the tail) at its maximum, continue breathing in, and tie with the dorsal pass section of the exercise

20.
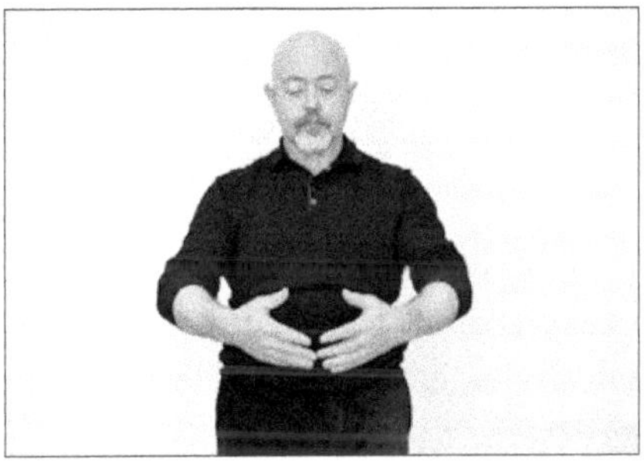

**Activating the thoracic pass** (second pass). Like in the previous part of the exercise, movements and breathing are done slowly with coordination between specific movements during inhalation and exhalation.

Continue inhaling, lifting the arms in a relaxed manner from the shoulders up to when the hands reach about the level of Ren17 (middle of the chest). Continue breathing in and extend the arms to the sides with the palms facing forwards (Fig. 21). Continue taking air in and stretch the arms with the palms facing out to the sides (Fig. 22), as though you were pushing two far away walls (Fig. 23), thus opening your interscapular area while doing this, your eyes continue opening. Pay attention to avoid tension in your shoulders when stretching the arms. When you reach a maximum extension and you are almost full of air, continue your inhalation and tie with the activation of the cervical pass.

**Activating the cervical pass** (third pass). Like in the previous opart of the exercise, the breath and movements are slow and coordinated.

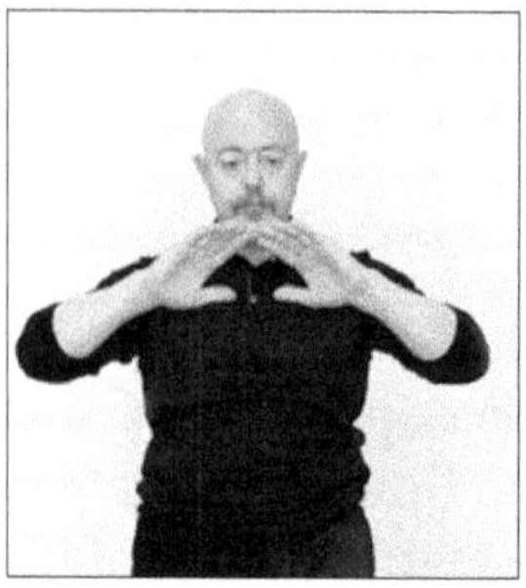

21.

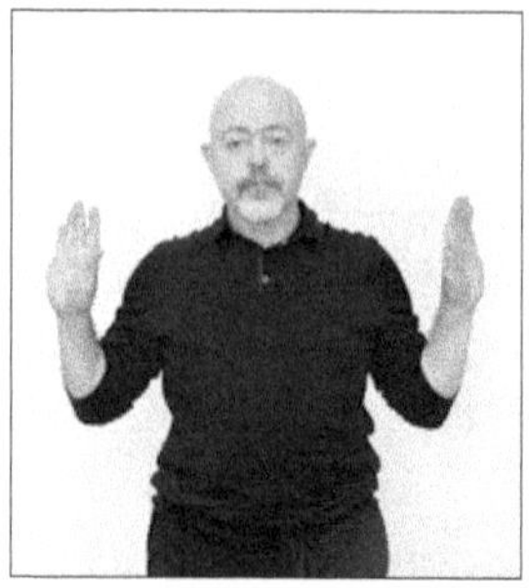

22.

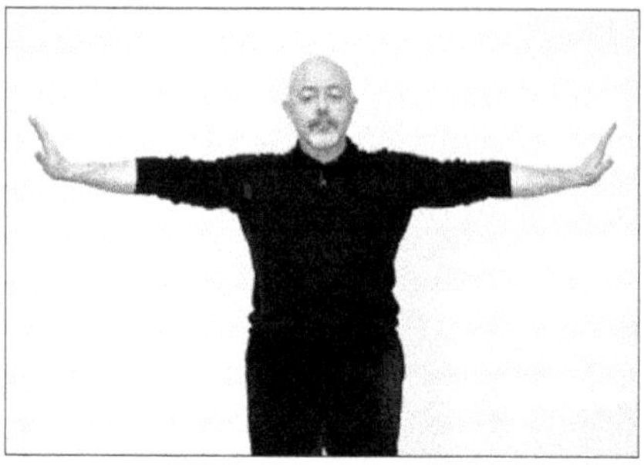

23.

Continue breathing in, lifting your hands from the laterally extended position, tilting the head backwards and following the hands with your sight up to when you are fully vertically extended (Fig. 24), with the palms looking to the heavens and the points of your fingers touching, your eyes looking to the dorsum of your hands, feeling at the same time fully extended upward and deeply rooted from your feet. Now start exhaling, breathing out smoothly via the mouth while relaxing the arms (Fig. 25) from the shoulders, elbows and wrists when descending in front of the body, bringing the head back to its natural position. When the elbows are about throat's level, relax the thoracic pass, and with it the elbows and knees, which will bend a bit more than when we started. The arms continue descending, always within the same exhalation, and the eyes follow the hands, so the head starts also tilting slightly forward as

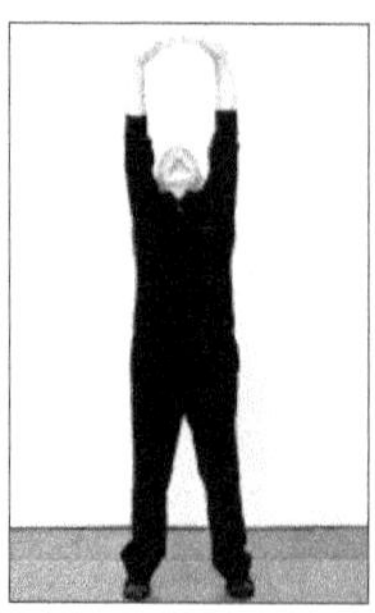

24.

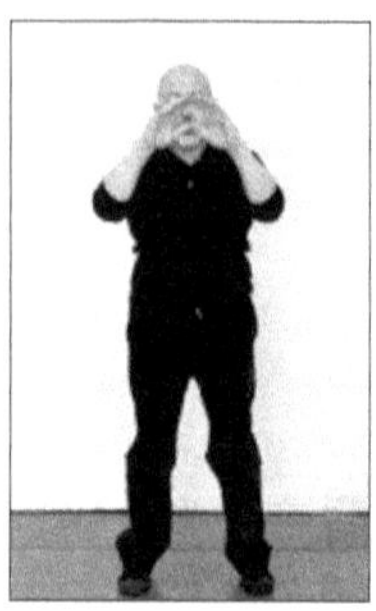

25.

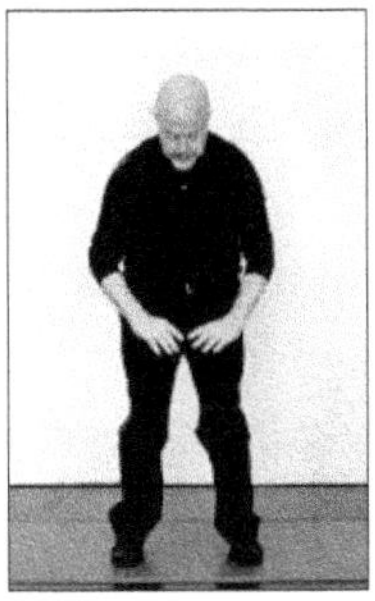
26.

the hands, relaxing the wrists, and with the palms pointing to the body, pass the level of dantian. The eyes follow the muscular movement, becoming more and more alive with the inhalation and progressively going inwards with the exhalation. When the exercise is finished, you will be collected, empty and relaxed (Fig. 26). From this Yin posture, we start breathing in again, and repeat the whole exercise the number of times you feel is adequate.

After the repetitions you have decided to do in your session, straighten your body, adopt the basic standing working posture, put your hands over your navel (Fig. 27 + Fig. 28) and make about three smooth and calm breaths, feeling how the qi moves and how the qi of your hands communicate with the qi inside your abdomen.

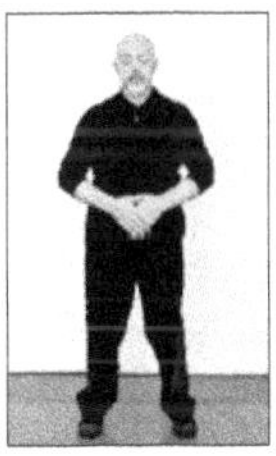
27.

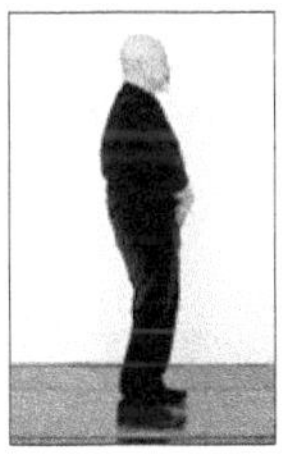
28.

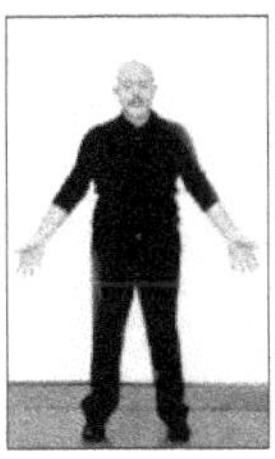
29.

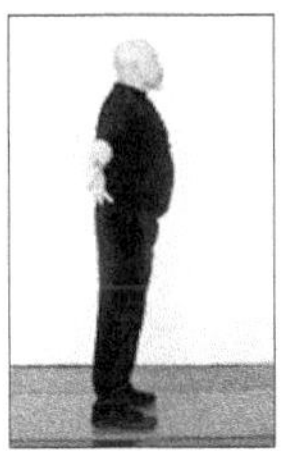
30.

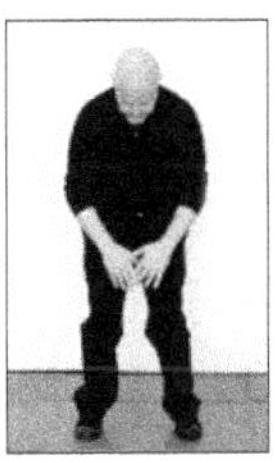
31.

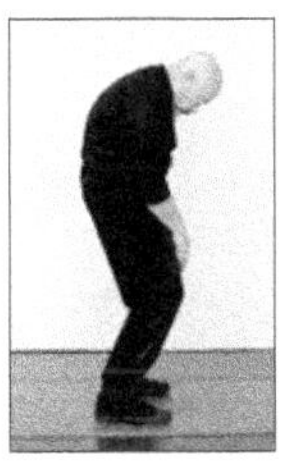
32.

Make a deep inhalation opening wide your eyes and presenting your palms to the front (a Yang attitude) (Fig. 29 + Fig. 30). When you feel full of air, let your breath out smoothly from your mouth while relaxing the whole body, the hands and the eyes (a Yin attitude) (Fig. 31 + Fig. 32).

Tips (for the whole exercise):

- Each step (opening each pass) is supported by the former, which is continuously present throughout the whole exercise.
- Maximum expansion is achieved together with maximum grounding.
- Each pass is more related with some specific physical and mental attitudes. You can use also these exercises to work consciously with them.
- Grounding: abdominal breathing, lumbar Pass, feeling of weight and descent.
- Individual consciousness: thoracic and costal breathing, thoracic pass (T3 approx.), feeling of expansion of the thoracic cage and the shoulder blades
- Expansion: clavicular breathing, cervical pass, feeling of elevation, expansion and integration.
- Integration: Grounding + individual consciounesss + expansion. Feeling heavier from the waistdown, feeling lighter from the waist up. Grounded feet, light head. Feeling of integration within oneself and with the environnement.

## 1.3 Movement

The previous task of aligning our posture and opening up our joints, together with the combination of mind-body in standing meditation, can help us along the path to maintaining a relaxed body and stillness within movement, or action.

Here we move the arms in simple rotations while rotating quietly from the waist, keeping grounded and centred in the body. The simple exercise is called the "cloud-hands" movement.

### *Cloud-hands movement*

In this movement, we listen to how we rotate from side to side. In this exercise the axis of movement is at the waist; the turning of the whole body is initiated at the waist. The arms do not turn; it is the whole body that moves as one unit, using the waist as a pivot. It is important to remember that when we raise our arms, we do not move our shoulders; we use our elbows as a pivot.

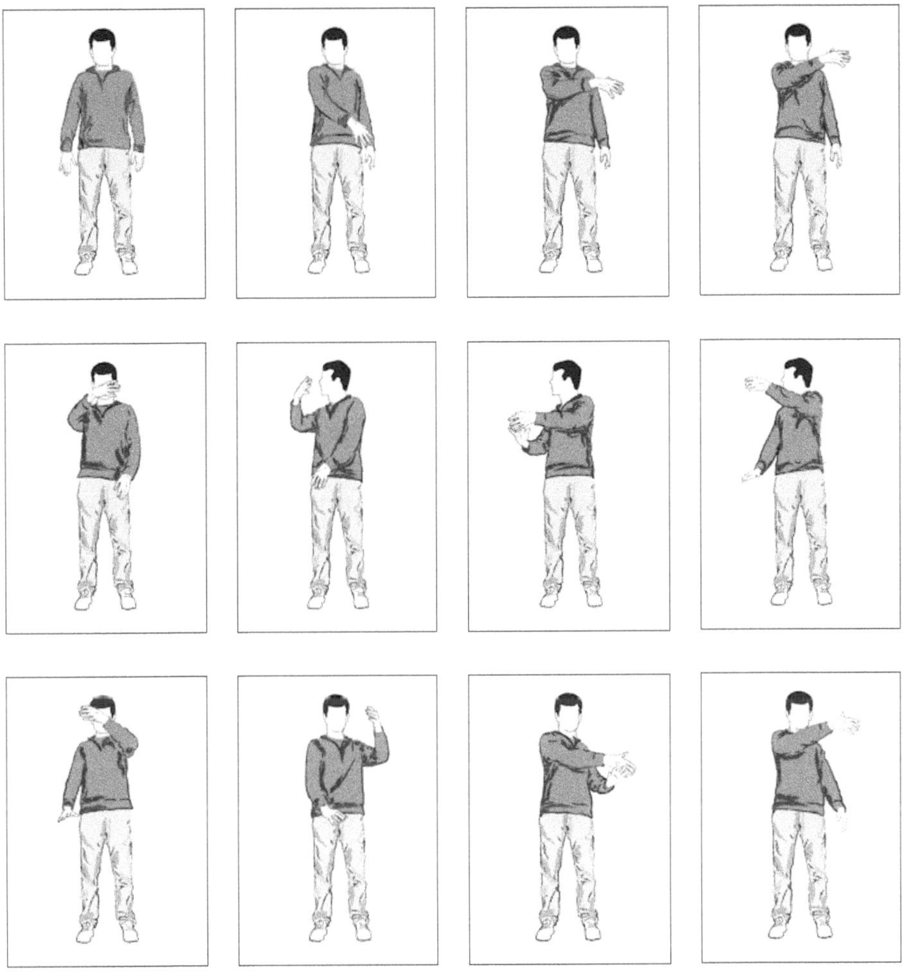

**Exercise**

Standing as shown in the first picture, slowly raise one arm up so that the palm of the hand is roughly in front of the face, then in a continuous movement, rotate from the waist towards the side of the arm that is raised. Keep your eyes comfortably focused on the hand in front of you. When you have rotated a comfortable amount to that side, in a fluid movement, slowly stop rotating, while lowering the hand down back to the side and simultaneously bringing the other hand up so that it has its palm in front of you. Continuing this fluid movement, slowly start rotating to the side of the raised arm. When you have rotated a comfortable amount, then, in the same fluid motion as on the other side, stop the rotation, lower the arm and raise the hand of the other arm and start to rotate slowly to the other side... Continue this back and forth rotating from side to side with alternate arms raised at least ten times to each side. Remember that once raised the arms are still, movement comes from the waist, and try to hold everything in a calm, quiet relaxed posture as you move slowly and with even rhythm.

### *Forward and backward movements*

In this movement, we listen to how we move forwards and backwards. Important points to remember are: We do not move backwards from the upper part of the back; when we move backwards, the weight of our body is not to go into our heels, rather it should stay near the centre of the foot, and when we move forwards, we do not put our weight into the tips of our toes, again keep the weight more around the centre of the foot; the arm movements are performed from the elbows; there is no intention of extending the arms from the shoulders. The exercise consists of a slow forward-backing rocking movement of the body, staying centred over the feet while the arms and hands follow the forward-backward movements in a broad gentle sweep backwards and a gentle push forwards.

**Exercise**

Start by placing one foot comfortably forward of the other. Raise the hands so that they are held in front of the body, facing forward with fingers slightly flared (picture lower left). Then slowly shift the weight of the body to lean

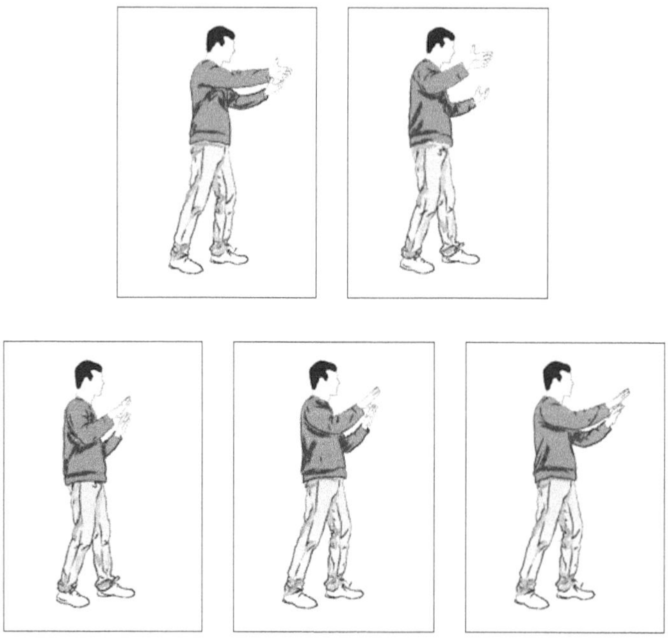

slightly forward whilst at the same time gently pushing the hands forward. After comfortably moving the body and pushing the hands forward, stop that movement and in a fluid motion, start moving the body backwards whilst at the same time bringing the hands, now palms facing slightly inwards, backwards in a comfortable wide sweep, stopping with the hands roughly in front of the shoulders at the time that you have stopped the comfortable movement backwards. Then continuing in the same fluid motions, start to move the body forward again, and at the same time face the palms slightly forward and start pushing the hands gently forward. Continue this till full forward motion again and reverse. Repeat this slow forward-backward rocking of the body while the arms push and pull gently backwards at least ten times. Make sure to breathe quietly and rhythmically throughout, make sure to keep the shoulders relaxed and make sure to move equally back and forth over the centre of gravity so that the weight is not placed on the feet too far forward (onto the toes) or too far back (onto the heel).

## 1.4 Touching/Adherence

In acupuncture and Taiji quan, our sense of touch is an important element. In the art of Taiji quan, we work on our sense of touch through the practice of tuishou. The art of tuishou does not seek to develop techniques based on power and speed; its objective is to awaken a kind of listening, which allows us to be aware of the slightest indication of change.

In acupuncture, and especially in Japanese acupuncture, feeling the pulse, the abdomen or the meridians are essential tools when making a diagnosis. Looking for the points and using needles also depend on our sense of touch.

The sense of touch we are seeking in the practice of tuishou can be compared to when we are taking a pulse. In both cases, we want to perceive the signs that will allow us to carry out a change without much effort, an action that causes the maximum change with the minimum effort.

Awakening a new sense of touch is one of the objectives of practicing tuishou. Using only words, it is impossible to define and learn the type of touch that we are trying to awaken. It is necessary to have direct experience with a person who has already acquired this sense of touch and can transmit it in action. The exercises that are proposed below are an introduction to this sensitivity, which is awakened through the practice of tuishou, a new way of sensing which needs the support of the previous movements.

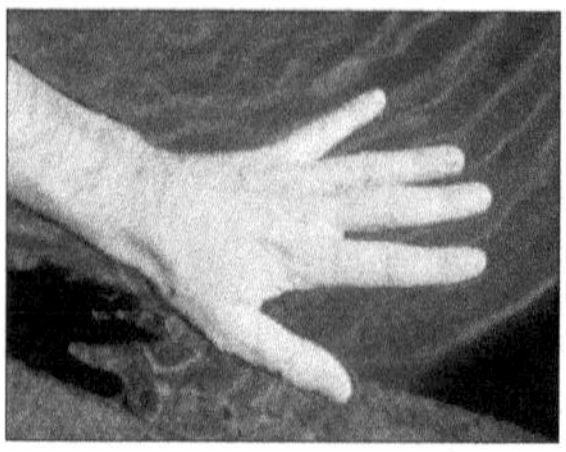
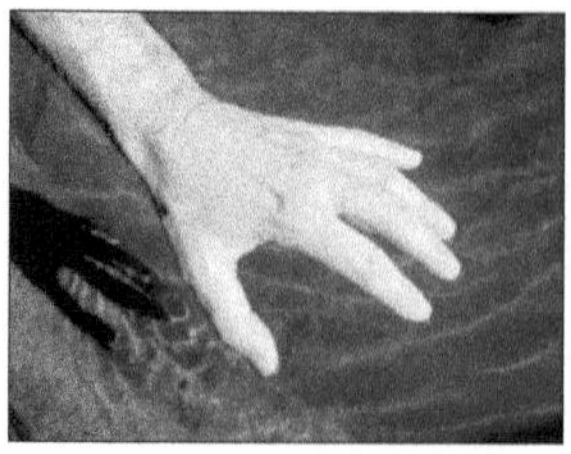
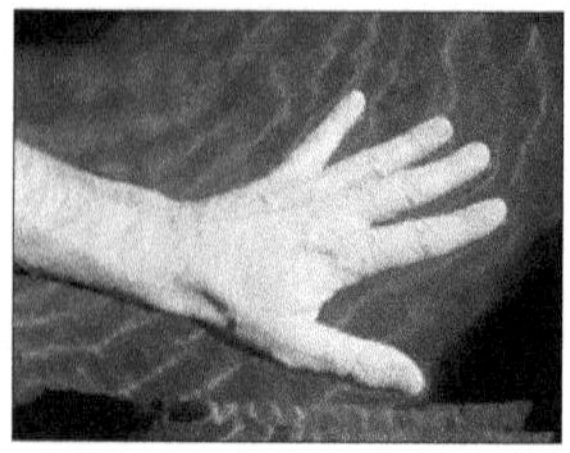

### A New Sense of Touch: exercises with water

Touching, adherence in acupuncture, is performed using the hands. The object of the exercise that follows is to awaken more sensitivity in our hands when we come into contact with the other person:

Place a bowl with water at a height where your shoulders are not tense and your knees are slightly bent. Place a hand so it is just in contact with the water. Stay in contact with the water for five minutes, perceiving the touch of your hand in contact with the water. You can then start to perform the following movements:

1- Softly push downwards but without submerging your hand; you have to perceive the texture of the water, its pressure on your hand.
2- Move your hand laterally without losing contact with the water.

We can use the running check from the standing meditation to help our body relax. Then, observe what perception you have of the side you have worked with, and compare it to the other. Then perform the same actions with the other hand. In these exercises we create minimal movements of the water, so as you hold your hand still touching try to make sure to not create the ripples that are an indication of movement. Also, when moving the hand try to do this with minimal disturbance of the water.

## 2. Putting all that to work in acupuncture practise

### Practical Exercises

If you are an acupuncturist it is not possible to tell you the specifics of how better to perform the needling techniques you have studied and apply within the system of practice you use, I (SB) only know about the needling techniques that I use. If you are another form of practitioner that utilises treatments on the body surface based upon TEAM models of practice such as massage traditions, what is described here may also be helpful. In this final section we refer back to the beginning section of chapter nine where we listed the details pertaining to the following for stages in our actions:

1- Decisions.
2- Engagement.
3- Enactment.
4- Completion.

It might be helpful to review that section before beginning the following exercises.

In acupuncture, as we have seen in the chapters above, diversity of methods is normal and to be expected within the field. Thus the processes of your decision making will need to be studied and refined within the context of the system you practice, using appropriate methods. The processes of enactment and completion, the application of the specific needling techniques you use within your system of practice will also need to be studied and refined within the context of that system of practice using methods developed for training and improving them. However, there is a common ground for us all: *we must all find the acupoint and apply the needling technique, whatever it is, to that acupoint*. It is here that treatment begins. It starts with paying attention to your body and preparing to treat the acupoint. Then it includes how you touch as you start to look for the acupoint. These actions begin the treatment so that the qi of the patient starts to be engaged. Indeed, these two aspects lay the foundation for the rest of the treatment. This happens **before** one applies the needle. In this sequence of actions the next things is how one further prepares oneself so that when the needle starts to be applied, it comes into an already active treatment context where there is an on-going interaction or communication between yourself and the patient, which we refer to and describe using the language of qi. These various stages are precisely those that we wish to target with exercises in order to help develop them so that you can maximise their effects during treatment.

*How to get feedback?*

Before describing the two practical exercises, we need to set the stage a bit further. It is one thing to apply certain techniques in one's practice, and to try to learn simply by doing with only a clinical sense of judging how well performed they were. It is quite another to have direct feedback to what you have done, so that it is no longer subject only to your imagination, but becomes observable to you and others when you practice with others. Having more direct feedback beyond only a clinical sense, especially when working with others in a group can greatly increase one's confidence in judgment and considerably accelerate one's learning process.

How can you observe changes to the condition of the qi of the person you are working on? Of course, in chapter one we argued that qi is related to our experiences of the world, thus through the senses we can make observations. But of these which are discussed in the historical literature and which found useful in modern practice? Lingshu chapter ten is the oldest treatise that describes the twelve jingmai and the fifteen luomai. At the end of the chapter the question naturally arises about how one can judge the xu-shi state of the jingmai and luomai. Of the luomai it states that they are visible and so looking with your eyes for changes in surface appearance will give you an indication about the xu-shi state of the luomai. But of the jingmai, it says that they are not visible, rather one must palpate the mai "pulses" to understand their xu-shi state. Since the time of the Neijing and especially the Nanjing, the radial arteries have been a major focus for making a diagnosis of a patient, with many treatises published over the centuries that are devoted to the art of pulse diagnosis. It is generally held that through the palpatory feelings of the radial arteries one can assess the state of qi and its various subsets in the body, both in healthy and abnormal conditions.

When we palpate the radial arteries, we find that in most people they are observable on both wrists, the arteries lie between the skin at the surface of the body and the underlying radial bone, with various soft-feeling anatomical structures around the arteries. What is felt with the fingers as one feels the arteries and the throbbing of the arteries that follow each heart contraction is described in a number of different ways with many "qualities" assigned to those different feelings/sensations. But, without paying attention to the specific "qualities", each usually associated with certain pathological states in the body, there are a number of core palpatory experiences that we can pay attention to:

–When we find the arteries they pulse at a certain rate, slower, faster or a "normal" range of rate.

–When we quest for the arteries with our fingers they can be felt with little pressure just under the skin or one needs to apply further pressure almost down to the bone in order to find the arteries, thus we can describe the feelings of depth, they are more superficial, more deep or in a more normal range of depth.

–Also, when we quest for the arteries, we sometimes feel them throbbing quite forcefully under our fingers with a lot of resistance as we press into them, while on others when we find the arteries the force of the pulsation and resistance of the artery wall is very mild and weak, thus we can speak of the pulses feeling stronger, weaker or a more normal range of strength.

These three aspects of the pulses, depth, strength and speed are also used to define what the "normal" or healthy pulse feels like: it is not too fast, not too slow, it is not to superficial and not too deep, it is not too strong and not too weak. These descriptions can form the foundation of pulse diagnosis before one attempts more complex observations and judgments with one's fingers.

Since the healthy pulse is in the mid-range of depth, strength and speed, then we might also expect that as we do something to the person whose arteries we are feeling, if that something has a positive influence on their qi, the pulse might move towards that mid-range state, in terms of the depth, strength and speed, and if what we do produces a not beneficial influence on the person's qi, the pulse might move away from that mid-range state in terms of depth, strength and speed.

For example if the pulse started out as being more floating, rapid and excess/hard, when something is done that produces a positive influence on the qi, the pulse will then be felt to be less floating, less rapid and less excess/hard, i.e. it will be felt to sink, slow and soften or one or more of these "normalizations" will be felt to occur. If the pulse had been felt to be in the mid depth, a little excess/hard and slightly slow, if something is done that creates a negative influence on the qi, the pulse might become more floating, more rapid and/or more hard.

By these means one can start to observe what kind of influences one has been able to produce with one's techniques during these practical exercises.

Of course it is never as simple as one can make it sound there are other aspects that may come into play as well. The feeling that the pulse becomes softer when it had felt stronger and harder before might be interpreted as a negative change if understood to be "too soft", but softening of the arteries with the feeling that the artery walls are clearly definable and have a kind of resilient light springiness to them is very different than if the artery walls become hard to feel (clearly hypotonic) and there is a loss or lack of this springiness. This takes some practice to understand. Luckily for us we have a number of teachers in Japan who have studied these changes quite extensively and have developed practice methods that can be used to train these observations and their judgments through repetitive practice.[2] For this kind of practice it is important to focus on what is felt in the pulse, putting aside the normal clinical judgments about the condition of the patient that arise with clinical use of pulse diagnosis. Of course this can be done with other colleagues also studying these methods, one or two people can palpate the radial arteries of someone laying on the practice table while you, for example, apply the practice exercises. Both radial arteries show the same basic pulse quality changes in terms of depth, strength and speed, and each person feeling a radial artery can feel the same changes and report them. This method comes from the study and practice of the Toyohari system of Japanese Meridian Therapy and is named after its developer, the "Kozato method". If you are able to get together with some colleagues (preferably 2 or 3 others) you can each try out the exercises below and give feedback to each other as to how you each influenced the qi of the person laid on the practice table.

The practice exercises can be practiced alone with someone to work on, or with colleagues to help give feedback. If you are attempting these exercises with a group of colleagues, when one of you lays down on the practice table and one or two others each take a wrist of that person to feel the radial arteries, as you practice the exercise those feeling the radial arteries can give you continuous feedback as to what changes are felt in the pulses. Both radial pulses show the same basic changes in terms of depth, strength and speed. If you do not have a group of colleagues to practice with, but instead you only have someone on whom you are practicing these exercises (such as a friend or relative), if you position yourself so that you can find the acupoint with one hand and feel the radial artery of the person on the practice table with the other, you can perform the exercises with some feedback. It is however easier if you have at least one other person to give feedback to the pulse changes rather than you. When you are alone judging the feedback it can be difficult to be doing the delicate techniques of the practice exercise with one hand, adjusting one's posture and mental state and at the same time feeling and noting the radial pulse changes. But as with any artisan's practice, the more you practice in either situation the easier it gets and the more you can start to get out of it.

## 2.1 Exercise one

The purpose of this exercise is to address three main factors:

–Your posture and position –both bodily and mental.

–How you touch –as both an act of touching another and an act of sensing that other.

–Your ability to sense the subtle changes and aspects –both through the direct sense of touch (tactile sensory stimulation) and the felt sense of change (not so clearly localised to any particular sensory system).

The questions to address are:
When you ready yourself for touching, can your initial touch create a positive change?
As you maintain your touch and start to move your finger-tip to look for the acupoint, can you produce incremental improvements through that movement, movement on the channel, touching of the acupoint?

*Preparation –body work*
As is clearly described above, it has been found that you need to be very relaxed in order to be able to create the positive changes you seek and so that you are still enough to be able to start sensing these subtle phenomena.

*Recommendations:*
(You will see many of the recommendations and exercises described above, put into practice here)
–It helps to stand with feet about shoulder width apart, knees relaxed and maybe even slightly bent.
–Position yourself so that when you touch the channel on which the point you will be looking for is located, you can pull the left index finger gently along the flow of the channel (if you are right handed) or the right index finger gently along the flow of the channel (if you are left handed).
–Practice on leg points such as SP-3, KI-7, SP-6 (this frees up both radial arteries for feedback).
–Look for acupoints that feel slightly xu or weak, signs being a slight depression, skin softer, subcutaneous tissues softer.
–For every movement you perform, state out loud what you are doing: e.g. "placing my hand", "looking for the channel", "found the channel", "stroking along the channel", "finding the acupoint", "touching the acupoint", etc. This allows specific feedback to each action and movement.
–Make sure to not react defensively to comments, make sure to remain emotionally still as you hear the feedback, make sure to keep your ego out of the way and just "hear" the feedback.
–When the feedback is not positive, don't stop what you are doing and remove your finger and simply start again, rather adjust yourself, adjust your focus and touch, do this until you start to get better feedback, then go onto

the next action. If you are not on the channel and thus no clear positive feedback is elicited, you may need to start again, but once on the channel, work with what you have by adjusting yourself and your actions until you get the positive feedback you are seeking.

Prepare yourself, making sure to relax your shoulders and arms, release tension in the inter-scapular region, don't crane your neck forward to look at what you are doing, once you have placed your finger so that you think it is on the channel, raise your head and relax your neck/shoulders.

Once you feel relaxed make sure also to quiet your mind and adopt a quietly looking focus.

### *Touching –initial engagement*

When ready, quietly, slowly and gently place our hand on the limb on which you will look for the acupoint. Touch lightly, gently and quietly, placing the index finger-tip on the area where the channel should be located and just distal to the acupoint you will locate. Pay attention to what you feel both in local sensory terms and in more general global terms.

*Recommendations:*

–When you place the hand, don't place only your index finger-tip, but gently let the hand and other fingers settle as well.

–Make sure that the touch is light so as not to cause visible depressions in the skin.

–Use the contact of the rest of the hand (besides the index finger-tip) as a fulcrum from which you can pivot your movements and maintain a smooth contact and pressure/contact of the index finger-tip.

**Questions**

–How does the pulse react as you place your hand and finger-tip?

–If you get more negative pulse changes, what do you feel? –remember that.

–If you get negative pulse changes –what do you need to do to start getting more positive feedback? remember that.

–When you get positive pulse changes, what do you feel? –remember that.

### *Moving –deepening engagement*

Next slowly and gently move the index finger-tip to find the channel and slowly pull the index finger along the channel flow, paying attention to what you feel both in local sensory terms and in more general global terms.

*Recommendations:*

–When you move the hand, pull as though from the elbow.

–Make sure to keep the finger contact on the skin constant and with no change in pressure.

–Move slowly, and at the same time paying attention to any change in bodily tension and release that.

**Questions**

–As you move your hand and index finger-tip, how does the pulse react?

–If you get more negative pulse changes, what do you feel? –remember that.

–If you get negative pulse changes, what do you need to do to start getting more positive feedback? –remember that.

When you get positive pulse changes, what do you feel? –remember that.

### *Locating the point –deeper engagement*

As you move the index finger-tip along the flow of the channel, carefully and slowly locate the acupoint you have selected to look for, as you find the acupoint, stop moving and hold the tip of the index finger gently touching the acupoint, all the while paying attention to what you feel both in local sensory terms and in more general global terms.

*Recommendations:*

–When moving the hand, do so slowly, softly with unvarying lightness of touch.

–Pay careful attention to what you are feeling.

–Once you have found the acupoint, remain completely still as you touch it.

**Questions**

–As you move your finger onto the acupoint how does the pulse react?

–When you maintain a constant touching of the acupoint, how does the pulse react?

–Throughout all these steps have you been able to create positive incremental changes in the pulses?

–If you get more negative pulse changes, what do you feel? –remember that.
–If you get negative pulse changes, what do you need to do to start getting more positive feedback? –remember that.
–When you get positive pulse changes, what do you feel? –remember that.

This is a relatively simple exercise, but you will find it is very difficult at first to create positive changes through your touch, movements and what you think was locating the acupoint, touching the acupoint. With practice you learn what kind of posture works better, how best to hold and release tension, how best to touch, what kind of touch and movement works best, what the acupoint feels like where qi is said to enter and exit.

It has been our experience and the experience of many colleagues and teachers that we have to get it wrong before we start to get it right, regardless of how "good" we think we may already be. It has been our experience that the softest, most quiet touch and movements seem to produce the best changes. With careful attentive practice we can all improve. Even if we have physical problems, we find the way that works for us in order to create these positive changes. Stillness, quietness, slow but gentle, firm but careful all with a quiet focal attention are important for this practice.

## 2.2 Exercise two

This exercise builds on the previous and brings into play the fact that once you have located the acupoint and are touching it, you will then begin a specific action (needling) of that point. The first exercise is about training how to engage the qi of the patient and how to increase that engagement before you start the more explicit act of treating it (by needles or for example massage techniques), this second relates to how you now get ready for that enactment, the treatment.

For this exercise, repeat all aspects of exercise one to locate and touch the acupoint that is the focus of your "treatment." Make sure that as you do this you now make specific adjustments to your posture, tension, touch, pressure, stabilising of the engagement and so on, so that you have clearly positive pulse feedback as you are touching the acupoint.

*Then:*

While trying to maintain your touch of the acupoint and maintain that positive change that you have already produced, with the other hand prepare the needle for treatment. This could involve picking up the needle or moving the hand holding the needle handle over to the acupoint you are touching as you might just before you insert the needle. DO NOT insert the needle, the purpose is only to prepare yourself for doing the needling.

What often happens as your focus shifts towards the other hand that is picking up and/or holding the needle is that your focus on the acupoint changes, and if your posture is not still, relaxed and stable, the physical contact at the point varies, even only very slightly. Either of these things can start to create negative influences with less positive or even negative changes in the pulses. Ideally you should be able to find the acupoint with the incremental improvements that reflect in the pulses and then hold/place the needle without detracting from that.

**Questions:**

–Can you maintain the improvements that you produced in the pulses while your other hand is engaged in these preparatory actions?

–What do you feel in your contact as you begin these actions with the other hand? –remember that

–What do you need to do in order to maintain the stability of those positive changes as you bring the other hand (with needle) into play?

–Can you feel something specific related to this? –remember that

–Can you reproduce it?

Eventually with practice and being open to change and feedback, you can improve each different aspect of these actions so as to create a clear positive engagement of qi with the patient and start to maintain a positive sway over these things, regardless of the other actions you perform. We believe that these different aspects represent the foundation for improved needling abilities, regardless of style of practice. Not being massage therapist we can only imagine how to modify this; for example in exercise two, rather than bringing the needle to the acupoint, moving say the thumb or finger of the other hand and placing it in preparation for beginning a specific technique of stimulation could substitute, or perhaps adjusting the body posture in preparation for starting to press the acupoint?

## 3. Postscript

It has been my (SB) observation, as someone who started out as a very intellectual person and had to learn the hard way to silence the mind at the appropriate times, and, as a person that has done a lot of teaching, many people will remain stuck in their heads as they attempt these kinds of actions. It is very easy to be distracted from what one feels and the very subtle nature of that and it's even more subtle changes by focusing on things that seem easier to grasp, like thinking... "What is this?" "What kind of qi am I feeling?" "How can I explain this in the terms of the model of practice I use?" And so on. These mental activities distract from the physical action, your perception of your experiences and cause you to lose the quiet focus you have when the mind is still and not asking these questions.

All I can say is that we should not stop our questioning, but we need to find the right times to ask the questions. It is all too easy to cite the first line of the Daode Jing [道可道，非常道] "the dao that can be spoken of is not the dao" (or something like that) which is really a way of avoiding the greater issue. But questions are not just words and relate not only to ideas they form a much more substantial layer of our understanding of things. I prefer to cite Guo Yu, the Han dynasty physician who said about the consummate skill required to practice acupuncture well:

"A kind of spirit connects the physician's heart with his hand, and that is something I can know but cannot explain"

Understanding lies not in the words we can use to explain things (though that too can be very important), understanding lies more in our actions and our ability to perform our actions with maximum impact. Perform the acts well, obtain the feedback that articulates how well the actions were performed and you have demonstrated a profound understanding, whether there are words to explain it or not. This is the art of practice. This is a very important part of understanding about qi and its conveyors, the jingmai. The piano teacher understands this, so too does the dance instructor, the expert sculptor, the master carpenter, the master martial artist. But in medicine, especially in this modern period, there is a strong need to have an explanation, even when the action cannot be carried out yet, nor is the action itself clear yet. To develop a better understanding of qi and the jingmai, focus on your practice. Let the explanations, if they are ever to be revealed, reveal themselves through that practice (but not during) –don't make the mistake of trying to force the practice and the experiences you have in practice through the narrow holes of the theories and conceptual frameworks that inform that practice.

We hope as somewhat experienced practitioners of different disciplines that are engaged in qi related activities (acupuncture, Taiji quan, qigong, aikido, herbal medicine, and etc.) that our trying to pry open these important understandings have made some impact on you and contributed something to your own understanding of and practice of things related to qi and their related jingmai.

## Endnotes

1. It must be said that the tree metaphor is not completely apt, because we are looking for a root that is mobile. For this reason, we prefer "grounding" to "rooting", a term that is used a lot by some teachers. We need to be conscious not only of our base, but also of its mobility. Once again, our base is more like the self-possession of a warrior than the solidity of a meditator.

2. The feedback method is called "Kozatohoshiki", the Kozato method after Mr Katsu-yukiKozato who developed the feedback method within the framework of studying and teaching Toyohari and especially training subtle needling techniques.

# INDEX

# Also by Sayoshi Books

Exceptional books on acupuncture, moxibustion, and East Asian medicine

Sayoshi Books is dedicated to publishing high-quality books for practitioners and students of East Asian medicine. Our books bridge traditional knowledge with modern clinical insights, offering practical guidance and deep expertise.

## Our Titles

***Moxa in Motion with the Ontake Method: Rhythmic Moxibustion Methods from Japan for Mind-Body Healing* – Oran Kivity**

A groundbreaking exploration of rhythmic moxibustion methods from Japan using Ontake Warm Bamboo, integrating traditional knowledge with innovative applications for pain relief and systemic balance.

*Also available in Chinese and Polish. Translations into Bahasa Indonesia, French, Portuguese, Spanish and Japanese will be available in late 2025.*

***Hirata Zone Therapy with the Ontake Method: Repurposing the Lost Art of Japanese Dermatome Moxibustion for Contemporary Practice* – Oran Kivity**

An exploration of the dermatome moxibustion system developed by twentieth century Japanese masters Kurakichi Hirata and Yoshio Manaka, repurposed for contemporary practice with Ontake Warm Bamboo. This practical guide will teach you to create immediate and powerful therapeutic effects.

*Also available in French.*

***The Moon Over Matsushima: Insights into Moxa and Mugwort (Second Edition)* – Merlin Young**

The definitive book about moxibustion, exploring its history and linking traditional East Asian practices with emerging scientific research on transient receptor potential ion channels.

***Restoring Order in Health and Chinese Medicine: Studies of the Development and Use of Qi and the Channels* – Stephen Birch, Miguel Angel Cabrer Mir, Manuel Rodriguez Cuadras**

An in-depth study of the dynamics of qi, the development of the channels, and how to apply classical principles to contemporary acupuncture practice.

***The Lost Art of Jôsetsu-Hô Moxibustion: Finding Effective Moxa Points with String Measuring* – Felip Caudet, Hideo Shinma**

The first translation into English of Caudet's seminal work in Spanish. A detailed exploration of the Jôsetsu-Hô string-measuring method, detailing ways to locate effective moxa points for enhanced therapeutic results.

***Manaka Made Simple: A Step-by-Step Guide to Dr Manaka's System of Japanese Acupuncture and Moxibustion* – Oran Kivity, Stephen Birch, Marian Fixler, Brenda Loew, Paul Movsessian**

A practical manual on Dr. Manaka's four-step protocol, demystifying his unique diagnostic and treatment system for modern practitioners.

**Other Titles by Sayoshi Books**

While Sayoshi Books primarily focuses on East Asian medicine, we also took the opportunity to republish this deeply personal memoir.

***Daughter of the Waves: Memories of Growing Up in Pre-War Palestine* – Ruth Jordan**

Ruth Jordan's award-winning autobiography is a vivid, witty, and poignant account of her childhood in British Mandate Palestine. Growing up in a seaside suburb of Haifa, she captures a nation in its formative years, navigating its struggles and transformation into statehood. Originally published in 1982, this timeless memoir is today more relevant than ever, providing a fresh perspective on Palestine through the eyes of someone who was actually there.

---

*Discover more at* **sayoshibooks.orankivity.com**

www.ingramcontent.com/pod-product-compliance
Ingram Content Group UK Ltd.
Pitfield, Milton Keynes, MK11 3LW, UK
UKHW051118290926
15471UKWH00010B/1742